MW01716218

Institutional Review Boards: A Primer

Third Edition

EDITORS
Gary W. Eiland
Richard G. Korman
Janet M. Lis
Teresa A. Williams

AUTHORS
Haley N. Bavasi
Valerie H. Bonham
Kate Bowen
Eve Brunts
Dale H. Cowan
Payal P. Cramer
Amy K. Dow
Heather L. Fields
Jennifer S. Geetter
Kimberly H. Gillespie
Gabrielle Goldstein
Michele R. Goodman
Igor Gorlach
Ann T. Hollenbeck
Jacqueline A. Holz
Beverly H. Lorell
Alice K. Marcee
Ernessa B. McKie
Melinda G. Murray
Katayoun (Kat) Neal
Laura M. Odwazny
David Peloquin
Mary Holloway Richard
Martha C. Romney
Chelsea M. Rutherford
Thomas D. Shrack
Lynn E. Smith
Katherine B. Steuer
Gelvina Rodriguez Stevenson
Sarah E. Swank
Leslie Thornton
Leah A. Voigt

AHLA

American Health
Lawyers Association

AMERICAN HEALTH LAWYERS ASSOCIATION
1620 Eye Street, NW, 6th Floor
Washington, DC 20006-4010
Website: www.healthlawyers.org
E-Mail: info@healthlawyers.org

Printed in the United States of America
ISBN: 978-1-5221-6666-5
978-1-5221-6667-2 (Members)

"This publication is designed to provide accurate and authoritative information with respect to the subject matter covered. It is provided with the understanding that the publisher is not engaged in rendering legal or other professional services. If legal advice or other expert assistance is required, the services of a competent professional person should be sought."

— from a declaration of the American Bar Association

AHLA Diversity+Inclusion Statement In principle and in practice, the American Health Lawyers Association values and seeks to advance and promote diverse and inclusive participation within the Association regardless of gender, race, ethnicity, religion, age, sexual orientation, gender identity and expression, national origin, or disability. Guided by these values, the Association strongly encourages and embraces participation of diverse individuals as it leads health law to excellence through education, information, and dialogue.

(2018–Pub.26885)

Recent Titles From American Health Lawyers Assocation

Fundamentals of Health Law, Seventh Edition

False Claims Act & the Health Care Industry: Counseling & Litigation, Third Edition

The Law of Digital Health, First Edition

Telehealth Law Handbook: A Practical Guide to Virtual Care, First Edition

Best Practices Handbook for Advising Clients on Fraud and Abuse Issues, First Edition

AHLA's Guide to Health Care Legal Forms, Agreements, and Policies, Second Edition with 2017 Cumulative Supplement

Federal Health Care Laws and Regulations, 2017-2018 Edition

The Fundamentals of Behavioral Health Care Law, First Edition

Enterprise Risk Management Handbook for Health Care Entities, Third Edition

Peer Review Guidebook, Fifth Edition

The Medical Staff Guidebook: Minimizing Risks and Maximizing Collaboration, Fourth Edition

Representing Hospitals and Health Systems Handbook, First Edition

Representing Physicians Handbook, Fourth Edition

Health Care Provider and Supplier Audits Practice Guide, First Edition

Health Plans Contracting Handbook: A Guide for Payers and Providers, Seventh Edition

Health Plan Disputes and Litigation Practice Guide, First Edition

Health Care Finance: A Primer, Third Edition

Data Breach Notification Laws: A Fifty State Survey, Second Edition

Health Care Compliance Legal Issues Manual, Fourth Edition

For more AHLA titles published with LexisNexis,
visit https://store.lexisnexis.com/ahla.

For more information on AHLA's ePrograms, webinar recordings and PDFs,
visit www.healthlawyers.org/store.

Acknowledgments

The contributors to this Third Edition sincerely thank the contributors to the two previous editions for their important work on this cumulative and updated text:

First Edition

Teresa A. Williams
Richard G. Korman
Janet M. Lis
Melinda G. Murray

Second Edition

Teresa A. Williams
Richard G. Korman
Janet M. Lis
Melinda G. Murray
Kate Bowen
Amy L. Bradshaw
Tara R. Cowell
Amy K. Dow
Kimberly H. Gillespie
Jennifer R. Henderson
Marta J. Hoffman
Veronica A. Marsich
Tamara J. O'Black
Kay M. Perry
Carol A. Poindexter
Stacey A. Ries
Martha C. Romney
Jennifer Sharp
Sarah E. Swank
Alexandra Trinkoff
Leah A. Voigt
Catherine M. With

Preface

The American Health Lawyers Association is pleased to bring you the revised and expanded third edition of *Institutional Review Boards: A Primer*. This publication outlines the regulatory requirements and legal challenges associated with human subjects research, and presents a thorough discussion of both the role that institutional review boards (IRBs) serve and the changing rules under which they operate.

Readers will find updated analysis exploring fundamental issues such as what constitutes research, the participation of special populations, conflicts of interest, privacy, and payment and billing. Several all new chapters address situations faced by today's IRBs, which function in an increasingly complex research environment: investigator responsibilities, secondary findings in genomic research, compliance and internal audits, and scientific misconduct.

Most critically, you will find clear explanations of the distinctions between the longstanding "Common Rule" regulatory scheme and the revised requirements scheduled to come into effect in January 2019. These include changes in regulatory applicability and exemptions, requirements for IRB policies and procedures, use of test articles outside of clinical trials, handling of identifiable private information and identifiable biospecimens, and the very definition of research. Every participant in the IRB process needs to be aware of these changes.

The American Health Lawyers Association commends this publication to IRB participants and the attorneys who will advise them. *Institutional Review Boards: A Primer, Third Edition* will prove a valuable resource to many.

About the Editors and Authors

About the Editors

Gary W. Eiland has provided legal services to health care industry clients for more than 40 years, focusing on the special regulatory and organizational problems faced by academic medical centers and other health care providers. Mr. Eiland's work includes handling sophisticated business transactions, government investigations, regulatory enforcement, clinical research compliance, self-disclosures, and pursuit of Office of Inspector General (OIG) Advisory Opinions. Mr. Eiland is a past President of the American Health Lawyers Association, and speaks at national programs sponsored by AHLA and other health care trade associations, including serving as a frequent speaker at the Health Care Compliance Association's Annual Compliance Institute.

Richard G. Korman is Executive Vice President and General Counsel for Avera Health, located in Sioux Falls, SD. Mr. Korman is responsible for all legal, public policy, compliance, government relations, internal audit, insurance and risk management activities for Avera. Avera is the Catholic health ministry of the Benedictine Sisters of Yankton, SD and the Presentation of the Blessed Virgin Mary Sisters of Aberdeen, SD. Avera delivers health care services through more than 350 locations in a five-state region made up of South Dakota, Minnesota, Iowa, Nebraska and North Dakota. Mr. Korman graduated from the University of Minnesota with a Bachelor's degree in political science and from William Mitchell College of Law with a law degree. He is admitted to the South Dakota Bar, the Minnesota Bar and is a member of the American Health Lawyers Association, where he is currently on the planning committee for the annual In-House Counsel Program. He has spoken at numerous regional and national conferences related to health care law and compliance issues.

Janet M. Lis practices health care law in Media, Pennsylvania. For over 20 years, she has provided legal services to institutional review boards in the Philadelphia metropolitan area related to structure, function, policies and procedures, and legal/regulatory compliance. Prior to practicing law, Ms. Lis worked as a registered nurse. Ms. Lis received undergraduate degrees from Bucknell University (B.A.) and Georgetown University (B.S.N.), and her law degree from Georgetown University Law Center (J.D.). She is admitted to the Pennsylvania Bar, and is a member of local and state bar associations, as well as the American Health Lawyers Association and Public Responsibility in Medicine and Research, which focuses on promotion of ethical standards in human subjects in research. She is a member of the Pennsylvania Bar Association Health Law Committee Bioethics Subcommittee and the Delaware County Health Literacy Coalition.

Teresa A. Williams is Vice President of Regulatory Services at INTEGRIS Health, Inc. She oversees Legal Services, Corporate Compliance, and Legislative Affairs, also serving as the system Corporate Compliance and Privacy Officer. She is a graduate of Rose State College (A.A. 1986), the University of Central Oklahoma (B.B.A., cum laude, 1987) and the University of Oklahoma (J.D., with distinction, 1991). Ms. Williams was formerly a director in the Oklahoma City law firm of Crowe & Dunlevy. She is a former member of the Board of Directors of the American Health Lawyers Association (AHLA) and a past Chair of the AHLA In-Counsel Practice Group. She is a past President of both the Oklahoma Health Lawyers Association and Oklahoma Bar Association Health Law Section. Ms. Williams serves on the Board of Directors of The C.A.R.E. (Child Abuse Response and Evaluation) Center and the Financial Development Team for the Oklahoma General Assembly of the Church of God. Ms. Williams is an adjunct professor at the University of Oklahoma College of Law in a Master of Legal Studies Program - Healthcare. She serves as an Advisory Committee Member at Mid-America Christian University and an Advisory Board Member for the Management Department at the University of Central Oklahoma. Ms. Williams is a frequent author and speaker on health law related topics at local and national seminars for continuing legal and compliance education.

About the Authors

Haley N. Bavasi is an attorney in the Boston office of Wilson Sonsini Goodrich & Rosati, where she is a member of the firm's life sciences technology transactions practice. She brings to her current role regulatory and transactional experience from Ropes & Gray LLP, where she was a member of the firm's health care and life sciences practices focused on advising clients in the areas of clinical research and health data privacy, with an emphasis on these issues in a global context. She now represents life sciences companies in a variety of domestic and international engagements, including collaboration agreements, research and development agreements, clinical trial management, university licenses, and intellectual property licenses. Ms. Bavasi attended law school at the University of California, Berkeley School of Law. Prior to attending law school, she worked as a research associate in HIV vaccine clinical trials in San Francisco. Ms. Bavasi co-authored Chapter 9, *Understanding Research Informed Consent*.

Valerie H. Bonham is Senior Advisor in the Office of Legislative Policy and Analysis at the National Institutes of Health (NIH), part of the U.S. Department of Health and Human Services. She previously served as Senior Attorney in the Office of General Counsel, DHHS/NIH, as well as Deputy Director of the NIH Office of Research Support and Compliance and Executive Director of the Presidential Commission for the Study of Bioethical Issues under President Obama. She advises on a range of issues, including clinical research and bioethics, Congressional oversight, investigations, statutory construction, federal grants, privacy, data sharing, risk management, and intragovernmental relations. She has published widely in all of these areas. She received her undergraduate degree from Rice University, and her law degree from the University of Virginia School of Law.

Kate Bowen is General Counsel at Texas Oncology, P.A., the nation's largest independent, physician-led oncology practice, delivering leading-edge technology and treatment options through more than 420 physicians at over 175 sites in Texas. Her work involves Phase I through III oncology trials offered in the community setting, allowing patients to access innovative therapies close to home. She received her law degree from SMU Dedman School of Law.

Eve Brunts is a partner in the Health Care Practice at Ropes & Gray LLP. Her practice focuses on regulatory compliance and reimbursement issues. Ms. Brunts regularly advises research sponsors and clinical sites on clinical research compliance and contracting issues, including human subjects protection requirements, FDA requirements for clinical trials, clinical trial funding, clinical trial agreements, and HIPAA research requirements. For research sponsors and clinical sites, Ms. Brunts has participated in research compliance reviews; assisted with the development of research policies, procedures, and template documents; negotiated research collaboration agreements and/or provided advice in connection with government investigations. Ms. Brunts graduated from Yale University and Yale Law School and received a master in law from Cambridge University. She is listed in *Chambers USA: America's Leading Lawyers for Business* (2006-2018) and *LMG Life Sciences Star* (2012-2017).

Dale H. Cowan is retired from the practice of medicine and health law in Cleveland, Ohio. During the course of his 45 years of practice in hematology and medical oncology he was affiliated with MetroHealth Medical Center, University Hospitals of Cleveland, the Cleveland Clinic, and Case Western Reserve School of Medicine. He served as Chair of the Institutional Review of MetroHealth Medical Center. Additionally he served as Chair of the Ethics Advisory Committee of the Eastern Cooperative Oncology Group during which time he drafted the Conflict of Interest policies for the Group. Dr. Cowan also served on the faculty of the Case Western Reserve Law School at which institution he initiated the first courses in health care regulation. Dr. Cowan authored an article on IRBs in the Spring, 1975, issue of the Case Western Reserve Law Review, several articles on the ethics of research with human subjects with cancer and alcoholism, and a book chapter on the issues of reviewing clinical trials by IRBs. Dr. Cowan also served on the Editorial Board of the journal IRB published by the Hastings Center. He is a Fellow of the American College of Physicians, the American College of Legal Medicine where he served on the Board of Governors and as President, and the American Health Lawyers Association (AHLA) where he served two terms on the Board of Directors. He is a recipient of the David J. Greenburg Service Award from the AHLA. Dr. Cowan is a graduate of Harvard College, Harvard Medical School, and Case Western Reserve School of Law. He is licensed in medicine in California, Florida, and Ohio, and is a member of the Bar in Ohio. Dr. Cowan authored Chapter 12, *Conflict of Interest Issues*.

Payal P. Cramer is counsel in the law firm of Baker Hostetler LLP. She focuses her practice on health care and regulatory compliance. She counsels clients on matters related to clinical research programs, including human subject protection and institutional review boards, contract negotiation, Food and Drug Administration (FDA) compliance, research-related billing, and federal grant compliance. She has significant experience advising clients on matters related to data use in research, including HIPAA compliance. She received her undergraduate degree from Emory University, her Master's in Public Health from Boston University, and her law degree from Emory University School of Law.

Amy K. Dow is in private practice with the Health Care and Life Sciences Practice of Epstein Becker & Green, P.C. She advises entities engaged in clinical and preclinical research activities, including health systems, IRBs, sponsors and contract research organizations. Ms. Dow also counsels clients regarding the manufacture, sale and promotion of pharmaceuticals, biologics and medical devices, including topics relating to fraud and abuse, FDA compliance, corporate compliance and state law issues, and drafts and negotiates clinical research, consulting, and other services agreements. She received her undergraduate degree from the University of Arizona and her law degree from Northwestern University School of Law. Ms. Dow co-authored Chapter 11, *Payment to Research Subjects*.

Heather L. Fields is a shareholder at the Chicago, IL and Milwaukee, WI offices of Reinhart Boerner Van Deuren SC, where she chairs the firm's Hospitals and Health Care Systems group. She is also a member of the firm's Corporate Compliance and White Collar Litigation and Hospice and Palliative Care and Tax-Exempt Organizations groups. For more than 20 years, Ms.

Fields has assisted clients with a wide variety of regulatory, transactional and compliance-related matters. She has extensive experience conducting internal investigations and advising clients in connection with compliance and fraud and abuse issues that arise in the context of operations and various health care provider relationships and transactions. Ms. Fields also deals regularly with patient safety and quality-of-care issues, peer review matters and medical staff issues, including investigations, corrective actions, fair hearings and drafting and review of medical staff bylaws and other governance documents. She advises clients on designing and implementing corporate compliance programs and assessing compliance program effectiveness, all aspects of HIPAA compliance, and clinical research compliance. Ms. Fields has served as interim associate general counsel on an in-house basis for extended periods for clients, and is Certified in Healthcare Compliance (CHC), as well as a Certified Compliance and Ethics Professional (CCEP). Ms. Fields co-authored Chapter 10, *HIPAA Compliance in Clinical Trials.*

Jennifer S. Geetter is a Partner in the law firm of McDermott Will & Emery LLP. Ms. Geetter advises global life sciences, health care, and informatics clients on legal issues attendant to biomedical innovation, research compliance, financial relationship management, digital health practices, and global privacy and data security laws. Ms. Geetter represents a broad range of clients, including pharmaceutical, device, and biologics companies; health plans institutional health care providers, and other enterprises; mobile app, mHealth, and other digital health technology companies and platform providers; research institutes; and informatics, data broker, and data aggregator companies. She assists these clients with a range of projects, including Health Insurance Portability and Accountability Act (HIPAA), Federal Trade Commission (FTC), and state and federal privacy, security and breach response preparedness and response; research compliance, research program structure, and operational and compliance infrastructure; complex research affiliation agreements and arrangements; scientific review and research misconduct proceedings and investigations; biobanking and registry development and compliance, including emerging issues in the future, unspecified use of biospecimens, and genomic data; development and implementation of data-sharing strategies and platforms to achieve business objectives, particularly in connection with biomedical innovation, health care reform, electronic health record implementation, and quality assurance requirements; and data privacy, data mapping, and data use strategies for mobile apps and other mHealth and digital technologies. Ms. Geetter co-authored Chapter 1, *Distinguishing Research from Other Activities.*

Kimberly Gillespie is Chief Legal Counsel for University of California San Diego Health (UCSDH). In this capacity, Ms. Gillespie is responsible for managing the legal affairs of the UCSDH and advising leadership in all aspects of health care law. Areas of specialty for Ms. Gillespie include corporate governance, health care compliance, health care fraud and abuse laws (Stark, Anti-Kickback Statute, the Civil Monetary Penalties Statute, and the False Claims Act), state and federal privacy laws, medical staff and peer review matters, hospital and physician transactions, regulatory affairs, research compliance, and conflict of interest. Ms. Gillespie also oversees the UCSDH Risk Management Office. Prior to serving as Chief Legal Counsel, Ms. Gillespie served as Principal Counsel in the UC Office of the General Counsel, Chief Compliance, Privacy and Risk Officer at UCSDH, and in-house counsel for UCSDH and Virginia Commonwealth University Health System. Ms. Gillespie earned her undergraduate and master's degree from Virginia Commonwealth University (B.A. 1992, M.P.A. 1994) and her law degree from the University of Richmond, T.C. Williams School of Law (J.D. 2003). She is licensed to practice in California, North Carolina, and Virginia. Ms. Gillespie previously served as a member of the Virginia State Bar, Health Law Section, Board of Governors and writes on a variety of health law topics. Ms. Gillespie co-authored Chapter 10, *HIPAA Compliance in Clinical Trials.*

Gabrielle Goldstein is Counsel at Nixon Peabody, where she provides regulatory and transactional advice to IRBs, hospitals, research institutions, academic medical centers and biotechnology companies. Her practice includes a wide range of issues, including federal and state requirements for the protection of human subjects, stem cell research, storage and use of biospecimens, research misconduct and financial conflicts of interest in research. She also provides transactional support to her clients through structuring collaborative arrangements between industry, government and health care institutions. Ms. Goldstein is currently completing her PhD in Health Policy at UC Berkeley, where her dissertation explores variation in biomedical research oversight operations in the U.S. and Canada. Ms. Goldstein has a B.A. from UC Berkeley, a J.D. from Boston University School of Law, and is a PhD Candidate at UC Berkeley. She is a frequent lecturer and author on issues relating to domestic and international clinical research regulation. Ms. Goldstein co-authored Chapter 14, *Use of Biospecimens and Private Information in Research and Research Repositories.*

Michele R. Goodman is an Associate in the Health Care and Life Sciences Practice of Jones Day. She advises clients on compliance, regulatory, and transactional matters throughout the health care and life sciences industries. Ms. Goodman counsels clients on fraud and abuse and transparency laws, and a diverse range of federal and state regulatory compliance issues. She also focuses on clinical trials and research programs and collaborations, including negotiating agreements, reviewing informed consent forms, and advising on regulatory and ethical issues. Prior to her legal career, Ms. Goodman was a certified clinical research professional at the National Cell Repository for Alzheimer's Disease, where she coordinated the participation of over thirty academic medical centers, including the collection of biospecimens and data from participating families and the distribution thereof to researchers across the country. She received her undergraduate degree from Indiana University and her law degree from the Maurer School of Law at Indiana University. Ms. Goodman co-authored Chapter 14, *Use of Biospecimens and Private Information in Research and Research Repositories.*

Igor Gorlach is a health care associate at King & Spalding LLP. He advises health systems, life sciences companies, pharmacies, laboratories, and device suppliers on complex Medicare and Medicaid compliance and reimbursement issues as well as privacy and data protection. Prior to joining King & Spalding, Mr. Gorlach served in various legal and policy positions in Washington, DC, and Boston, MA. During 2014-2015, he served on the George Washington University institutional review board. Igor received his JD degree from Harvard Law School and his MPH degree from Harvard School of Public Health. Mr. Gorlach co-authored Chapter 6, *Roles and Responsibilities of Investigators.*

Ann T. Hollenbeck is a Partner in the Health Care and Life Sciences Practice of Jones Day. She advises entities engaged in clinical research activities, including health systems, IRBs, sponsors, research consortia, and unique research collaborations. Ms. Hollenbeck provides legal advice on a wide range of issues including research compliance, governance and corporate law, reimbursement and funding, and fraud and abuse. She received her undergraduate degree from Butler University and her law degree from Indiana University School of Law, and is licensed to practice law in Michigan, Indiana, and Illinois. Ms. Hollenbeck authored Chapter 15, *Secondary Findings in Genomic Research: Ethics, Law, and Practicality.*

Jacqueline A. Holz currently is a Contract Specialist providing legal support to U.S. Oncology Research within McKesson Specialty Health for patient participation in community based oncology research and clinical trials. Prior to arriving at McKesson Specialty Health in January 2017, she received a Masters of Law degree from Loyola University, Chicago School of Law while serving as senior legal advisor and U.S. compliance officer at Chugai Pharma. At Chugai starting in 2008, she provided for the legal counsel and management associated with both the corporate and the clinical research portions of a global pharmaceutical company. She received her Bachelor's Degree from Rutgers University and her Juris Doctor degree from Touro College, Jacob D. Fuchsburg Law Center. Ms. Holz edited and expanded Chapter 16, *Typical Areas of IRB Noncompliance.*

Beverly H. Lorell is the Senior Medical and Policy Advisor for the FDA and Life Sciences group at King & Spalding in Washington, D.C. Dr. Lorell was a Professor of Medicine at Harvard University, interventional cardiologist, and heart failure specialist. She was a clinical investigator in many pharmaceutical and medical device clinical trials. She also served on FDA Cardiovascular and Renal Drugs Advisory Committee. Before joining King & Spalding, she was vice president and the global chief medical and science officer of Guidant Corporation. In her practice at King & Spalding, she advises many manufacturers as well as health care systems on issues regarding clinical trial conduct, data integrity, and the protection of human subjects—including IRB matters— related to the Common Rule and FDA regulations. Dr. Lorell represents King & Spalding's membership in the Clinical Trials Transformation Initiative (CTTI), a public-private partnership with FDA, and she was the lead author of a recent publication on the reform of informed consent. Ms. Lorell co-authored Chapter 6, *Roles and Responsibilities of Investigators.*

Alice K. Marcee is an Assistant Vice Chancellor & Counsel for Academic and Health Affairs at the University of Texas System (UTS). Dr. Marcee provides strategic, legal, and operational advice regarding the development of two new medical schools in UTS and health care matters that include physician alignment and aggregation, governance, public-private partnerships, and value-based care models. While serving as in-house counsel at The University of Texas Southwestern Medical Center (UTSW), she was a non-voting, *ex-officio* member of the institution's IRB panels for approximately four years. Prior to law school, Dr. Marcee was on faculty in the Department of Family & Community Medicine at UTSW, engaged in health services research, supporting physicians with the integration of electronic health records into practice, and telemedicine program development and implementation. She received a Doctor of Veterinary Medicine, *magna cum laude,* from the Texas A&M College of Veterinary Medicine and a Juris Doctor from Southern Methodist University Dedmen School of Law. Dr. Marcee authored Chapter 8, *Special Categories of Review* and co-authored Chapter 14, *Use of Biospecimens and Private Information in Research and Research Repositories.*

Ernessa B. McKie is an associate at BakerHostetler in Atlanta. She focuses her health care practice on licensure applications and recovery audit work. She has a wealth of previous experience in working with the Centers for Medicare and Medicaid Services and in assisting hospitals in quality reporting, regulatory drafting, and reconsideration requests for quality reporting programs, as well as working with clients in litigation. Ms. McKie serves as an advisor to institutional review boards on a variety of matters, including but not limited to informed consent review, policy and procedure review, and operational guidance. Well-versed in government policy, analysis, and alternative dispute resolution, Ms. McKie also has experience working as a pharmaceutical sales representative, which provides her with additional insight regarding the pharmaceutical and health care industry.

Melinda G. Murray is Associate General Counsel at Holy Cross Health in Silver Spring, MD where she advises on regulatory matters, contracts, privacy issues, clinical research and bioethics, medical staff, risk, and compliance issues. Prior to 2008, she served as In-House Counsel to several hospitals and hospital systems. She served for 3 years on the Health Law Steering Committee for the D.C. Bar and has presented and written on a variety of health care issues for health care groups and the community. She received her undergraduate degree from Wheaton College (MA), and her law degree from Georgetown University Law School. Ms. Murray co-authored Chapter 10, *HIPAA Compliance in Clinical Trials.*

Katayoun (Kat) Neal is Staff Counsel at McKesson Corporation, headquartered in The Woodlands, TX. Ms. Neal supports McKesson's specialty pharmacy businesses focusing on health care contracting, legal, and regulatory matters. Prior to focusing on specialty pharmacies, Ms. Neal supported the U.S. Oncology Research clinical trial program. She dedicated eight years to the clinical trial research program, where she managed clinical trials, assisted with process improvements, and negotiated clinical trial agreements. She received her undergraduate degree from the University of Houston, and her law degree from the University of Houston Law Center. Ms. Neal co-authored Chapter 3, *Understanding the Clinical Trial Process.*

Laura M. Odwazny is a Senior Attorney with the Office of the General Counsel, U.S. Department of Health and Human Services, where she is a subject matter expert in human subject protections, research compliance, and administrative law pertaining to rulemaking. Ms. Odwazny's primary client is the Office for Human Research Protections, which interprets and enforces the HHS regulations that provide protections for human research subjects. Ms. Odwazny also currently advises the HHS Office of Global Affairs. Throughout her 18 years with the Office of the General Counsel, Ms. Odwazny has provided legal advice to various other agencies within HHS, including the Presidential Commission for the Study of Bioethical Issues, the Office of the Assistant Secretary for Health, the Program Support Center Division of FOIA Services, the Health Resources and Services Administration, and the Substance Abuse and Mental Health Administration. Prior to her employment with HHS, Ms. Odwazny served as a law clerk to the Superior Court of Pennsylvania and the Supreme Court of Pennsylvania. Ms. Odwazny is a graduate of the University of Chicago and the University of Pittsburgh School of Law, and received a M.A. in Bioethics through the History and Philosophy of Science Department at the University of Pittsburgh.

Ms. Odwazny speaks frequently on issues of human subjects research protection as applied to biomedical and behavioral research. Ms. Odwazny served as an adjunct professor at American University Washington College of Law, teaching "The Law and Ethics of Human Subjects Research," and currently teaches "Compliance in Research" at the University of Pittsburgh School of Law Health Care Compliance Certificate program. Ms. Odwazny serves as a member of the IRB for the Walter Reed Army Institute of Research (WRAIR), U.S. Department of Defense. Ms. Odwazny has served on the Core Conference Planning Committee of the Public Responsibility in Medicine & Research (PRIM&R) Advancing Ethical Research conference since 2013 and is the past committee co-chair (2015-17). Ms. Odwazny also serves as a member of the Model Agreements and Guidelines International (MAGI) Advisory Board. Ms. Odwazny co-authored Chapter 9, *Understanding Research Informed Consent.*

David Peloquin is an attorney at Ropes & Gray LLP where he practices in the firm's health care group. He focuses his practice on advising academic medical centers, life sciences companies, and information technology companies on issues related to human subjects and animal research, Medicare/Medicaid and other third-party payer reimbursement, and data privacy. Mr. Peloquin frequently writes and speaks on topics related to each of these areas. He also serves as a community member of the Institutional Review Board at Partners Healthcare in Boston. Mr. Peloquin received his undergraduate degree from Carleton College and his law degree from the Yale Law School. He clerked for the Honorable Diana E. Murphy of the United States Court of Appeals for the Eighth Circuit. Before attending law school, Mr. Peloquin worked as a project manager for Epic Systems, a leading provider of electronic medical records.

Mary Holloway Richard, of Counsel with Phillips Murrah PC in Oklahoma City, represents hospitals, clinics, group practices and individual providers across Oklahoma on a broad range of issues—transactions, reimbursement audits and appeals, OIG investigations, and compliance. She works with clients to develop business strategies in this highly regulated industry and to minimize their exposure to risks. She lectures and publishes on topics including nonprofit operations, responses to the opioid epidemic, clinical research, telehealth, HIPAA, employment and management agreements, and behavioral health law topics. She was formerly in house counsel assigned to the system's IRB. Mary has been in leadership of the American Health Lawyers Association's Behavioral Health Task Force since its inception. She is past Chair of the Health Law Section of the Oklahoma Bar Association where she inaugurated a vulnerable population webcast series for state lawyers and is past president of the Oklahoma Health Lawyers Association. She is a graduate of George Washington University law school and teaches at Oklahoma City University School of Law.

Martha C. Romney is an Assistant Professor at the Jefferson College of Population Health (JCPH), Thomas Jefferson University. Ms. Romney's research focuses on issues related to obesity, cancer, population health, employee wellness, and health disparities in research and implications for policy, which has been disseminated through publications and presentations. Ms. Romney teaches Public Health Policy and Advocacy, Cultural Humility & Competency in Population Health and Bioethics, as well as lectures on legal/regulatory, ethical and policy issues in the JCPH Master of Public Health (MPH) and Doctoral Population Health Sciences programs, in the University and at professional conferences. Ms. Romney also has pharmaceutical product litigation support and regulatory policy experience. Ms. Romney earned her BSN from Duke University, MS in Nursing from Columbia University, JD from the Antioch School of Law, MPH from Drexel University School of Public Health. Ms. Romney co-authored Chapter 3, *Understanding the Clinical Trial Process.*

Chelsea M. Rutherford is an associate in McDermott Will & Emery's Washington, DC office. Ms. Rutherford advises health care clients on a wide range of transactional and regulatory issues, including physician practice management, fraud and abuse enforcement and investigations, and research compliance. Prior to law school, she worked in clinical genetics laboratories and co-authored peer-reviewed research in the field. Ms. Rutherford received a Bachelor of Arts in Human Biology from the University of Virginia, a Masters of Bioethics from Columbia University, and a Juris Doctor from Boston University, where she also served as the editor in chief of the *American Journal of Law and Medicine.* Ms. Rutherford co-authored Chapter 1, *Distinguishing Research from Other Activities.*

Thomas D. Shrack is the Practice Area Senior Attorney-Clinical Research for Ascension, in Indianapolis, Indiana. Ascension is the largest non-profit health system in the U.S. and the world's largest Catholic health system and operates more than 2,600 sites of care in 22 states and the District of Columbia. Previously, Mr. Shrack was a shareholder at Hall, Render, Killian Heath & Lyman, P.C., where he focused his practice on the legal and ethical issues involved in clinical research activities and clinical research compliance, as well as on general clinical services, patient care issues, corporate counsel services, medical staff relations, and general regulatory and compliance issues. Mr. Shrack has served as a voting member on two hospital institutional review boards and, prior to practicing law, participated in clinical research as ultrasonographer for a group of peripheral vascular surgeons. Mr. Shrack received his undergraduate degree from Miami University in Oxford, Ohio, law degree from Indiana University School of Law, Indianapolis, and is a member of the Indiana Bar. Mr. Shrack authored Chapter 18, *Scientific Misconduct in Clinical Research.*

Lynn E. Smith is a Director with Huron Consulting Group and has 20+ years of experience in research administration and regulatory compliance. Her areas of expertise include transformation of Human Research Protection Programs (HRPP), Institutional Review Boards (IRB) and assisting clients achieve accreditation of their HRPP. Other areas of expertise include research compliance assessments, investigations of investigator non-compliance, management of research compliance and clinical trial offices, conflicts of interest (COI), scientific misconduct, and export controls.

Katherine B. Steuer is Senior Associate Counsel at St. Jude Children's Research Hospital, in Memphis, Tennessee. Ms. Steuer advises the institution and its clinical departments and committees on legal, regulatory, and strategic matters, including clinical research, bioethics, genomics, pathology and pharmaceutical regulation, medical staff, graduate medical education, managed care, compliance, reimbursement, and fraud and abuse. She is counsel to the IRB and the human subjects' protection program, and also drafts health care and affiliation agreements, consent forms, and policies and procedures. Ms. Steuer is a member of the board and past chair of the Memphis Bar Association Health Law Section, and a member of state and federal bar associations. Having graduated from Wesleyan University in Connecticut, she obtained her law degree from Harvard Law School. More recently, Ms. Steuer obtained a Certificate in Pediatric Bioethics from Children's Mercy Bioethics Center, Children's Mercy Hospital in affiliation with the University of Missouri – Kansas City. Ms. Steuer co-authored Chapter 15, *Secondary Findings in Genomic Research: Ethics, Law, and Practicality.*

Gelvina Rodriguez Stevenson is an Associate General Counsel at the Children's Hospital of Philadelphia. In her role at CHOP, Ms. Stevenson advises the hospital on the legal aspects of medical research and scientific innovation. Ms. Stevenson also provides legal support in the areas of privacy, contract negotiation, conflicts of interests, controlled substances and other matters. Prior to working at CHOP, Ms. Stevenson was an Associate University Counsel at Weill Cornell Medical College, a Legislative Attorney for the New York City Council, an associate at Chadbourne & Parke LLP and a law clerk to The Honorable Audrey B. Collins, U.S. District Court, Central District of California. Ms. Stevenson holds a JD from New York University School of Law, a Master's degree from the Woodrow Wilson School at Princeton University and a Bachelor of Arts from New York University. Ms. Stevenson serves as a Vice Chair of the AHLA Teaching Hospitals and Academic Medical Centers practice group and as Co-chair of the Hispanic National Bar Association Health and Life Sciences Committee. Ms. Stevenson is Adjunct Clinical Faculty at Drexel University School of Medicine Masters in Clinical Research Program. Ms. Stevenson co-authored Chapter 7, *Children in Research.*

Sarah E. Swank is an experienced attorney who has worked as in house counsel in two national health care systems and as a Shareholder in a nationally recognized law firm. Ms. Swank was Senior Counsel at Dignity Health in Pasadena, California supporting five hospitals, laboratory services and six CINs and a Shareholder in Ober|Kaler's Health Law Group in the Washington, DC office providing advice and guidance on health care transactions, governance, ACOs, telehealth, compliance, EMTALA, clinical research, IRBs and health care reform. Before joining Ober|Kaler, Sarah was an Associate General Counsel for Trinity Health in the metro-DC area, where she managed the local legal team and assisted in system-wide initiatives. She started her career as a managed care attorney and government affairs associate in New York State. Sarah works with clients to navigate the complex legal framework facing the health care industry today and to promote access to high quality and safe care by breaking down silos through innovation, technology, clinical research and patient-centeredness.

About the Editors and Authors

Leslie Thornton is an attorney at Ropes & Gray LLP, practicing in the firm's health care group. Dr. Thornton advises academic medical centers, pharmaceutical and device manufacturers, research institutes, health technology companies, and other health care organizations on a broad range of research issues, including preclinical and clinical matters, federal grants and contracts, research misconduct, and government audits and investigations. She also advises her clients regarding health care privacy and security matters, both U.S. and ex-U.S. Before law school, Dr. Thornton gained experience as an academic researcher in both public health and psychiatric settings, including extensive training in advanced statistical and epidemiologic methods. She received her J.D. from the University of California, Berkeley School of Law, her Ph.D. from the Johns Hopkins Bloomberg School of Public Health, and her undergraduate degrees from the University of California, Los Angeles.

Leah A. Voigt is Chief Privacy & Research Integrity Officer at Spectrum Health System in Grand Rapids, Michigan. Prior to joining Spectrum Health, Ms. Voigt was an attorney in private practice in the Washington, DC office of the global firm, Squire Sanders & Dempsey (now Squire Patton Boggs). She was a member of both the Health Care and Life Sciences practice groups, and her clients included a diverse range of organizations, from large academic medical centers, health systems, and health insurance companies, to start-up health information technology companies and global medical device and pharmaceutical manufacturers. Before graduate school, Ms. Voigt served as an administrator for a biomedical research institute in Los Angeles, California. Ms. Voigt is currently Chair of the Academic Medical Centers & Teaching Hospitals Practice Group of the American Health Lawyers Association. She received a Bachelor of Arts from Smith College, a Masters of Health Policy from University of Michigan, and her Juris Doctor from Loyola Law School in Los Angeles. Ms. Voigt co-authored Chapter 7, *Children in Research.*

About the American Health Lawyers Association

Leading health law to excellence through education, information, and dialogue, the American Health Lawyers Association (AHLA) is the nation's largest nonpartisan 501(c)(3) educational organization devoted to legal issues in the health care field, with nearly 14,000 members.

The mission of the American Health Lawyers Association is to provide a collegial forum for interaction and information exchange to enable its members to serve their clients more effectively; to produce the highest quality non-partisan educational programs, products, and services concerning health law issues; and to serve as a public resource on selected health care legal issues.

AHLA provides resources to address the issues facing its active members who practice in law firms, government, in-house settings, and academia and who represent the entire spectrum of the health industry: physicians, hospitals and health systems, health maintenance organizations, health insurers, life sciences entities, managed care companies, nursing facilities, home care providers, and consumers.

Table of Contents

Chapter 8 Special Categories of Review

Alice K. Marcee

Chapter 9 Understanding Research Informed Consent

Laura M. Odwazny
Haley N. Bavasi

Chapter 1

Distinguishing Research from Other Activities

Chelsea M. Rutherford

Jennifer S. Geetter

Introduction

HUMAN SUBJECTS RESEARCH is conducted at a range of settings—teaching hospitals, academic medical institutions, community hospitals, regional health care delivery systems, large group health practices, biotech companies, and other health care provider organizations. Millions of individuals participate in research each year.[1] Large-scale national research initiatives, such as the Precision Medicine Initiative, are aiming to engage a historic number of research participants.[2] As a result, in-house counsel employed by health care organizations are often looked upon to provide legal advice about research or to serve as a member on an institutional review board (IRB).

In-house counsel may have the responsibility of proactively addressing research compliance within the organization. The first step for in-house counsel is to acquire a working knowledge of the current regulations promulgated by the Department of Health and Human Services (HHS) and the Food and Drug Administration (FDA), the two primary federal agencies that regulate the majority of human subjects research. In-house counsel must also understand the requirements of the Health Insurance Portability and Accountability Act of 1996 and its implementing regulations[3] (HIPAA) with respect to research activities involving a Covered Entity's use and disclosure of an individual's protected health information (PHI).[4] This foundation is necessary to identify potential issues and maintain a well-functioning research program.

[1] *See* Battelle Technology Partnership Practice for the Pharmaceutical Research and Manufacturers of America (PhRMA), *Biopharmaceutical Industry-Sponsored Clinical Trials: Impact on State Economies* (Mar. 2015), *available at* http://phrma-docs.phrma.org/sites/default/files/pdf/biopharmaceutical-industry-sponsored-clinical-trials-impact-on-state-economies.pdf.

[2] *See* NIH, All of Us Research Program, *available at* https://allofus.nih.gov/.

[3] *See* 45 C.F.R. Parts 160 and 164.

[4] The term "Covered Entity" refers to a health plan, a health care clearinghouse, and a health care provider who transmits any health information in electronic form in connection with a covered transaction and would include all providers. Researchers may also be Covered Entities if they meet the definition above. HIPAA also applies to Business Associates of Covered Entities, though we only use the term Covered Entity for purposes of this memorandum. The term "Business Associate" includes entities that perform a variety of functions, including

This primer provides an overview of these regulatory requirements and legal challenges associated with research and IRB matters, but should not be the exclusive source of reference. Nevertheless, it provides a good starting point for in-house counsel and outside counsel who may be called upon to advise health care organizations about research-related matters.

1.1 Distinguishing Research from Other Activities

In-house counsel is often called upon by the IRB to help determine whether a proposed project is research or is some other type of activity (*e.g.*, one undertaken as part of the organization's quality assurance, quality improvement activities, or other operational activities (collectively referred to herein as QI)). To be effective, in-house counsel must be able to help IRBs distinguish which activities constitute research subject to regulation and which activities do not. Determining whether an activity is research is critical. If an activity is research, IRBs must also be able to discern whether it involves human subjects. Researchers and research entities generally need to obtain consent and/or HIPAA authorization from human research subjects before engaging them, or using their identifiable information, in research. Even when human subjects research projects are exempt from consent/authorization requirements or such requirements are waived, IRB oversight is still necessary. If institutions are conducting research involving human subjects and do not realize it, the institution and its IRB will not meet applicable compliance requirements and may face other consequences, including restrictions on using any collected data.

Determining whether an activity is research is not always an easy task. IRBs must be familiar with the definitions set forth in the applicable federal and state laws and guidance, and must be able to ascertain which research regulations apply to a given project. Lastly, IRBs must be able to determine whether the proposed research is exempt from one or more research regulations or otherwise eligible for an expedited or streamlined review process.

1.2 "Research" Defined

Unless an exemption applies, research that requires IRB review under federal law is generally any activity that either (i) meets the definition of "research" and involves "human subjects" under the "Common Rule,"[5] and is an entity or project subject to the Common Rule's requirements; (ii) meets the definition of "research" under HIPAA;[6] or (iii) meets the FDA definition of a "clinical investigation" and involves "human subjects" as defined by the FDA.[7] Note that, even when IRB oversight does not apply by operation of federal law, state law and long-standing ethics and norms will counsel for following Common Rule approaches.

---

an entity that, on behalf of a covered entity, creates, receives, maintains, or transmits PHI for a function or activity regulated by HIPAA, such as claims processing or administration, data analysis, process, or administration, utilization review, quality assurance, and practice management services. 45 C.F.R. § 160.103.

[5] 45 C.F.R. § 46.102(d), (f).

[6] 45 C.F.R. § 164.501.

[7] 21 C.F.R. § 56.102(c), (e).

The Federal Policy for the Protection of Human Research Subjects "Common Rule," is the main source of federal protections for individuals participating in federally funded research. It is enforced by the Office of Human Research Protections (OHRP) at HHS, and has been adopted by more than 15 federal departments or agencies. Although the Common Rule generally only applies to human subjects research that is conducted or funded by a Common Rule-adopting department or agency, many institutions who receive federal funds have elected to subject all of their human subjects research to the Common Rule requirements and HHS oversight.[8] The Common Rule may also apply to an entity that contributes to a federally funded study, for example, and is thus "engaged" in human subjects research.[9] Moreover, the Common Rule requirements are seen as a guidepost for appropriate human subjects research requirements and may be used by private funding groups or institutions even when the regulations would not otherwise apply.

The Common Rule defines "research" as "a systematic investigation, including research development, testing and evaluation, designed to develop or contribute to generalizable knowledge."[10] Examples of systematic investigations include:

- interventions and procedures;
- surveys and questionnaires;
- interviews and focus groups;
- analyses of existing identifiable data or biological specimens;
- epidemiological studies;
- evaluations of social or educational programs;
- cognitive and perceptual experiments; and
- medical chart review studies.

Research results *do not* have to be published or presented at a professional meeting to qualify the activity as research. From HHS's perspective, the *intent* to contribute to "generalizable" or scholarly knowledge makes an experiment or data collection research, and extends protections to research participants, regardless of publication.

The Common Rule's definition of research highlights the pursuit of *generalizable knowledge* as the element that distinguishes research from other activities.[11] Unlike a straightforward

[8] This option is sometimes referred to as a 4(b) election. Notably, this option was removed by the 2018 Common Rule, discussed *infra*; while institutions may still voluntarily choose to conduct all of their human subjects research in accordance with the Common Rule, research that is not federally funded or supported will no longer be subject to HHS oversight. 82 Fed. Reg. 7180 (final §__.101(a)).

[9] *See generally* HHS OHRP, *Guidance on Engagement of Institutions in Research involving human subjects*, Oct. 16, 2008, *available at* https://www.hhs.gov/ohrp/policy/engage08.html.

[10] 45 C.F.R. § 46.102(d), (f).

[11] Baily, Mary Ann; Bottrell, Melissa; Lynn, Joanne; Jennings, Bruce, *The Ethics of Using QI Methods to Improve Health Care Quality and Safety,* The Hastings Center Special Report, S11 (July–Aug. 2006) (hereafter "Hastings").

QI activity, in which a problem in a particular clinical department or setting is analyzed only to improve outcomes in that limited setting, the goal of research is to intentionally seek conclusions that are generalizable to a larger group. For example, generalizable knowledge has been defined as "results that will be shared with others for learning purposes."[12] Activities that are *designed* on the front end to examine or test the efficacy of a QI intervention, in addition to improving the quality of care, might qualify as research under the Common Rule (assuming the other elements of the definition were met) since the primary purpose of the project is an assessment of the efficacy of the QI intervention, not the provision of validated QI approaches. QI studies who merely end up sharing their results, but were not designed or completed with the aim to do so, would likely not. Research within a clinical setting is usually conceived, funded, and managed as discrete projects, each led by a principal investigator who is responsible for the study's conduct. The resources often come from outside of the organization in which it is carried out—from a federal agency, private foundation, pharmaceutical corporation, etc. (though research can also be unfunded). To be considered research, the activity should be designed to produce generalizable knowledge, not to immediately improve individual patient care.[13]

FDA regulations define a "clinical investigation" as any experiment that involves a "test article" and one or more "human subjects" and that is either subject to requirements for prior submission to the FDA, or is not subject to requirements for prior submission to the FDA under the Federal Food, Drug, and Cosmetic Act (FDCA), but the results of which are intended to be submitted later to, or held for inspection by, the FDA as part of an application for a research or marketing permit.[14] Examples of clinical investigations include, but are not limited to:

- investigational drug clinical trials;
- studies involving medical treatment with an investigational device; and
- studies of medical outcomes comparing approved drugs/devices.

A "test article" means any drug (including a biological product for human use), medical device for human use, human food additive, color additive, electronic product, or any other article subject to regulation under the FDCA.[15]

1.3 Research with "Human Subjects" Defined

The term "human subject" is defined differently under the Common Rule and FDA regulations, and is also separately analyzed for HIPAA purposes (which is only concerned with the use and disclosure of PHI[16]). The pre-2018 Common Rule considers a "human subject" to be

[12] *See, e.g.*, McGraw and Leiter, *Risk-Based Regulation of Clinical Health Data Analytics*, COLO. TECH. L.J. 435 (2014).

[13] *Id.*

[14] 21 C.F.R. § 56.102(c).

[15] 21 C.F.R. § 56.102(l).

[16] HIPAA, notably, also protects the individually identifiable health information of a decedent for 50 years following the date of death of the decedent. Both the Common Rule and FDA regulations require an individual to

"a living individual about whom an investigator conducting research obtains (i) data through "intervention" or "interaction" with the individual; or (ii) identifiable "private" information."[17] "Intervention" includes both physical procedures by which data are gathered (*e.g.*, venipuncture) and manipulations of the subject or the subject's environment that are performed for research purposes. "Interaction" includes communication or interpersonal contact between an investigator and subject. "Private information" includes information about behavior that occurs in a context in which an individual can reasonably expect that no observation or recording is taking place, and information which has been provided for specific purposes by an individual and which the individual can reasonably expect will not be made public (*e.g.*, a medical record). Private information must be individually identifiable (*i.e.*, the identity of the subject is or may readily be ascertained by the investigator or associated with the information) in order for obtaining the information to constitute research involving human subjects. Under the pre-2018 Common Rule, then, research encompasses communication of private information without any physical procedure, like a retrospective chart review of patients with a particular medical condition.[18]

After a five-plus-year rulemaking process, HHS promulgated final updates to the Common Rule on January 19, 2017, to be implemented in 2019 (referred to in regulations and here as the 2018 Requirements, or 2018 Common Rule). Among other changes, the 2018 Common Rule revised the definition of a "human subject" to explicitly include identifiable biospecimens and built in a process to reassess and update the meaning of identifiability in the context of the Common Rule.[19] This pathway is of particular importance as all biospecimens could ultimately be reclassified as "identifiable" for Common Rule purposes, outside of additional notice and comment rulemaking. This would make all federally funded research with biospecimens fall under the Common Rule's definition of research with human subjects, and would be a dramatic shift in the research oversight paradigm. The majority of the changes were initially scheduled to go into effect on January 18, 2018, but have since been delayed until January 21, 2019.[20]

FDA regulations define "human subject" as an individual who is or becomes a participant in research, either as a recipient of the "test article" or as a "control." A subject may be either a healthy human or a patient. FDA regulations expressly exclude research limited to data analysis from its definition of research.[21] De-identification of data, however, does not terminate an individual's legal status as a "subject" under FDA regulations. For example, the FDA does not require informed consent for studies of *in vitro* diagnostic devices that use leftover

---

be living to be considered a human subject. 45 C.F.R. § 160.103(2)(iv).

[17] 45 C.F.R. § 46.102(f).

[18] *Id.*

[19] 82 Fed. Reg. 7149, 7179 (Jan. 19, 2017) (final §__.102(e)).

[20] 83 Fed. Reg. 28497 (Jun. 19, 2018). Despite the delay, institutions may voluntarily implement three "burden-reducing" provisions contained in the 2018 Common Rule: the revised definition of "research," the elimination of the requirement that IRBs review grant applications or proposals, and the elimination of certain annual continuing review requirements. *Id.*; *see also* 83 Fed. Reg. 17595 (Apr. 20, 2018).

[21] 21 C.F.R. § 56.102(c).

biospecimens that are not individually identifiable (provided the study meets other additional requirements), though IRB review of the study is still generally required.[22] More recently, the FDA has also issued guidance regarding waivers of informed consent for FDA-regulated minimal risk research, including research with de-identified data.[23] While additional regulations appear forthcoming, this guidance confirms the FDA won't object to an IRB approving a waiver or alteration of informed consent, for the use and/or disclosure of de-identified data, when the applicable Common Rule waiver or alteration requirements are met.[24]

As described above, HIPAA governs a Covered Entity's use and disclosure of an individual's protected health information (PHI) for research purposes.[25] HIPAA defines research as "a systematic investigation, including research development, testing and evaluation, designed to develop or contribute to generalizable knowledge."[26] This definition mirrors the Pre-2018 Common Rule. Unlike the Common Rule, however, HIPAA expressly designates QI activities as health care operations, and <u>not</u> research. As discussed *infra,* the "primary purpose" of these activities is evaluated to determine whether they are health care operations or research (mutually exclusive definitions under HIPAA). As applicable, research involving PHI must be conducted in accordance with HIPAA (in addition to following FDA and/or Common Rule requirements, when required). HIPAA supplements FDA and Common Rule regulations by requiring specific data protection measures. For more information on HIPAA and research, see **Chapter 10**, *HIPAA Compliance in Clinical Trials*.

1.4 Research Distinguished from Therapeutic Patient Care

As stated above, the purpose of research is to develop or contribute to generalizable (scholarly) knowledge. Research can be distinguished from individual care or treatment which is directed toward diagnostic or therapeutic goals of a specific patient. Patients expect that medical treatment will be personalized to treat their specific condition(s) in a manner that is consistent with their individual needs. Therapeutic treatment is for the benefit of the specific patient and usually does not produce generalizable knowledge that can be applied to other patients.

Research itself is not a per se therapeutic intervention, although in certain cases, enrolling in a research study may be essential to a person's medical care, for example, if standard treat-

[22] FDA, *Informed Consent for In Vitro Diagnostic Device Studies Using Leftover Human Specimens that are Not Individually Identifiable*, April 25, 2006, *available at* https://www.fda.gov/downloads/MedicalDevices/DeviceRegulationandGuidance/GuidanceDocuments/ucm071265.pdf.

[23] FDA, *IRB Waiver or Alteration of Informed Consent for Clinical Investigations Involving No More Than Minimal Risk to Human Subjects*, July 25, 2017, *available at* https://www.fda.gov/downloads/RegulatoryInformation/Guidances/UCM566948.pdf. Minimal risk is defined in applicable FDA regulations as "the probability and magnitude of harm or discomfort anticipated in the research are not greater in and of themselves than those ordinarily encountered in daily life or during the performance of routine physical or psychological examinations or tests." 21 C.F.R. §§ 50.3(k), 56.102(i).

[24] *Id.*

[25] 45 C.F.R. § 160.103.

[26] 45 C.F.R. § 164.501.

ments have failed. For patients, research activities may or may not be beneficial or contribute to their care. Study participants often (mistakenly) believe, however, that therapy and research are governed by the same primary goal—advancing the individual patient's interests. This is often referred to as the "therapeutic misconception." The therapeutic misconception occurs when a research subject fails to appreciate the distinction between the goals of research and those of treatment, and therefore inaccurately attributes therapeutic intent to research interventions. The therapeutic misconception is an ethical challenge in research because it presents the concern that some patients may volunteer as research participants with a distorted notion of the benefits and risks, despite explicit efforts by the researchers to explain that there is no anticipated benefit for the patients/subjects. Institutions should strive to address this issue during the informed consent process (addressed further in **Chapter 9**, *Understanding Research Informed Consent*).

1.5 Research Distinguished from Quality Assurance / Quality Improvement Activities

Distinguishing research from QI is often more challenging than distinguishing research from therapeutic patient care activities, as both activities can share similar characteristics. For instance, both QI and research activities may involve living participants, both may be systematic investigations, and both may collect and analyze data to generate information. There are, however, important distinctions between the two.

A QI activity might begin with a review of aggregate data at the patient, provider, clinical unit or organizational level to identify a clinical or management change expected to improve care.[27] QI can look like a type of practical problem solving, an evidence-based management style, or the application of a theory-driven science of how to bring about system change.[28] QI activities generally are intended to monitor quality issues for specific institutional operations. Although they often involve human participation, QI activities typically are not designed to produce the "generalizable knowledge" for application outside of a specific department or operations that are the focus of the QI activity.[29] They are generally designed to bring about immediate improvements in care in a particular localized health care setting. The participants are therefore not human subjects.

In considering revisions to the pre-2018 Common Rule, HHS proposed to exclude certain QI activities from the Common Rule's jurisdiction, proposing to designate them as non-research activities. These changes were proposed in direct response to industry questions, to help clarify HHS's position on QI activities constituting research under the Common Rule.[30] HHS declined to finalize these proposals in its 2018 Common Rule, however, stating that certain QI and internal monitoring activities do "involve research and deserve the protections" of the Com-

[27] Hastings at S11.

[28] *Id.* at S5.

[29] Murray, Jan E., *Clinical Research: A Primer for In-House Counsel,* American Health Lawyers Association In-House Counsel Program, San Francisco, California (June 30, 2002).

[30] 80 Fed. Reg. 53931, 53947 (Sept. 8, 2015).

mon Rule.[31] This decision confirms there is no bright line for determining when an activity may qualify as research, and such activities should be evaluated on a case-by-case basis.

1.6 Research Distinguished from Health Care Operations

In contrast to FDA and the pre-2018 Common Rule's definition of research, HIPAA defines "health care operations" to generally cover QI activities, including "quality assessment and improvement activities [and] outcomes evaluation and development of clinical guidelines, *provided* that the obtaining of generalizable knowledge is *not the primary purpose* of any studies resulting from such activities."[32] HIPAA also expressly includes "population-based activities relating to improving health or reducing health care costs, protocol development, case management and care coordination"[33] in its health care operations definition, as well as the creation of de-identified data sets and limited data sets (provided that such activities are not undertaken as part of research). In practice, activities are generally either health care operations or research, and these terms are generally treated as mutually exclusive for HIPAA purposes.

Analyzing whether a QI activity is a health care operation or research under HIPAA turns on whether the *primary purpose* of the activity is to obtain generalizable knowledge.[34] If the primary purpose is to obtain generalizable knowledge, then the activity *cannot* be a health care operation. As a result, the primary purpose test is relied upon to help distinguish health care operations from research under HIPAA. Historically, HIPAA-regulated entities have sometimes struggled to distinguish between QI activities and research in certain cases, and it has been unclear at times whether QI activities that met HIPAA's definition of health care operations could nevertheless constitute research activities under the pre-2018 Common Rule. The 2018 Common Rule, however, included a new exemption category for the secondary research use (information collection and analysis) of identifiable private information and/or identifiable biospecimens regulated as health care operations under HIPAA.[35] This exemption seeks to align the Common Rule and HIPAA in treating health care operations as distinct from research activities, despite HHS's decision not to finalize the QI-specific exclusion in the 2018 Common Rule.

1.7 Other Activities That Are Not Considered Research

Below are examples of other activities that generally are not classified as research. These activities may involve aspects which are similar to research, but do not rise to the level of

---

[31] 82 Fed. Reg. 7149, 7179 (Jan. 19, 2017).

[32] 45 C.F.R. § 164.501 (emphasis added).

[33] *Id.*

[34] *See* 65 Fed. Reg. 82608. Notably, this analysis is generally limited to data-related activities. Clinical interactions or interventions with patients are nearly always considered research activities.

[35] 82 Fed. Reg. at 7262 (final §__.104(d)(4)(iii)). Notably, despite the exemption, a researcher may still need to work with an IRB and seek limited review if HIPAA would require a waiver of authorization to perform the research.

research. It is always advisable to refer back to the applicable definition(s) of research when evaluating a specific intervention.

1.7.1 The Case Report or Case Series

Physicians frequently access a patient's medical records to prepare a "case report" for publication in a medical journal. It is important to analyze such access and use to determine if it meets the regulatory definition of research—the *systematic investigation* element and the intent to contribute to *generalizable knowledge*. Case reports usually fall under the category of an educational activity as the preparation of a case report does not usually constitute a systematic investigation. A case report from a research study involving only one subject (sometimes called an "N-of-1" trial), however, in which there was systematic manipulation of an intervention to produce generalizable results, may constitute a research activity.

1.7.2 Education

If an activity is undertaken for the specific purpose of teaching something it does not automatically transform the activity into research, even though the purpose of most educational activities is to disseminate or "generalize" knowledge. Again, it is important to conduct an analysis to determine whether the project contains both elements from the regulatory definition of research—the systematic investigation and the intent to contribute to generalizable knowledge. In addition, the 2018 Common Rule expressly deems "[s]cholarly and journalistic activities (*e.g.*, oral history, journalism, biography, literary criticism, legal research, and historical scholarship), including the collection and use of information, that focus directly on the specific individuals about whom the information is collected" not to be research.[36]

1.7.3 Medical Practice for the Benefit of Others

In such situations, the objective of the medical practice is to benefit people other than those who are directly affected by the health care intervention. Blood donations and some vaccine programs are examples of medical practices for the benefit of others, and the goal is to benefit a well-defined group of people in a predictable way.

1.7.4 Public Health Practice

Similar to medical practice for the benefit of others, a public health practice generally involves individuals who do not directly benefit from the intervention and can include the review of private, identifiable information about health status. Examples include surveillance (*e.g.*, monitoring of diseases) and program evaluation (*e.g.*, immunization coverage or use of clinical preventive services such as mammography). As HHS has noted, however, "[t]he line between public health surveillance and epidemiological research can be difficult to draw, as the same epidemiological techniques may be used in both. Generally, the difference between the

---

[36] 82 Fed. Reg. at 7261 (final §__.102(*l*)(1)).

activities is the purpose or context in which the investigation is being conducted . . ."[37] and the research entity conducting or directing the activity (*e.g.*, surveillance systems maintained by the Centers for Disease Control and Prevention (CDC)). In the 2018 Common Rule, necessary public health surveillance activities that are conducted, supported, required, or authorized by a public health authority are expressly excluded from the definition of research.[38]

[37] 82 Fed. Reg. at 7176.

[38] 82 Fed. Reg. at 7261 (final §__.102(*l*)(2)).

Chapter 2

Regulations that Govern Clinical Research in the United States

David Peloquin

Leslie Thornton

Introduction

Our current clinical (or human subject) research protection system was developed in response to research projects that offered subjects no direct benefit and exposed them to substantial harm.[1] Since the implementation of the federal regulations, significant advances have been made in protecting human research subjects. The regulatory body that has oversight responsibilities over a particular clinical research study depends on the type of study that is being conducted and the funding source for the study. Clinical trials involving investigational products regulated by the U.S. Food & Drug Administration (FDA), including drugs, devices and biologics, are regulated by the FDA.[2] Clinical studies that are conducted or supported by federal government agencies may be subject to regulation by the U.S. Department of Health & Human Services (HHS)[3] or other governmental agencies that conduct or support the research.[4] Human subjects research that is neither regulated by the FDA nor conducted nor supported by HHS or another federal government agency that has adopted regulations governing human subjects research may not be subject to direct federal oversight. Nevertheless, as a practical matter, in most instances research either will be subject to oversight by one or more federal agencies, such as HHS or FDA, or it will be subject to institutional policies that are based upon federal regulations.[5] The Health Insurance Portability and Accountability Act of 1996 (HIPAA) Privacy Rule[6] supplements federal human research regulations by imposing specific requirements for the protection of human research subject privacy in research studies that take

[1] Baily, Mary Ann; Bottrell, Melissa; Lynn, Joanne; Jennings, Bruce, *The Ethics of Using QI Methods to Improve Health Care Quality and Safety,* The Hastings Center Special Report, S11 (July–Aug. 2006) (hereafter "Hastings").

[2] 21 C.F.R. § 56.102(c).

[3] 45 C.F.R. § 46.101(a).

[4] For example, the requirements for the Department of Veterans Affairs are codified at 38 C.F.R. Part 16.

[5] Malinowski, Michael J., *Institutional Conflicts and Responsibilities in an Age of Academic-Industry Alliances,* 8 Widener Law Symposium Journal 47 (2001).

[6] 45 C.F.R. Parts 160 and 164 (Subparts A & E).

place at entities that are "covered entities" subject to HIPAA, which includes most U.S. health care providers.

2.1 National Research Act/The Belmont Report

Following revelations about the Public Health Service's "Tuskegee Study of Untreated Syphilis in the Negro Male," Congress passed the National Research Act in 1974.[7] This Act created the National Commission for the Protection of Human Subjects of Biomedical and Behavioral Research (National Commission). The National Commission was charged with identifying the basic ethical principles that should govern the conduct of biomedical and behavioral research. The principles were presented in 1979 in a document called "The Belmont Report: Ethical Principles and Guidelines for the Protection of Human Subjects of Research," so named because the National Commission met in the Belmont Conference Center of the Smithsonian Institution.[8]

The Belmont Report is the cornerstone statement of ethical principles upon which federal regulations for the protection of human subjects are based.[9] The Belmont Report describes three basic ethical principles that are particularly relevant to the ethics of research involving human subjects: (i) respect for persons; (ii) beneficence; and (iii) justice.

Respect for persons involves recognition of the personal dignity and autonomy of individuals, and protection of those persons with diminished autonomy, such as minors, persons with mental disorders, or prisoners. Respect for persons is manifested in the informed consent process in which potential subjects are provided information about the study[10] in a manner that is understandable and comprehensive to allow the individual to make a reasoned decision about whether or not to participate in the research.

Beneficence entails an obligation to protect persons from harm by maximizing anticipated benefits and minimizing possible risks of harm. Beneficence requires that investigators and IRB members engage in an analysis of the risks and benefits of the research to the subjects, making sure that anticipated risks are proportional to the potential benefits. Risks should be minimized as much as possible.

---

[7] Pub. L. No. 93-348, 88 Stat. 342, codified at 42 U.S.C. §§ 289–300aaa-13.

[8] National Commission for the Protection of Human Subjects of Biomedical and Behavioral Research, The Belmont Report: Ethical Principles and Guidelines for the Protection of Human Subjects of Research. GPO Pub. No. 887-809 (1979) (hereafter "The Belmont Report").

[9] Dunn, Cynthia McGuire and Gary Chadwick, Pharm.D., M.P.H., *Protecting Study Volunteers in Research: A Manual for Investigative Sites,* CenterWatch, Inc., 11 (1999).

[10] This information includes, but is not limited to, study purpose, duration, procedures, reasonably foreseeable risks or discomforts, reasonably expected benefits, alternative procedures or courses of treatment, the extent to which confidentially of records will be maintained, compensation and treatments available in the event of injury, and right to refuse or discontinue participation at any time without penalty or loss of benefits to which the individual is otherwise entitled. *See* 21 C.F.R. § 50.25; 45 C.F.R. § 46.116.

Justice requires that the benefits and burdens of research be distributed equitably. The principle of justice instructs IRBs that subjects should not be chosen simply because they are available and easy to manipulate and that research should not unduly involve persons from groups who are unlikely to be among the beneficiaries of treatments developed through the research. In addition, the principle of justice requires that subjects who are likely to benefit from a study should not be excluded.

The three ethical principles presented in The Belmont Report guided the development of the federal regulations for protecting research subjects. In response to The Belmont Report, both HHS and FDA promulgated regulations that are discussed in more detail below.

2.2 Federal Policy/Pre-2018 Requirements

Until 1991, the federal agencies that conducted, supported, or regulated research each used a variety of policies and procedures to protect human research subjects. To eliminate confusion and promote uniformity, these departments adopted as regulation a common federal policy for the protection of human research subjects known as "The Federal Policy for Protection of Human Subjects," which now referred to as the "Pre-2018 Requirements" or "Pre-2018 Common Rule" as it was adopted "in common" by certain federal department and agencies and applies to research involving human research subjects that is conducted, supported, or otherwise subject to regulation by these federal departments and agencies. The Pre-2018 Requirements were based on the regulations first issued by HHS and FDA in 1981 and is codified in HHS regulations at Title 45, Part 46, Subpart A.[11]

Because the Pre-2018 Requirements apply to "research" involving "human subjects," to understand the scope of the Common Rule one must examine the Rule's definitions of each of these terms. The Pre-2018 Requirements define "research" as "a systematic investigation, including research development, testing and evaluation, designed to develop or contribute to generalizable knowledge," and it defines a "human subject" as "a living person about whom an investigator (whether professional or student) conducting research obtains: (1) data through

[11] In addition to HHS, the Common Rule (now referred to as "Pre-2018 Requirements") was adopted by 14 other federal departments and agencies in 1991, each of which codified it in their own set of federal regulations: Departments of Agriculture, Energy, Commerce, Housing and Urban Development, Justice, Defense, Education, Veterans Affairs, Transportation, National Aeronautics and Space Administration, Consumer Product Safety Commission, Agency for International Development, Environmental Protection Agency, and National Science Foundation. In addition to those departments and agencies that have codified the Common Rule in their own regulations, the Central Intelligence Agency, Office of the Director of National Intelligence, the Social Security Administration, and the Department of Homeland Security have historically followed the Common Rule as a matter of internal policy. In January 2017, with the issuance of a final rule revising the Common Rule, the Department of Labor announced that it would codify the Common Rule in its own regulations. The Consumer Product Safety Commission, which was not a party to the 2018 Requirements, adopted the changes found in the 2018 Requirements through separate rulemaking on September 18, 2017. Also in the 2018 Requirements, the Social Security Administration and the Department of Homeland Security announced that they are codifying the rule in their own regulations for the first time, despite having historically followed the Common Rule as a matter of policy. *See* 82 Fed. Reg. 7149, 7154 (Jan. 19, 2017).

intervention or interaction with the individual; or (2) identifiable private information."[12] Under the Rule, "interventions" include both procedures by which data are gathered and manipulations of the subject or the subject's environment, whereas "interactions" include communication or interpersonal contact between the investigator and the subject. "Identifiable private information" is information about behavior that occurs in a context that the individual can reasonably expect not to be observed or recorded by others, or information that the individual can reasonably expect will not be made public (*e.g.*, a medical record), but only when "the identity of the subject is or may readily be ascertained by the investigator or associated with the information."[13] The Rule's focus on information being "identifiable" is important, because it means that secondary research involving information or biospecimens collected for a purpose other than the present research study can be taken outside of the ambit of the Rule by stripping them of information that would permit the investigator readily to ascertain the subject's identity.[14]

The central requirements of the Pre-2018 Requirements are (i) that individuals who participate as subjects in covered research are selected equitably and give their fully informed, fully voluntary written consent;[15] (ii) that proposed research be reviewed by an independent oversight group referred to as an institutional review board (IRB), and approved only if risks to subjects have been minimized and are reasonable in relation to anticipated benefits, if any, to the subjects, and the importance of the knowledge that may reasonably be expected to result; and (iii) that each institution engaged in federally supported human subjects research file an assurance of compliance. An assurance formalizes the institution's commitment to pro-

[12] 45 C.F.R. § 46.102.

[13] *See id.*

[14] Note that the concept of "identifiable private information" under the Pre-2018 Requirements differs from the concept of "de-identified" information under the HIPAA Privacy Rule. Under the HIPAA Privacy Rule, information can be rendered de-identified only by: (i) adhering to a Safe Harbor through which 18 specific identifiers are removed from the information, or (ii) obtaining from a statistical expert an opinion that there is a "very small" risk of re-identification. *See* 45 C.F.R. § 164.514. Under the Pre-2018 Requirements, the standard of identifiability is more flexible, meaning that certain information that must be removed in order for information to be considered "de-identified" under the HIPAA Privacy Rule Safe Harbor (*e.g.*, treatment or admission dates) generally do not need to be removed in order for the information no longer to be considered "identifiable" under the Pre-2018 Requirements, since dates alone typically do not permit an investigator readily to ascertain the identity of a subject. The 2018 Requirements issued in January 2017 provide that the Common Rule agencies will revisit at least every four years the definition of "identifiable" given changes in technology that may render additional information, *e.g.*, genetic information, identifiable. In addition, these agencies will undertake a parallel process of evaluating certain technologies to determine whether the information generated by such technologies is inherently identifiable for purposes of the Rule, placing technologies deemed to generate inherently identifiable information on a list after providing notice and an opportunity for public comment. *See* 82 Fed. Reg. 7149, 7169 (Jan. 19, 2017).

[15] An IRB can alter certain elements of, or waive entirely, the informed consent requirement if the following criteria are satisfied: (i) the research involves no more than minimal risk to subjects; (ii) the research could not practicably be carried out without the requested waiver or alteration; (iii) the waiver or alteration will not adversely affect the rights and welfare of the subjects; and (iv) whenever appropriate, the subjects or legally authorized representatives will be provided with additional pertinent information after participation. 45 C.F.R. § 46.116(d). The 2018 Requirements added a new required element for an IRB to grant a waiver of informed consent, *i.e.*, that the research could not practicably be carried out without using the information or biospecimens in an identifiable format. *See* § __.116(f)(3), 82 Fed. Reg. at 7267.

tect human subjects. Thus, the Pre-2018 Requirements have established three main protective mechanisms: (i) institutional assurances of compliance; (ii) review of research by an IRB; and (iii) requiring informed consent of human subjects.[16] These requirements continue to guide IRB reviews today.

As referenced in **Chapter 1**, the Pre-2018 Requirements were the subject of an extensive rulemaking process to revise the Rule that included an Advance Notice of Proposed Rulemaking issued in July 2011, a Notice of Proposed Rulemaking issued in September 2015, and a Final Rule issued in January 2017, which were scheduled to take effect in January 2018, but have been delayed until January 2019 (referred to here as 2018 Requirements).[17] The 2018 Requirements maintain the same core processes and protections as the Pre-2018 Requirements, but make several modifications to account for the changes in the nature of research that have occurred since the initial adoption of the Rule in 1991. These changes include the increase in the amount of research conducted outside of academic medical centers as well as the increasing prevalence of "secondary research" involving existing information and biospecimens that were collected during the course of clinical care or earlier research studies. This chapter discusses some of these changes below.

2.3 Department of Health and Human Services

In addition to the Pre-2018 Requirements (45 C.F.R. Part 46, Subpart A), HHS has adopted regulations that offer additional protections to certain sub-populations involved in HHS-conducted or -supported research. These include Subparts B (Pregnant Women, Human Fetuses and Neonates), C (Prisoners), and D (Children). These regulations embody the principles of The Belmont Report regarding protecting subjects with diminished autonomy.[18] Some, but not all, of the other Common Rule agencies have adopted these additional subparts. Accordingly, when conducting research supported by a non-HHS Rule department or agency that involves one of the sub-populations covered by Subparts B–D, it is important to verify whether the department or agency in question has adopted the relevant subpart. Taken together, The Belmont Report and 45 C.F.R. Part 46 articulate the minimal ethical and legal obligations of those

[16] Dunn, *supra*, at 9.

[17] 82 Fed. Reg. 7149 (Jan. 19, 2017). The effective date and general compliance date of the 2018 Requirements were delayed until July 19, 2018 by an interim final rule published in January 2018. 83 Fed. Reg. 2885 (Jan. 22, 2018). The Common Rule departments and agencies issued a notice of proposed rulemaking on April 20, 2018 proposing to delay further the general compliance date of the 2018 Requirements until January 21, 2019 while permitting institutions voluntarily to implement as of July 19, 2018 three "burden-reducing" provisions contained in the 2018 Requirements: the revised definition of "research," the elimination of the requirement that IRBs review grant applications or proposals, and the elimination of certain annual continuing review requirements. 83 Fed. Reg. 17595 (Apr. 20, 2018). The proposed delay was later implemented in a final rule. 83 Fed. Reg. 28497 (Jun. 19, 2018).

[18] The Belmont Report, *supra* at 8; *see also*, Wichman, Alison, *Protecting Vulnerable Research Subjects: Practical Realities of Institutional Review Board Review and Approval,* 1 Journal of Health Care Law & Policy 88 (1998).

who conduct, review, and oversee research that is conducted or supported, in whole or in part, by HHS, including the National Institutes of Health.[19]

In June 2000, the Office for Human Research Protections (OHRP)[20] was formed. The primary purpose of OHRP is to develop and implement policies and procedures to protect human subjects participating in HHS-sponsored research, maintain regulatory oversight of such research, and provide advice on ethical and regulatory issues in biomedical and behavioral research.

2.3.1 Institutional Assurances

Historically, there were four types of institutional assurances: Single Project Assurances (SPA), Cooperative Project Assurances (CPA), Multiple Project Assurances (MPA), and, beginning in 2001, Federalwide Assurances (FWA). Effective December 31, 2005, all MPAs and CPAs were to be deactivated and replaced by an FWA. Then-approved SPAs were to remain in effect for the duration of the project and through all non-competitive award renewals.

OHRP now requires an institution to execute a written FWA before it will allow the institution to engage in any non-exempt human subjects research that is conducted or supported by HHS or by any other U.S. federal department or agency that has adopted the Common Rule and relies upon the FWA. The FWA is an agreement between the organization and OHRP through which the organization commits itself and the IRBs upon which it relies to abide by certain standards of conduct in research, including the Pre-2018 Requirements and a statement of principles (*e.g.*, The Belmont Report, The Declaration of Helsinki, or other similar code, declaration, or statement of ethical principles).[21] The institution agrees to submit all federally funded research from a Common Rule department or agency to an IRB registered with OHRP and designated on its FWA, and assure that such research will adhere to HHS regulations.[22] The FWA also sets forth requirements for institutional policies and procedures for the review and monitoring of research activities, including IRB responsibilities.[23]

At present, U.S. institutions voluntarily may extend their FWAs to agree that all human subjects research conducted at or by the institution, regardless of funding source, will be conducted in accordance with HHS regulations, including reporting requirements. However, the 2018 Requirements eliminate this "check the box" option for research institutions with an

---

[19] Wichman, *supra,* at 18.

[20] Formerly the Office of Protection from Research Risks (OPRR).

[21] HHS, Federalwide Assurance (FWA) for the Protection of Human Subjects, Terms (hereafter "FWA Terms"), https://www.hhs.gov/ohrp/register-irbs-and-obtain-fwas/fwas/fwa-protection-of-human-subjecct/index.html.

[22] IRB registration is discussed in **Chapter 4**.

[23] FWA Terms, *supra* at 21; 45 C.F.R. § 46.103; *see also* Wichman, *supra* at 18.

FWA, reasoning that this change will eliminate an unnecessary administrative burden while also enabling institutions to examine flexible approaches to oversight of low risk research.[24]

The FWA extends to the institution's employees and agents, including students, who are performing institutionally designated activities, acting on behalf of the institution, or otherwise exercising institutional authority or responsibility in carrying out research covered by the FWA. The institution may extend its FWA to cover collaborating independent investigators and collaborating institutional investigators, and the arrangement should be documented with an Individual Investigator Agreement or similar agreement.[25]

The institution must review its FWA every five years, even if no changes have occurred, and within 90 days after any changes related to the legal name of the institution or certain other institutional officials. If the institution fails to renew or update its FWA appropriately, OHRP may restrict, suspend, or terminate approval of the institution's FWA.

2.3.2 HHS Exempt Research

The Common Rule, as it existed prior to the issuance of the 2018 Requirements (which we refer to herein, consistent with the federal regulators, as the "Pre-2018 Requirements"), contains six specific categories of research that are exempted from HHS regulations. Exempt research, while meeting the definition of "research" involving "human subjects," does not need to comply with most requirements of the Rule, including obtaining full IRB review of the research or the informed consent of the subject.[26] The categories of exempt research underwent significant revisions in the 2018 Requirements, and thus, in describing them below, we discuss both the exemption categories as they exist in the Pre-2018 Requirements and the changes made in the 2018 Requirements. It is beneficial for in-house counsel to maintain a checklist of exempt categories for handy reference when presented with this inquiry. Sample checklists are attached at **Exhibits 2.3.2(a)** and **2.3.2(b)**. OHRP also maintains decision charts to assist in-house counsel in its decision-making process when determining whether a proposed activity is exempt.[27]

Research activities are exempt from the Pre-2018 Requirements when the only involvement of the human subject falls within one or more of the categories below (within each category, any changes made by the 2018 Requirements are discussed):

---

[24] The preamble to the 2018 Requirements states that "this voluntary extension will no longer be part of the assurance process and such research will not be subject to OHRP oversight." 2018 Requirements, 82 Fed. Reg. at 7181.

[25] HHS, Extending an FWA to Cover Collaborating Investigators, http://www.hhs.gov/ohrp/regulations-and-policy/guidance/extension-of-institutional-fwa-via-individual-investigator-agreement/index.html.

[26] 45 C.F.R. § 46.101(b)(1)–(6). In the 2018 Requirements, the exemption categories are moved to § __.104, *see* 82 Fed. Reg. at 7261.

[27] *See* HHS, Regulations & Policy, http://www.hhs.gov/ohrp/humansubjects/guidance/decisioncharts.htm. Note that as of July 2017, these charts had not been updated to reflect the changes made in the 2018 Requirements.

- Research conducted in established or commonly accepted educational settings, involving normal educational practices, such as (i) research on regular and special education instructional strategies, or (ii) research on the effectiveness of or the comparison among instructional techniques, curricula, or classroom management methods. The 2018 Requirements added a requirement that this exemption category be applied only when the research is not likely to impact adversely (i) students' opportunity to learn required educational content or (ii) the assessment of educators who provide instruction. The 2018 Requirements preamble explained that this change was made based on concerns about whether the conduct of some research projects could draw enough time and attention away from the delivery of the regular educational curriculum that the research could have a detrimental effect on student achievement.[28]
- Research involving the use of educational tests (cognitive, diagnostic, aptitude, achievement), survey procedures, interview procedures, or observation of public behavior, unless: (i) information obtained is recorded in such a manner that human subjects can be identified, directly or through identifiers linked to the subjects; and (ii) any disclosure of the human subjects' responses outside the research could reasonably place the subjects at risk of criminal or civil liability or be damaging to the subjects' financial standing, employability, or reputation. The 2018 Requirements additionally provide that identifiable information may qualify for this exemption if an IRB performs a "limited IRB review," a new concept introduced by the 2018 Requirements that requires that the IRB's review be limited to determining that there are adequate provisions to protect the privacy of subjects and maintain the confidentiality of data. The 2018 Requirements provide that the Rule agencies will issue further guidance to assist IRBs in making this assessment.[29]
- The 2018 Requirements eliminated a provision of the Pre-2018 Requirements that permitted research not exempt under the exemption immediately above to be exempt if: (i) the human subjects are elected or appointed public officials or candidates for public office; or (ii) federal statute(s) require(s) without exception that the confidentiality of the personally identifiable information will be maintained throughout the research and thereafter (*e.g.*, Department of Justice or National Center for Educational Statistics). The 2018 Requirements preamble noted that this type of research is likely to be covered by other exemptions without needing a separate exemption category.
- Research involving the collection or study of existing data, documents, records, pathological specimens, or diagnostic specimens, if these sources are publicly available or if the information is recorded by the investigator in such a manner that subjects cannot be identified, directly or through identifiers linked to the human

---

[28] § __.104(d)(1), 82 Fed. Reg. at 7186.

[29] § __.111(a)(7), 82 Fed. Reg. at 7264.

subjects. According to the OHRP, to qualify for this exemption, the data, documents, records or specimens must be in existence before the project begins. The 2018 Requirements made significant revisions to this exemption. First, it removed the requirement that the information or specimens be in existence before the project begins. Accordingly, under the revised exemption, any "secondary research," *i.e.*, research involving identifiable private information or identifiable biospecimens *collected during some other primary or initial activity*, such as clinical care or other research projects, can qualify for the exemption, if the other requirements of the exemption are met. Second, the 2018 Requirements expanded this exemption to apply in two additional scenarios: (i) secondary research use of identifiable health information that is regulated under the HIPAA Privacy Rule, and (ii) research that is conducted by, or on behalf of, a federal department or agency using government-generated or government-collected information obtained for nonresearch activities, if the information is stored in a manner that complies with certain federal government standards.[30] The expansion of the exemption to include information subject to the HIPAA Privacy Rule is important, as it means that investigators performing *secondary research* involving identifiable health information at entities subject to the Privacy Rule need only comply with the HIPAA Privacy Rule's requirements for research as opposed to complying with both the Privacy Rule and the Rule. The HHS Secretary's Advisory Committee on Human Research Protections (SACHRP) issued a lengthy guidance document in December 2017 that discusses the application of this new "HIPAA exemption" in more detail.[31] Notably, the SACHRP guidance interprets the HIPAA exemption to be available only for research involving identifiable private information and not for research involving identifiable biospecimens.

- Research and demonstration projects which are conducted by, supported by, or subject to the approval of department or agency heads, and which are designed to study, evaluate, improve or otherwise examine: (i) public benefit or service programs; (ii) procedures for obtaining benefits or services under those programs; (iii) possible changes in or alternatives to those programs or procedures; or (iv) possible changes in methods or levels of payment for benefits or services under those programs. The 2018 Requirements added an additional requirement that each federal department or agency conducting research and demonstration projects qualifying for this exemption establish on a publicly available website a list of all such research and demonstration projects.[32]

---

[30] § __.104(d)(4), 82 Fed. Reg. at 7262.

[31] SACHRP, December 12, 2017 Letter to the HHS Secretary, Attachment B – Recommendations on the Interpretation and Application of § __.104(d)(4) the "HIPAA Exemption," https://www.hhs.gov/ohrp/sachrp-committee/recommendations/attachment-b-december-12-2017/index.html.

[32] § __.104(d)(5), 82 Fed. Reg. at 7262.

- Taste and food quality evaluation and consumer acceptance studies, (i) if wholesome food without additives are consumed or (ii) if food is consumed that contains a food ingredient at or below the level and for a use found to be safe, or agricultural chemical or environmental contaminant at or below the level found to be safe by the FDA or approved by the Environmental Protection Agency (EPA) or the Food Safety and Inspection Services of the U.S. Department of Agriculture.

The 2018 Requirements introduced the following three new exemption categories that did not appear in the Pre-2018 Requirements:

- Benign behavioral interventions in conjunction with the collection of information from an adult subject through verbal or written responses or audiovisual recording if the subject prospectively agrees to the intervention and information collection and at least one of the following criteria is met: (i) the information obtained is recorded by the investigator in such a manner that the identity of the human subjects cannot readily be ascertained; (ii) any disclosure of the human subjects' responses outside the research would not reasonably place the subjects at risk of criminal or civil liability or be damaging to the subjects' financial standing, employability, educational advancement, or reputation; or (iii) the information obtained is recorded in an identifiable format, but an IRB conducts a review limited to determining that there are adequate provisions to protect the privacy of subjects and maintain the confidentiality of data. A "benign behavioral intervention" is defined as an intervention that is brief in duration, harmless, painless, not physically invasive, not likely to have a significant adverse lasting impact on the subjects, and the investigator has no reason to think the subjects will find the intervention offensive or embarrassing. This exemption cannot be used for research involving deception, unless the subject authorizes the deception through a prospective agreement to participate in research in which the subject is informed that he or she will be deceived.[33]
- Storage or maintenance for secondary research for which broad consent is required. This exemption permits identifiable private information or identifiable biospecimens *to be stored for secondary research uses*, such as storage in a data repository or biobank, provided that the subject provides "broad consent" to the storage and the IRB conducts a "limited IRB review" to determine that (i) a broad consent has been obtained; (ii) a broad consent is appropriately documented; and (iii) if a change is made for research purposes in the way the identifiable private information or identifiable biospecimens are stored or maintained, there are adequate provisions to protect the privacy of the subject or to maintain the confidentiality of data.[34]
- Secondary research for which broad consent is required. This exemption permits identifiable private information or identifiable biospecimens *to be used for second-*

[33] § __.104(d)(3), 82 Fed. Reg. at 7262.

[34] § __.104(d)(7), 82 Fed. Reg. at 7262-63.

ary research purposes if (i) the subject provided broad consent for the secondary research use of identifiable private information or identifiable biospecimens, (ii) an IRB conducts a "limited IRB review" to determine that there are adequate provisions to protect the privacy of subjects and maintain the confidentiality of data and to determine whether the research is within the scope of the broad consent obtained from the subject; and (iii) the investigator does not include returning individual research results to subjects as part of the study plan.[35] This exemption could be used, for example, to permit the *use* of information or biospecimens stored pursuant to the exemption immediately above, though it could also be used to permit use of information and biospecimens stored under other mechanisms.

The concept of "broad consent" included in the last two exemption categories discussed above is a regulatory flexibility added by the 2018 Requirements that can be used to obtain consent for "secondary research" both in conjunction with the exemptions discussed above or as part of non-exempt secondary research. It is described as a "regulatory flexibility" because broad consent is only one option that an investigator may use to enable secondary research use of identifiable private information or identifiable biospecimens—the investigator can instead obtain study specific informed consent or obtain a waiver of informed consent from an IRB to permit such research. "Broad consent" consists of the following core elements, in addition to certain of the elements contained in traditional consent: (i) description of general types of research that may be conducted; (ii) description of identifiable private information or identifiable specimens covered and types of potential recipients; (iii) period of time during which identifiable private information and identifiable biospecimens will be maintained/used; (iv) statement that subjects will not be given details of individual research projects, and that they might have chosen not to consent to some of those specific research studies; (v) statement that clinically relevant results may not be disclosed (unless results will always be returned); and (vi) information about whom to contact with questions.[36] One aspect of "broad consent" that differs from regular consent is that if a subject is offered a broad consent but refuses to provide consent, an IRB cannot later waive the consent requirement with respect to the identifiable private information or identifiable biospecimens that were the subject of the broad consent request.[37] Nevertheless, a researcher presented with a refusal of the subject to provide broad consent could presumably still use the information and/or biospecimens in question for research if the researcher first shed them of identifiers. SACHRP issued a lengthy guidance document in April 2018 discussing in detail the application of broad consent.[38]

At the time the Pre-2018 Requirements were promulgated, HHS regulations stated that the exemptions did not apply to research involving pregnant women, fetuses, human in vitro

---

[35] § __.104(d)(8), 82 Fed. Reg. at 7263.

[36] *See* § __.116(d), 82 Fed. Reg. at 7266–67.

[37] *See* § __.116(f), 82 Fed. Reg. at 7267.

[38] SACHRP, April 11, 2018 Letter to the HHS Secretary, Attachment A – FAQs Relating to Recommendations on Broad Consent, https://www.hhs.gov/ohrp/sachrp-committee/recommendations/attachment-a-faqs-relating-to-recommendations-on-broad-consent/index.html.

fertilization (Subpart B) and prisoners (Subpart C). On November 13, 2001, HHS published a revised version of 45 C.F.R. Part 46, Subpart B (Additional Protections for Pregnant Women, Human Fetuses and Neonates Involved in Research). The revised Subpart B became effective on December 13, 2001 and stated that the exemptions at 45 C.F.R. 46.101(b)(1) through (6) were applicable to this Subpart. The exemption for research involving educational tests, surveys, interviews, or observations of public behavior does not apply to children (Subpart D) except when the investigator does not participate in the activities being observed.[39] The 2018 Requirements modify the application of the exemptions slightly by providing that the exemptions may be applied to research involving prisoners (Subpart C) if the research is aimed at a broader population and only incidentally includes prisoners. The 2018 Requirements continue to take the position that the exemption for research involving educational tests, surveys, interviews, or observations of public behavior may apply to research involving children (Subpart D) only if the investigator does not participate in the activities being observed, and adds that the application of this same exemption for instances in which identifiable information is collected and the IRB conducts a "limited review" is not available for research involving children.[40] Moreover, the 2018 Requirements do not permit use of the new exemption for benign behavioral interventions in research involving children.

The Pre-2018 Requirements do not specify who within an institution may determine that research is exempt. However, OHRP guidance suggests that to minimize conflict of interest, the determination should generally be made by someone other than the investigator conducting the research. Different institutions take different approaches to this issue: Some have the IRB issue exemption determinations and others assign the task to research administration personnel. Familiarity with these exemptions will be beneficial to in-house counsel assisting those responsible for determining exempt status in making these determinations. The 2018 Requirements preamble states that OHRP may in the future issue an "exemption decision tool" that could be used by an investigator and/or other institution personnel to determine whether research qualifies for an exempt category.[41]

2.3.3 HHS Enforcement

OHRP derives compliance authority from The Public Health Service Act and from HHS regulations.[42] The HHS OIG recently analyzed OHRP compliance activities over the period 2010 through 2015. While OIG found that "OHRP generally conducted its compliance activities independently," OIG recommended certain changes to strengthen such independence, including that HHS (i) issue guidance to clarify OHRP's role, (ii) evaluate OHRP's position

[39] 70 Fed. Reg. 36328 (June 23, 2005); 45 C.F.R. § 46.101, footnote 3.

[40] *See* § __.104(b), 82 Fed. Reg. at 7261.

[41] *See* 82 Fed. Reg. at 7184.

[42] 45 C.F.R. Part 46; *See also* OHRP Compliance Oversight Procedures for Evaluating Institutions (Oct. 14, 2009) (hereafter "2009 OHRP Compliance Oversight"), http://www.hhs.gov/ohrp/compliance/ohrpcomp.pdf.

within HHS as a whole, and (iii) evaluate OHRP's resources and determine ways in which to "elevate the prominence of its budget."[43]

For-cause evaluations occur at OHRP's discretion[44] and in response to its receipt of substantive written allegations or indications of noncompliance with HHS regulations. Such allegations or indications may come from research participants and their family members, individuals engaged in the conduct of research (*e.g.*, investigators and study coordinators), institutional officials, and peer-reviewed publications, among others.[45] OHRP accepts anonymous complaints, but asks those complainants who identify themselves whether OHRP may disclose their identity to the institution at which noncompliance is alleged to have occurred. If OHRP has jurisdiction to evaluate the possible noncompliance,[46] it informs the complainant (if he/she/it has provided contact information) regarding whether OHRP will open a compliance oversight evaluation and, in such case, sends an initial inquiry letter to the institution, with copy to principal investigator(s), informing it that OHRP is evaluating research protections at the institution. The initial letter: (i) describes the allegations or indications of noncompliance and potential regulatory violations; (ii) asks the institution to conduct an investigation regarding the same; (iii) asks for a written response to the allegations and for supporting documentation (*e.g.*, research records) by a certain date; (iv) asks the institution to submit a corrective action plan if the institution's investigation finds any noncompliance; and (v) provides an explanation of OHRP's compliance oversight evaluation process.

Before taking action against an institution, OHRP provides the institution an opportunity to bring forth further information that could rebut the allegations or indications of noncompliance. However, OHRP may not afford an institution such opportunity to present other evidence when serious concerns about subject safety are at issue and thus require immediate suspension of affected research activities. OHRP may present additional questions and concerns to the institution; may conduct interviews (remotely or in person) with institutional employees, IRB members or investigators; and may engage external experts. Based on the institution's response and any relevant information received from the complainant or other sources, OHRP issues a letter (or letters) to the institution with OHRP's determinations regarding (i) the specific allegations or indications of noncompliance with HHS regulations; and (ii) the institution's program for protecting human subjects, including IRB policies and procedures.

OHRP also conducts not-for-cause compliance oversight evaluations, in which case there are no substantive allegations or indications of noncompliance. Institutions are selected to undergo not-for-cause evaluation based on many factors, including: (i) the volume of

[43] The OIG Summary is available at https://oig.hhs.gov/oei/reports/oei-01-15-00350.asp. The full OIG Report is available at https://oig.hhs.gov/oei/reports/oei-01-15-00350.pdf.

[44] OHRP may address allegations or indications of noncompliance through mechanisms other than a for-cause evaluation.

[45] 2009 OHRP Compliance Oversight *supra* at 42.

[46] OHRP jurisdiction is based upon whether the possible noncompliance involves non-exempt human subjects research that is conducted or supported by HHS or otherwise covered by an applicable OHRP-approved FWA.

institutional research that is conducted or supported by HHS; (ii) a relatively low frequency of reporting to OHRP under applicable HHS regulations (*e.g.*, reporting unanticipated problems involving risks to subjects or others); (iii) whether implementation of corrective actions (stemming from a prior for-cause compliance oversight evaluation) requires further examination; (iv) geographic location; (v) the status of accreditation by professionally recognized human subjects protection program accreditation groups; and (vi) the status of any recent human subjects protection evaluation or audit conducted by other regulatory agencies, such as the FDA, or recent participation in quality improvement programs, such as OHRP's Quality Improvement Program.[47] As with for-cause evaluations, OHRP advises the institution in writing that it intends to conduct an evaluation, requests that the institution provide to OHRP certain relevant information concerning the institution's human subjects protection program (including, but not limited to, IRB policies and procedures and minutes from recent IRB meetings), may conduct interviews and on-site evaluations of institutional protections, and may engage external experts as needed.

Upon conclusion of for-cause and not-for-cause evaluations, OHRP issues a letter to the institution with OHRP's determinations regarding the institution's compliance with HHS regulations. If OHRP makes findings of noncompliance, it describes in its letter any corrective actions proposed or implemented by the institution. If OHRP finds these corrective actions to be inadequate, OHRP requires the institution to submit an appropriate written corrective action plan by a certain date.[48] Corrective action plans must address the specific facts under evaluation, as well as OHRP's conclusions regarding the strength of the institution's human subjects protection program.[49]

If OHRP finds no noncompliance, or finds noncompliance but also finds that the institution has addressed the issue adequately through corrective action, OHRP then concludes its evaluation and so informs the institution in writing. In the case of for-cause evaluations, OHRP informs the complainant (if he/she/it has provided contact information) in writing of OHRP's determinations and any corrective actions taken. The institution or complainant may request that the OHRP Director reconsider any determinations stemming from a for-cause or not-for-cause evaluation.

When noncompliance is found, OHRP's enforcement powers range from advising an institution of needed reforms (*e.g.*, improvements to relevant policies and procedures) to government-wide debarment of the institution or investigators. OHRP may impose administrative actions for violations of the federal regulations or the terms and conditions of an institution's FWA and, as appropriate, may refer the matter to another federal department or agency for further review. If OHRP finds that a particular researcher or the IRB has not adhered to applicable federal guidelines, it may (i) limit the types of research protocols that the FWA

[47] *Id.* at 4–5.

[48] In-house counsel can be an invaluable resource in assisting the institution with drafting an appropriate response letter and corrective action plan.

[49] *Id.* at 2–4.

covers; (ii) suspend the FWA; or (iii) recommend that an individual researcher or an institution be temporarily or permanently forbidden from conducting federally supported research (*i.e.*, suspension or debarment).[50] When an organization or individual is debarred, it may not receive any federal funding for research.

2.4 Food and Drug Administration

The FDA regulations pertaining to human subjects protections are found at 21 C.F.R. Parts 50 (Protection of Human Subjects) and 56 (Institutional Review Boards). Part 50 was adopted in May 1980, while Part 56 became final in January 1981. The FDA regulates research, but does not typically support or conduct research. Its regulatory mandate differs substantially from other HHS agencies and departments that conduct and support a significant amount of research, such as the National Institutes of Health. FDA regulations apply to research involving products regulated by the FDA, which include research and marketing authorizations for drugs, biological products, or medical devices for human use; food and color additives; or electronic products. When used in research, these items are referred to as "test articles."

There are some key differences between the role of the FDA and the other federal agencies that regulate research. In its role as the regulator of drugs and medical devices, the FDA is concerned with human subjects protection and data integrity, and is charged with monitoring other parties to the research process, *e.g.*, sponsors. The agency is concerned not only with the protection of human subjects, but also with the integrity of data generated by clinical trials. The FDA will only approve for marketing those drugs and devices that are proven safe and effective in clinical trials. Thus, the FDA monitors and regulates the design of clinical trials to ensure that the trials will yield meaningful, reliable data.

Unlike HHS regulations, federal funds do not need to be involved for FDA regulations to apply. However, when research involving products regulated by the FDA is funded by HHS, both HHS and FDA regulations apply. Nonetheless, the FDA largely has adopted standards found in the Pre-2018 Requirements in its regulatory approach to the protection of human subjects.[51]

2.4.1 FDA Exempt Research

The FDA provides only three types of exemption from IRB review:

- Research which started before July 27, 1981, and either did not require FDA approval before that date, or, was subject to requirements for IRB review prior to that date, and remains subject to review by an IRB which meets FDA requirements in effect before July 27, 1981;

[50] *Id.* at 5–7; *see also* Wichman, *supra* at 18.

[51] Murray, Jan E., *Clinical Research: A Primer for In-House Counsel,* American Health Lawyers Association In-House Counsel Program, San Francisco, California (June 30, 2002).

- Emergency use of a test article, provided any such use is reported to the IRB within five working days and any future use of the test article at the institution is subject to IRB review; or
- The taste and food quality evaluation provided for in category six of HHS regulations.[52]

2.4.2 FDA Enforcement

The FDA developed its Bioresearch Monitoring (BIMO) Program to ensure the protection of the rights, welfare, and safety of human subjects involved in FDA-regulated research, as well as the quality and integrity of data submitted to the FDA in support of new products. The BIMO Program organizes on-site visits to IRBs, clinical investigators, sponsors, monitors, contract research organizations, nonclinical (animal) laboratories, and bioequivalence analytical laboratories.[53] As to IRBs specifically, the FDA seeks to determine whether IRBs are operating in compliance with then-current FDA regulations and statutory requirements and with their own written policies and procedures. FDA's IRB inspections typically can be categorized as (i) surveillance inspections or (ii) directed inspections. Surveillance inspections are periodic and scheduled, focused on an IRB's overall operations and procedures. Directed inspections are unscheduled inspections, focused on an IRB's review of one or more particular clinical trials, and often stem from a complaint, clinical investigator misconduct, or safety issues.[54]

The FDA's District Offices reach out to the institution, often to the IRB chairperson, to schedule a site visit. Before an inspection commences, FDA personnel issue a Notice of Inspection (Form FDA 482) and present their credentials to the institution. FDA personnel interview appropriate individuals at the institution, and often review and copy: (i) records of IRB membership; (ii) IRB procedures and guidelines; (iii) minutes of IRB meetings for the past year; (iv) IRB-held documents related to the studies, as provided by the clinical investigator to the IRB; (v) IRB-held documents related to the studies, as provided by the IRB to the clinical investigator; and (vi) any other materials about the studies. After the inspection, FDA personnel conduct an exit interview with institutional and IRB representatives, during which FDA personnel describe their inspection findings and, if appropriate, issue a written Form FDA 483 for any deficiencies. The IRB or institution may respond to any 483 observations verbally during the exit interview or in writing after the inspection.

After an inspection, FDA personnel prepare a written Establishment Inspection Record (EIR), and then forward to the appropriate FDA Center for further evaluation the EIR, form FDA 483 (if issued), any materials collected during the inspection, and any IRB response. After its review, the FDA Center usually sends to the IRB or institution one of the following:

---

[52] 21 C.F.R. § 56.104; 21 C.F.R. § 56.102(d).

[53] FDA Information Sheet: "FDA Institutional Review Board Inspection," (Jan. 2006), (hereafter "FDA Information Sheet Institutional Review Board Inspection"), https://www.fda.gov/downloads/RegulatoryInformation/Guidances/UCM126555.pdf.

[54] *Id.* at 2.

- A letter stating that the FDA observed no significant deviations from applicable statutes and regulations, although such a letter may not be sent when no significant deviations are found.
- An informational or untitled letter identifying deviations from applicable statutes and regulations, for which voluntary corrective action is sufficient, and (in certain cases) requesting a response from the IRB.
- A Warning Letter identifying serious deviations from applicable statutes and regulations and requesting prompt correction by the IRB and a formal written response to the FDA.

Letters also may be issued under "lesser administrative actions" (21 C.F.R. § 56.120), in which case the FDA describes the corrective action needed to achieve compliance and requires the IRB or institution to respond within a specified timeframe.[55] Based on the IRB's or institution's response, FDA may schedule a reinspection to confirm whether corrective actions were implemented by the IRB or institution appropriately. Until such appropriate corrective actions have been implemented, FDA may, for those studies that are subject to FDA's IRB regulations:

- Withhold approval of new studies conducted at the institution or reviewed by the IRB;
- Direct that no new subjects be on-boarded to ongoing studies; and
- Terminate ongoing studies when doing so would not endanger subjects.[56]

The FDA may notify relevant state and federal regulatory agencies and other parties with direct interest in the FDA's action of the deficiencies found "[w]hen the apparent noncompliance creates a significant threat to the rights and welfare of human subjects."[57] The FDA Commissioner also may commence proceedings to disqualify an IRB or an institution if the IRB has refused or repeatedly failed to comply with applicable regulations and such noncompliance adversely affects the rights or welfare of the human subjects involved.[58]

2.5 Distinctions Between HHS and FDA Regulations

While the structural and functional requirements for IRBs in the FDA regulations are identical to HHS regulations, there are a number of substantive differences between the FDA and HHS regulations. The regulations contain different requirements, based on statutory scope or requirements including, but not limited to, (i) enforcement of non-compliance (refusal to permit data to be used in support of application); (ii) financial disclosure by investigators versus institutional compliance; (iii) enforcement against IRBs versus the institution. Also,

[55] 21 C.F.R. § 56.120(a).

[56] 21 C.F.R. § 56.120(b).

[57] 21 C.F.R. § 56.120(c).

[58] FDA Information Sheet: Institutional Review Board Inspection, *supra* 53 at 2–4.

FDA regulations do not require a written FWA. The following is a listing of differences in these two sets of regulations:[59]

IRB Regulations

Section Numbers	Description
§ 56.102 (FDA) § 46.102 (HHS)	FDA definitions are included for terms specific to the type of research covered by the FDA regulations (test article, application for research or marketing permit, clinical investigation). A definition for emergency use is provided in the FDA regulations.
§ 56.104 (FDA) § 46.116 (HHS)	FDA provides exemption from the prospective IRB review requirement for "emergency use" of test article in specific situations. HHS regulations state that they are not intended to limit the provision of emergency medical care.
§ 56.105 (FDA) § 46.101 (HHS)	FDA provides for sponsors and sponsor-investigators to request a waiver of IRB review requirements. HHS exempts certain categories of research and provides for a Secretarial waiver.
§ 56.109 (FDA) § 46.109 (HHS) § 46.117(c) (HHS)	Unlike HHS, FDA does *not* provide that an IRB may waive the requirement for signed consent when the *principal* risk is a breach of confidentiality because FDA does not regulate studies which would fall in that category of research. (Both regulations allow for IRB waiver of *documentation* of informed consent in instances of minimal risk.)[60]
§ 56.114 (FDA) § 46.114 (HHS)	FDA does not discuss administrative matters dealing with grants and contracts because they are irrelevant to the scope of FDA regulation. (Both regulations make allowances for review of multi-institutional studies.)
§ 56.115 (FDA) § 46.115 (HHS) § 46.103 (HHS)	FDA has neither an assurance mechanism nor files of IRB membership. Therefore, FDA does not require the IRB or institution to report changes in membership whereas HHS does require such notification.

Table continues

[59] OHRP IRB Guidebook (1993), archived at https://wayback.archive-it.org/org-745/20150930181805/http://www.hhs.gov/ohrp/archive/irb/irb_guidebook.html; *see also* FDA Comparison of FDA and HHS Human Subject Protection Regulations (2000), https://www.fda.gov/ScienceResearch/SpecialTopics/RunningClinicalTrials/EducationalMaterials/ucm112910.html.

[60] Both FDA regulations and the Pre-2018 Requirements define the term "minimal risk" to mean that the "probability and magnitude of harm or discomfort anticipated in the research are not greater in and of themselves than those ordinarily encountered in daily life or during the performance of routine physical or psychological examinations or tests." 21 C.F.R. §§ 50.3(i), 56.102(i); 45 C.F.R. § 46.102.

Informed Consent Regulations, continued

Section Numbers	Description
§ 56.115(c) (FDA)	FDA may refuse to consider a study in support of a research or marketing permit if the IRB or the institution refuses to allow FDA to inspect IRB records. HHS has no such provision because it does not issue research or marketing permits.
§§ 56.120–56.124 (FDA)	FDA regulations provide sanctions for non-compliance with regulations.
§ 50.23 (FDA)	FDA, but not HHS, provides for an exception from the informed consent requirements in emergency situations. The provision is based on the Medical Device Amendments of 1976, but may be used in investigations involving drugs, devices, and other FDA regulated products in situations described in § 50.23.
§ 46.116(c), (d) (HHS)	HHS provides that an IRB may waive or alter the elements of informed consent under certain conditions. FDA regulations historically did not permit an IRB to waive or alter informed consent in research subject to FDA regulations. However, the 21st Century Cures Act, enacted in December 2016, provided FDA authority to revise its regulations to permit for waivers of informed consent for minimal risk research.[61] On July 24, 2017, FDA issued a guidance document with immediate effect stating that it would exercise enforcement discretion not to sanction IRBs that grant a waiver or alteration of informed consent for minimal risk research that meets the requirements for waiver of informed consent found in the Pre-2018 Requirements.[62]
§ 50.25(a)(5) (FDA) § 46.116(a)(5) (HHS)	FDA explicitly requires that subjects be informed that FDA may inspect the records of the study because FDA may occasionally examine a subject's medical records when they pertain to the study. While HHS has the right to inspect records of studies it funds, it does not impose that same informed consent requirement, though as a practical matter, investigators generally inform subjects in the informed consent form that HHS may inspect their records.
§ 50.27(a) (FDA)	FDA explicitly requires that consent forms be dated as well as signed by the subject or the subject's legally authorized representative. HHS regulations do not explicitly require consent forms to be dated.

[61] Pub. L. No. 114-255 § 3024.

[62] *See* FDA, *IRB Waiver or Alteration of Informed Consent for Clinical Investigations Involving No More than Minimal Risk to Human Subjects, Guidance for Sponsors, Investigators, and Institutional Review Boards* (July 24, 2017).

2.6 State Regulation

The federal regulations establish the basic protections for research that cannot be diminished by state law. However, federal law expressly preserves additional state law protections.[63] State law plays an important role in determining whether an individual has consented to research properly. States generally require the provision of informed consent prior to medical treatment either as a result of court decisions or legislative action. In addition, some states specifically regulate research or have special provisions related to informed consent for research that may vary from informed consent for treatment, particularly as it applies to minors and other vulnerable persons.[64] Other specific types of state laws that counsel should be familiar with are (i) confidentiality of patient records/medical research records; (ii) clinical research laws; (iii) investigational drug laws; (iv) laws governing communicable diseases (*e.g.*, HIV); (v) genetic testing and research laws; and (vi) public health data collection laws, *e.g.* tumor registries. Nonconformance with state laws can have implications at the federal level. For example, if a minor or incapacitated person is enrolled without proper authorization by a third party, the researcher and sponsor potentially have violated the informed consent requirements of the federal regulations. Additionally, nonconformance also may result in civil liability for the researcher, sponsor, and members of the IRB. It is imperative that counsel be familiar with both state and federal laws in the conduct of research trials.

---

[63] *See* 21 C.F.R. § 50.25(c) which states: "The informed consent requirements in these regulations are not intended to pre-empt any applicable federal, state or local laws which require additional information to be disclosed for informed consent to be legally effective;" 45 C.F.R. § 46.101(f) also states that the Common Rule does not pre-empt state or local laws which provide additional protection.

[64] Cal. Health & Safety Code § 24172 (sets forth a bill of rights for the subjects of medical experimentation that requires that those conducting the experiment to provide complete disclosure about the experiment and to follow specific requirements for securing informed consent); 105 CMR 700.009 (requires a person who is conducting research that involves investigational drugs to submit certain information to the Massachusetts Department of Public Health, including a statement of "Assurance of Compliance"); Minn. Stat. § 144.295 (health records may be released to an external researcher solely for purposes of medical or scientific research only after certain criteria have been met, including the provider's using reasonable effort to obtain the patient's written authorization); N.Y. Civ. Rights Law § 79-1 (no person may perform a genetic test on biological samples taken from an individual without obtaining the prior written informed consent of the individual, which must include (among other things) a general description of the test and statement that the individual may wish to obtain genetic counseling, with certain exceptions to this consent requirement, including, but not limited to, use of anonymized biospecimens); *see also* Murray, *supra* at 51, at 10–11.

Chapter 3

Understanding the Clinical Trial Process

Martha C. Romney

Katayoun (Kat) Neal

Introduction

Clinical trials are a form of research that employ the use of human subjects for the assessment of a drug, treatment, or device to evaluate its safety and effectiveness for humans.[1] Clinical trials follow strict scientific standards. There are several different types of clinical trials and some include: prevention trials, diagnostic trials, screening trials, quality of life trials, genetic trials, epidemiological trials, and treatment trials.[2] Prevention trials seek better ways to prevent disorders. Diagnostic trials seek better ways to identify a disorder or condition.[3] Screening trials seek better methods for detecting disorders or health conditions, while quality of life trials explore ways to improve quality of life in subjects with chronic illnesses. Genetic trials look at understanding how a subject's genes and illness may be related and can lead to tailor-made treatments based on the subject's genetic make-up, while epidemiological studies try to identify patterns, causes, and control of disorders. Finally, treatment trials seek better ways to treat diseases or conditions.[4]

A clinical trial is an organized study conducted with human subjects, who either have a particular disease or condition or who are in normal health, to answer specific questions about a new treatment or a new way of using a known treatment. Each study tries to increase medical knowledge and to find new and better ways to help humans. Besides studying new drugs, clinical trials study new combinations of drugs already used in treatment, new ways of giving treatment, and how changes in lifestyle can help people or prevent diseases from occurring. Other clinical trials compare the best known standard diagnostic products or therapy with newer diagnostic products or therapy. A study comparing the diagnostic accuracy of one type of imaging modality with another is an example of research involving diagnostic products. Clinical trials comparing drugs, devices, or different types of surgery are types of research involving therapy.

---

[1] The terms "clinical trial" and "clinical study" are synonymous.

[2] See, U.S. Food and Drug Admin. (FDA), *What Are the Different Types of Clinical Research?* https://www.fda.gov/ForPatients/ClinicalTrials/Types/default.htm.

[3] *Id.*

[4] *Id.*

Before the advent of the clinical trial, therapeutic effectiveness was judged on the basis of observation. However, clinical observation was a poor method by which to determine the effectiveness of an intervention. A clinical study, by definition, involves the use of intervention techniques. Central to the conduct of a modern clinical trial is the notion of the control group. The control group is a group against which the intervention group is compared. At the outset of the clinical trial it is essential that the control group be sufficiently similar in relevant respects to the intervention groups so that differences in outcome may reasonably be attributed to the action of the intervention.[5] Basically, a clinical study examines the efficacy of an intervention under controlled conditions.

The goal of the clinical trial is to provide scientifically meaningful results. Clinical trials must be carefully planned and are devised around a plan, or protocol, that specifies the parameters of the study. Trials must be described in detailed written protocols defining the treatment, eligibility criteria, evaluation process, and population to be studied. The study objectives, research design, and number of subjects required to answer the study questions also must be included in the protocol. New protocols involving an investigational drug must be submitted to the FDA for review and approved by an Institutional Review Board (IRB) prior to initiation.[6] Protocol amendments which "significantly affect" subject safety, study scope, or "scientific quality" must also be submitted to the FDA and the IRB.[7] The Investigational Device Exemption (IDE) regulations govern safety and effectiveness studies involving devices.[8]

Human subject clinical trials are conducted in distinct phases designed to test drugs or devices under different conditions until proven safe and effective enough to be taken to market. Post-market studies are frequently conducted to test the safety of drugs or devices over time in larger markets or to test them for use in different ways. For example, investigational new drugs must be tested in Phase I, II, and III clinical trials before they can be taken to market. Phase IV trials involve post-market studies. Phases are generally conducted sequentially. They may also overlap, however.[9]

3.1 U.S. Regulatory Drug Development Process

Pharmaceutical (prescription) drug products intended for use in the U.S. must be approved by the FDA prior to marketing. This regulated process requires the compilation and submission of preclinical, clinical and chemistry, manufacturing, quality control, and other types of data per specified standards.[10] The FDA regulations describing the different phases of studies and

[5] Freedman, Benjamin, *Equipoise and the Ethics of Clinical Research,* 317 NEW ENGLAND JOURNAL OF MEDICINE 141–45 (1988).

[6] Simon, Richard T., *Clinical Trials in Cancer,* Cancer Principles and Practice of Oncology 513–34 (Vincent T. DeVita, *et al.* eds., 5th ed. 1997); 21 C.F.R. §§ 312.23 and 312.30(a).

[7] 21 C.F.R. § 312.30(b)(i) and 2(a) and (b).

[8] 21 C.F.R. § 812.2(a).

[9] 21 C.F.R. § 312.21.

[10] 21 C.F.R. § 312 *et seq.*; 21 C.F.R. § 314 *et seq.*

data required for U.S. pharmaceutical drug applications are codified in 21 C.F.R. § 312 *et seq.* and 21 C.F.R. § 314 *et seq.*

3.2 Investigational New Drug Applications

An Investigational New Drug Application (IND) is submitted to the FDA prior to initiating certain drug studies in humans. The IND seeks exemption from the statutory prohibition of transporting unapproved drugs across state lines.[11] There are three types of INDs: (i) ones submitted by a sponsor investigator to propose studying an unapproved drug or an approved drug for a different indication or new patient population; (ii) Emergency Use IND that allows the use of an experimental drug for emergency situations where there is no time for submission of an IND to the FDA; and (iii) Treatment IND that is submitted for experimental drugs showing promise in clinical testing for serious or immediately life-threatening conditions as clinical work is being conducted and the FDA review takes place.[12] A sponsor must wait 30 calendar days to receive a response from the FDA regarding their IND submission before initiating a clinical trial. Some clinical trials are exempt from submitting IND applications. Clinical trials that involve approved marketed drugs, bioavailability or bioequivalence studies, or clinical trials involving radioactive drugs safe for certain research uses are exempt from the IND application requirement.[13]

Prior to initiation of clinical studies conducted under an IND, investigators must receive IRB review and approval unless the study meets the exemptions or waiver provisions cited in 21 C.F.R. §§ 56.104 and 56.105. Investigators are also responsible for prompt reporting of "... changes in the research activity and all unanticipated problems involving risk to human subjects or others," as well as submission of annual reports updating the IRB about the trials.[14] Additionally, clinical human drug studies must comply with FDA's human subject protection requirements (21 C.F.R. Part 50), Financial Disclosure by Clinical Investigators requirements (21 C.F.R. Part 54), and other applicable regulations.[15]

---

[11] 21 C.F.R. §§ 312.1 and 312.2; 21 C.F.R. § 312.3 b; *see also* FDA, *Investigational New Drug (IND) Application*, https://www.fda.gov/drugs/developmentapprovalprocess/howdrugsaredevelopedandapproved/approvalapplications/investigationalnewdrugindapplication/default.htm.

[12] *Id.*

[13] 21 C.F.R. § 312.2; *see also* FDA, *IND Application Procedures: Exemptions from IND Requirements*, https://www.fda.gov/Drugs/DevelopmentApprovalProcess/HowDrugsareDevelopedandApproved/ApprovalApplications/InvestigationalNewDrugINDApplication/ucm362743.htm.

[14] 21 C.F.R. § 312.66.

[15] *See* FDA, *Information Sheet Guidance For IRBs, Clinical Investigators, and Sponsors, Frequently Asked Questions About Medical Devices* (Jan. 2006), *available at* https://www.fda.gov/downloads/regulatoryinformation/guidances/ucm127067.pdf.

3.3 Phases of Drug Trials

Phase I clinical trials include the initial introduction of an investigational new drug into humans.[16] Phase I trials are typically closely monitored and generally utilize about 20 to 80 volunteers. Phase I trials may be conducted in patients or normal volunteer subjects.[17] Phase I trials are designed to determine the metabolic and pharmacologic actions of the drug in humans, the side effects associated with increasing doses and, if possible, to gain early evidence of effectiveness.[18] Sufficient information about the drug's pharmacokinetics and pharmacological effects should be obtained to permit the design of well-controlled, scientifically valid, Phase II trials.[19] Phase I trials may also include studies of drug metabolism, structure-activity relationships, and mechanisms of action in humans, as well as studies in which investigational drugs are used as research tools to explore biological phenomenon or disease processes.[20]

Phase II trials follow positive results from Phase I trials. While the emphasis in Phase I trials is on safety, the emphasis in Phase II is on effectiveness.[21] Phase II trials are typically well-controlled, closely monitored, and conducted in a relatively small number of patients, usually involving no more than several hundred subjects.[22] Phase II trials are structured to evaluate the effectiveness of the drug for a particular indication or indications in patients with the targeted disease or condition under the study and to determine the new drug's short term side effects and risks.[23] Since the goal of a Phase II trial is to test the drug for its efficacy, it is usually compared against control subjects who are similar to the patient but not receiving the study drug. Instead, these control subjects receive a different treatment, usually a placebo or a different drug.[24]

Phase III trials build from Phase I and Phase II trials if evidence of effectiveness is shown in Phase II.[25] They are expanded controlled and uncontrolled trials.[26] They are performed after preliminary evidence suggesting effectiveness of the drug has been obtained, and are intended to gather additional information about safety and effectiveness that is needed to evaluate the overall risk to benefit relationship of the drug and to provide an adequate basis for physician

---

[16] 21 C.F.R. § 312.21(a).

[17] *Id.*

[18] *Id.*

[19] *Id.*

[20] 21 C.F.R. § 312.21(a)(2).

[21] FDA, *The FDA's Drug Review Process: Ensuring Drugs Are Safe and Effective*, www.fda.gov/Drugs/ResourcesForYou/Consumers/ucm143534.htm.

[22] 21 C.F.R. § 312.21(b).

[23] *Id.*

[24] FDA, *The FDA's Drug Review Process: Ensuring Drugs Are Safe and Effective*, www.fda.gov/Drugs/ResourcesForYou/Consumers/ucm143534.htm.

[25] *Id.*

[26] 21 C.F.R. § 312.21(c).

labeling.[27] Phase III trials generally involve a much larger number of subjects (several hundred to several thousand) to monitor adverse reactions to long term drug use. Phase III trials may also compare the study drug to standard treatment or to alternative drugs or placebos to determine the efficacy of the new drug. These trials may also test the study drug at different doses or when administered in a different manner.

Phase IV clinical trials follow the approval of the drug by the FDA. Concurrent with marketing approval, the FDA may seek agreement from the sponsor to conduct Phase IV trials to delineate additional information about the drug's risks, benefits, and optimal use.[28] Phase IV trials can also be used to evaluate use of the drug as different doses or schedules of administration than were used in Phase II, in a different patient population, over a greater period of time, or in other stages of a disease.[29]

3.4 New Drug Application (NDA)

Sponsors may file an NDA with the FDA seeking approval to market the drug once the requisite clinical trials have been conducted that demonstrate significant evidence of effectiveness and safety and provide other required content. The NDA provides extensive data reflecting information across the spectrum of development from the initial stages of molecular development. The required content is delineated in 21 C.F.R. § 314 and includes: chemistry, manufacturing and controls, preclinical laboratory and animal data, human pharmacokinetic and bioavailability findings, clinical and safety data, description of the product and substance, relevant patents, packaging, claims, proposed labeling, and collected data.

3.5 Device Studies

A medical device is an instrument which is recognized in the official National Formulary, or the United States Pharmacopeia, or any supplement to them, used in the diagnosis of a disease or other condition, or in the cure, mitigation, treatment, or prevention of disease, or intended to affect the structure or any function of the body, and which does not achieve its primary intended purposes through bodily chemical action on the body and which is not dependent on being metabolized to achieve its intended purpose.[30] Examples of medical devices include wheelchairs, sutures, pacemakers, laparoscopes, urinary catheters, cardiac valves, orthopedic pins, and infusion pumps.[31] Medical devices may also be diagnostic products such

---

[27] *Id.*

[28] 21 C.F.R. § 312.85.

[29] *Id.*

[30] 21 U.S.C. § 321(h); *see also* FDA, *Information Sheet Guidance For IRBs, Clinical Investigators, and Sponsors, Frequently Asked Questions About Medical Devices* (Jan. 2006), *available at* https://www.fda.gov/downloads/regulatoryinformation/guidances/ucm127067.pdf.

[31] *See* FDA, *Information Sheet Significant Risk and Nonsignificant Risk Medical Device Studies* (Jan. 2006), *available at* https://www.fda.gov/downloads/RegulatoryInformation/Guidances/UCM126418.pdf (hereafter "Information Sheet Guidance for IRBs").

as pregnancy test kits and imaging systems such as magnetic resonance imaging (MRI).[32]

Investigational devices are those that are the object of a clinical investigation or research to determine the safety or effectiveness of the device.[33] The IDE regulations govern safety and effectiveness studies involving devices.[34] Additionally, clinical studies of medical devices must comply with FDA's human subject protection requirements (21 C.F.R. Part 50), IRB requirements (21 C.F.R. Part 56), Financial Disclosure by Clinical Investigators requirements (21 C.F.R. Part 54) and other applicable regulations.[35] Safety and effectiveness studies must be conducted before the FDA will approve an application to take the device to market.[36] The IDE regulations describe three types of device studies: significant risk, non-significant risk, and exempt device studies.[37]

3.6 Significant Risk Device Trials

A significant risk device poses a "potential for serious risk to the health, safety, or welfare of a subject."[38] A significant risk device is one that is intended for use as an implant, is intended for use in supporting or sustaining human life, is intended for use of substantial importance in diagnosing, curing, mitigating or treating disease, or for preventing impairment of human health.[39] Significant risk device trials may not be conducted until an IDE has been granted by the FDA.[40]

3.7 Non-significant Risk Device Trials

Devices that do not meet the significant risk criteria are non-significant risk devices.[41] Sponsors are initially charged with making this determination.[42] IRBs must then determine if this designation is appropriate. IRBs should evaluate the risks associated with the device as well as the risks associated with the procedure for using the device (*i.e.*, surgery to insert a device) when determining whether a device poses a significant or non-significant risk. Research can

---

[32] *See* FDA, *Information Sheet Guidance For IRBs, Clinical Investigators, and Sponsors, Frequently Asked Questions About Medical Devices* (Jan. 2006), *available at* https://www.fda.gov/downloads/regulatoryinformation/guidances/ucm127067.pdf.

[33] 21 C.F.R. § 812.3(g) and (h).

[34] 21 C.F.R. § 812.2(a).

[35] *See* FDA, *Information Sheet Guidance For IRBs, Clinical Investigators, and Sponsors, Frequently Asked Questions About Medical Devices* (Jan. 2006), *available at* https://www.fda.gov/downloads/regulatoryinformation/guidances/ucm127067.pdf.

[36] *See* 21 C.F.R. Part 814, which governs premarket approval of medical devices that have been shown to be safe and effective, and 21 C.F.R. Part 807, Subpart E, which governs premarket notification, or 510(k) submissions in which the device sought to be marketed is substantially equivalent to a legally marketed device.

[37] 21 C.F.R. § 812.2 and § 812.3(m); Information Sheet: Guidance for IRBs.

[38] 21 C.F.R. § 812.3(m).

[39] *Id.*

[40] 21 C.F.R. § 812.20.

[41] Information Sheet Guidance for IRBs, *supra.*

[42] *Id.*

proceed without an FDA-approved IDE if the IRB agrees with a non-significant risk classification. This is because an IDE is "considered approved" for non-significant risk devices under the FDA's abbreviated regulations without having to submit a formal application.[43] The FDA has authority to disagree with the IRB's determination of non-significant risk and can require submission of an application for an IDE before the device can be studied.[44]

The IRB must notify the investigator, or sponsor when appropriate, if it does not agree with the non-significant risk device classification so that an application for an IDE can be submitted to the FDA.[45] The FDA may agree or disagree with the IRB's determination. The FDA may approve an IDE if it finds that the device is significant risk and if it is assured that the study will be conducted in accordance with all other regulatory requirements.[46] The FDA may recommend that the study be returned to the IRB as a non-significant risk study if it does not believe the device is a significant risk device.[47]

The term "non-significant risk" should not be confused with "minimal risk," which is a term used in the IRB regulations[48] to assist in identifying studies that can be approved by IRBs through an expedited process. Device studies are not eligible for expedited review unless they are non-significant risk, present no more than minimal risk, and fall within an expedited review category.[49] IRBs must follow the IRB regulations[50] when considering whether to approve a device study regardless of whether the FDA has classified a device as significant or non-significant risk.

3.8 Exempt Device Studies

Certain device studies are exempt from IDE regulations and can be performed without significant risk and non-significant risk determination.[51] IRBs must still follow IRB regulations and perform a risk to benefit assessment before approving them.[52]

Devices studies exempt from FDA IDE regulations include those involving devices undergoing consumer preference testing, testing of a modification, or testing of a combination of two or more devices already in commercial distribution when the testing is not being done to test safety and effectiveness and does not put subjects at risk.[53] Other exempt devices studies

---

[43] 21 C.F.R. § 812.2(b)(1); *see also* Information Sheet Guidance for IRBs, *supra*.

[44] 21 C.F.R. §§ 812.20 and 812.42; *see also* Information Sheet Guidance for IRBs, *supra*.

[45] 21 C.F.R. §§ 812.66 and 812.20.

[46] 21 C.F.R. §§ 812.20 and 812.43(c)(4); 21 C.F.R. Parts 50 and 56.

[47] Information Sheet Guidance for IRBs, *supra*.

[48] *See* 21 C.F.R § 56.102(i).

[49] *See* 21 C.F.R, § 56.110.

[50] 21 C.F.R. Parts 50 and 56.

[51] 21 C.F.R. § 812.2(c).

[52] 21 C.F.R. § 56.111; *see also* 21 C.F.R. Parts 50, 56 and § 812.60.

[53] *See* 21 C.F.R. § 812.2(c) for an entire list of exempt devices studies.

include diagnostic devices including in vitro diagnostic products in compliance with 21 C.F.R. § 809.10(c) if the testing is non-invasive, does not require invasive sampling procedures that present significant risk, does not introduce electrical energy into the subject and is not used as a diagnostic procedure without confirmation of the diagnosis by another medically established diagnostic product or procedure.[54]

3.9 Phases in Device Trials

Once preclinical studies in non-humans have been completed, sponsors may wish to perform limited studies in humans for purposes of verifying the design and operating specifications of a device before engaging in more extensive clinical trials. These limited trials help to establish the parameters for larger clinical studies and are intended to provide data about a device's feasibility for diagnostic or clinical use.[55] These limited studies are referred to as feasibility studies. They may also be referred to as Phase I or pilot studies.[56] Feasibility studies are followed by phases of research in which the safety and effectiveness of a device is investigated.

The FDA may require device manufacturers to conduct post-market approval studies to help monitor the safety, effectiveness, and reliability of a device.[57] IRB approval or exemption may be required during the safety and effectiveness phases of research.[58]

3.10 Guidance Documents

In addition to promulgating regulations for governing the pharmaceutical and medical device development and promotional processes, the FDA issues Guidance Documents. Guidance Documents are not legally binding, but convey the agency's current thinking or interpretation of a regulatory issue, policy, or particular subject and identify ways to comply with regulations. The FDA publishes notices about guidance documents in the *Federal Register* (https://www.federalregister.gov) and on its website (www.fda.gov/RegulatoryInformation/Guidances).[59] Of particular relevance to clinical trials are the following Draft and Final Guidance Documents released by the FDA over the past five years:

- *IRB Waiver or Alteration of Informed Consent for Clinical Investigations Involving No More Than Minimal Risk to Human Subjects* (07/2017)

---

[54] *Id.*

[55] FDA, *Review of IDEs for Feasibility Studies #D89-1 (Blue Book Memo)* (May 17, 1989), *available at* https://www.fda.gov/medicaldevices/deviceregulationandguidance/guidancedocuments/ucm081405.htm.

[56] *Id.*

[57] 21 C.F.R. Part 822; *see also* FDA, *Postmarket Surveillance Under Section 522 of the Federal Food, Drug, and Cosmetic Act, Guidance for Industry and Food and Drug Administration Staff* (May 16, 2016), *available at* https://www.fda.gov/downloads/MedicalDevices/DeviceRegulationandGuidance/GuidanceDocuments/ucm268141.pdf.

[58] *Id.*

[59] Guidance documents are searchable at www.fda.gov/RegulatoryInformation/Guidances/ucm122046.htm.

- *IRB Responsibilities for Reviewing the Qualifications of Investigators, Adequacy of Research Sites, and the Determination of Whether an IND/IDE is Needed* (08/2013)
- *Final Guidance: Investigational New Drugs Determining Whether Human Research Studies Can Be Conducted Without an IND* (5/30/2012)
- *Considerations When Transferring Clinical Investigation Oversight to Another IRB* (05/2014)
- *IRB Continuing Review After Clinical Investigation Approval* (02/2012)

Chapter 4

Introduction to Institutional Review Boards

Payal P. Cramer

Ernessa B. McKie

Introduction

AN INSTITUTIONAL REVIEW BOARD (IRB) provides critical oversight, monitoring, and support for the research activity involving human subjects performed or contemplated within a health care organization. Federal regulations delegate authority for the review, approval, and monitoring of research to an IRB. Both in-house and outside counsel must have a working understanding of the purpose, scope, and regulatory requirements for the IRB to be able to advise the IRB, to respond to inquiries by the IRB members and the institution's administration or governing body, and, in some instances, to participate in the IRB process in an advisory capacity. IRBs have the important responsibility of ensuring that the proposed research activity meets the standards for human subjects research protection.

4.1 IRB Defined

The term "IRB" is commonly used to describe the group of individuals responsible for analyzing, approving, monitoring, and reviewing clinical research trials involving human subjects.[1] An IRB is a board, committee, or other group designated by an institution[2] to review, to approve the initiation of, and to conduct periodic reviews of clinical research studies involving human subjects. The IRB is considered an "agent of [its] own institution."[3] Whether the IRB organizes to serve a (i) single institution within its community; (ii) multiple institutions within a designated geographical area; (iii) a group of hospital systems or institutions in distant locations; or (iv) multiple institutions conducting the same research study, the IRB should be established and operate in conformance with the federal regulations, namely, regulations and guidance set forth by HHS/OHRP and FDA.[4] As discussed in greater detail below, IRBs must have certain policies and procedures in place when overseeing clinical research that has federal

[1] *See generally* 21 C.F.R. § 56.102(g); 45 C.F.R. § 46.102(g).

[2] Defined as "any public or private entity or agency (including federal, state, and other agencies)"; 21 C.F.R. § 56.102(f); 45 C.F.R. § 46.102(b). The 2018 Common Rule moved this definition to 45 C.F.R. § 46.102(f).

[3] Levine, Robert J., ETHICS AND REGULATION OF CLINICAL RESEARCH, 342 (1988).

[4] Historically, IRBs have been part of the institution where human subjects research is being performed. Increasingly this IRB structure is changing, as discussed below.

support. While HHS and FDA have many regulations in common, IRBs have an independent duty to understand where the regulations coincide and where they diverge.[5]

Practitioners who represent IRBs should understand the IRB's place within the overall organizational structure of the research entity. Given the sensitivity of clinical research data and participant information and the importance of human subjects protection, it is critical for institutions to monitor IRB compliance with federal regulations and institutional policies. In-house counsel and external counsel should be in communication with the IRB in order to evaluate overall risks to the institution and to ensure compliance with federal requirements.

The institution or organization within which it resides establishes the structure of an IRB. Though HHS/OHRP and FDA provide limited guidance to institutions regarding an IRB's reporting arrangements, it is critical that the IRB has independent authority to operate within the confines of its approved policies and procedures. Regulations require that each IRB designate a senior officer or head official to be responsible for oversight of IRB activities.[6] In some instances, the IRB will report to an administration liaison who reports directly to the governing board of the institution. In other cases, the IRB will be a medical staff committee, which reports indirectly to the governing board of the institution through the medical staff. This latter type of organization may present issues of real or perceived conflicts of interest. If such an organizational structure exists, significant consideration should be made to change the IRB to a governing board committee instead of a medical staff committee. This is, in part, due to concerns that an IRB that reports to a medical staff committee may feel pressure or a lack of autonomy in its decision-making.[7] Often in community-based settings where the research infrastructure is minimal, the IRB reporting structure may vary, but it still must operate in compliance with regulations that apply and in accordance with ethical standards for human subjects research.

As discussed in detail in **Chapter 10**, research activities must be performed in compliance with the federal privacy rule. Therefore, it is also important to distinguish between the role of an IRB and a Privacy Board. A Privacy Board is a review body that may be established to act upon requests for a waiver or an alteration of the Authorization requirement under the Privacy Rule of the Health Insurance Portability and Accountability Act of 1996, as amended, HIPAA for uses and disclosures of protected health information (PHI) for a particular research study.[8]

---

[5] The 2018 Common Rule introduces regulatory changes in the HHS regulations. The 21st Century Cures Act, Pub. L. No. 114-255 § 3023, 42 U.S.C. 289 note (Dec. 13, 2016), provides for harmonization of differences between HHS and FDA human subjects regulations as practicable and consistent with other statutory provisions, in order to avoid regulatory duplication and unnecessary delays. This harmonization is to be completed not later than three years after the date of the enactment of this law.

[6] 21 C.F.R. § 56.106(b); 45 C.F.R. § 46.502(a).

[7] Bankert, Elizabeth A. & Amdur, Robert J., INSTITUTIONAL REVIEW BOARD, MANAGEMENT AND FUNCTION, 32 (2006).

[8] 45 C.F.R. § 164.512(i); *see also* Nat. Insts. of Health, *Privacy Boards and the HIPAA Privacy Rule*, https://privacyruleandresearch.nih.gov/privacy_boards_hipaa_privacy_rule.asp and U.S. Dept. of Health & Human Svcs., *Health Information Privacy, Research*, https://www.hhs.gov/hipaa/for-professionals/special-topics/research/index.html.

A Privacy Board may waive or alter all or part of the Authorization requirements for a specified research project or protocol. A Covered Entity may use and disclose PHI without an Authorization, or with an altered Authorization, if it receives the proper documentation of approval of such alteration or waiver from a Privacy Board.[9] In some cases, the IRB may function as a Privacy Board. However, the two roles represent distinct functions with separate regulatory obligations.[10]

4.2 Primary Purpose of the IRB

The primary purpose of the IRB is to assure, both in advance and by periodic review, that appropriate steps are taken to protect the rights and welfare of humans participating as subjects in research.[11] The IRB is charged with balancing the risks and benefits of the research, ensuring an equitable selection of human subjects, obtaining valid informed consent of the human subjects, protection of subjects' privacy and data confidentiality, and providing appropriate safeguards for any vulnerable subject populations.[12] To accomplish this purpose, IRBs use a group process to review research protocols and related materials (*e.g.*, informed consent documents and investigator brochures) to ensure protection of the rights and welfare of human subjects of research.[13] IRBs offer a consistent approach to clinical trial review and an opportunity for community involvement in decisions related to the conduct of clinical research.

An IRB's authority to approve or disapprove a research proposal is vested by federal regulation and corresponding institutional guidelines.[14] Each IRB must develop clear and concise policies and procedures to address, among other things, the operational responsibilities of the board, administrative processes of the board, and methods for researchers to submit a study protocol for review. These policies and procedures should address the IRB's expectation of the initial review of a study, continuing review of an approved study, expedited review of a study, adverse event and deviation reporting, amendments to a study protocol, review of study

[9] *Id.*

[10] *Id.*

[11] FDA, *Institutional Review Boards Frequently Asked Questions - Information Sheet*, FAQ 1 (last updated Jan. 25, 2016), https://www.fda.gov/RegulatoryInformation/Guidances/ucm126420.htm (hereafter "FDA Information Sheet FAQ").

[12] 21 C.F.R. § 56.111; 45 C.F.R. § 46.111. The 2018 Common Rule made changes in 45 C.F.R. § 46.111(a)(3). The definition of vulnerable populations varies for research approved prior to the implementation of the 2018 Common Rule. Namely, for the pre-2018 Common Rule the definition of vulnerable populations includes pregnant women, children, mentally disabled persons, prisoners, and economically or educationally disadvantaged persons. The 2018 Common Rule removed pregnant women from the list of potentially vulnerable populations. It also replaced the term "mentally disabled persons" with the term "individuals with impaired decision-making capacity." The FDA regulations retain prior terminology and include pregnant women, physically disabled individuals, and "mentally disabled persons" in the category of vulnerable populations. Additionally, 45 C.F.R. Part 46 Subpart B, Additional Protections for Pregnant Women, Human Fetuses and Neonates Involved in Research, remains unchanged.

[13] FDA Information Sheet FAQ, FAQ 1.

[14] 21 C.F.R. § 56.109; 45 C.F.R. § 46.109. Further review may be done by the institution, but institutional officials may not approve research if it has not been approved by the IRB. 21 C.F.R. § 56.112; 45 C.F.R. § 46.112.

materials distributed to participants, as further described in **Chapter 5**, and the requirements for obtaining informed consent, as described in **Chapter 9**.

4.3 IRB Registration

HHS regulations require registration of IRBs prior to review of any human subjects research conducted or supported by HHS.[15] FDA regulations also require registration of IRBs that review FDA-regulated studies or studies intended to support research or marketing permits of FDA-regulated products.[16] The registration requirements for both HHS and FDA require that registration be submitted electronically (unless otherwise arranged with OHRP directly), which requires the following information for all registrations:

- the name, mailing address, and street address (if different from the mailing address) of the institution operating the IRB;
- the name, mailing address (if different from the institution above), phone number, facsimile number, and electronic mail address of the senior officer of that institution responsible for overseeing activities performed by the IRB;
- the name, name of institution and mailing address (if different from the institution information above), phone number, facsimile number, and electronic mail address of the contact person providing the registration information;
- the IRB's name, mailing address, street address (if different from mailing address), phone number, facsimile number, and electronic mail address;
- each IRB chairperson's name, name of institution and mailing address (if different from the institution information above) phone number, and electronic mail address.

For HHS registration, the following additional requirements apply:

- the approximate number of active protocols (defined as any protocol for which an IRB conducted an initial review or a continuing review at a convened meeting or under an expedited review procedure during the preceding 12 months);
- the number of active protocols conducted or supported by HHS;
- the approximate number of full-time equivalent positions devoted to the IRB's administrative activities; and
- a roster of IRB members (including alternate members).

FDA registrants must include the following additional information:

- the number of active protocols (defined as any protocol for which an IRB conducted an initial review or a continuing review at a convened meeting or under

[15] 45 C.F.R. Part 46, Subpart E, 45 C.F.R. § 46.501 *et seq.*

[16] 21 C.F.R. § 56.106. Registration of non-U.S. IRBs, or Independent or Research Ethics Committees (IECs/RECs), is voluntary. *See* FDA, *Guidance for Institutional Review Boards (IRBs) — Frequently Asked Questions — IRB Registration* (July 2009), http://www.fda.gov/downloads/RegulatoryInformation/Guidances/UCM171256.pdf.

an expedited review procedure during the preceding 12 months) involving FDA-regulated products; and

- a description of the types of FDA-regulated products (such as biological products, color additives, food additives, human drugs, or medical devices) involved in the protocols that the IRB reviews.

The registration form and on-line registration for the combined HHS and FDA registration requirements can be found on the OHRP website.[17] The registration must be renewed every three years.[18] IRBs must maintain an accurate registration record. Changes in the contact person or IRB chair must be updated within 90 days of the change, and any expansion in the type of FDA-regulated products (for FDA-registered IRBs), discontinuation of reviews of FDA-regulated studies, or disbanding of an IRB must be reported within 30 days.[19] Once approved by OHRP, IRBs receive an email confirming registration and the entity is included on the OHRP website as an active registrant.

Depending upon the type of research reviewed, an IRB may have oversight of human subjects research that has no federal support and involves no FDA-regulated products and, therefore, no corresponding federal oversight requirements. In such a case, there is no need to register the IRB on the OHRP website and no need for a Federalwide Assurance (FWA). If the institution does review federally supported research, or research involving FDA-regulated products, the IRB must be registered. If the institution reviews federally supported research it must also have an FWA. Through the FWA, an institution commits to HHS that it will comply with the requirements set forth in 45 C.F.R. Part 46, as well as the associated Terms of Assurance. Currently, if the institution "checks the box" on the FWA, it grants OHRP oversight over all of the research conducted by the institution, including research with no federal support and involving no FDA-regulated products. By limiting the FWA to federally supported research, that is the scope of OHRP's oversight.[20] IRBs are required to update the FWA at least every five years, or sooner if there are certain IRB changes. Making a change in the FWA will restart the five-year period. OHRP maintains a web page with a complete listing of institutions with active FWAs.[21]

Registration does not necessarily mean the IRB is in compliance with HHS and FDA regulations, nor does it mean that the IRB composition meets a particular standard of competence

---

[17] Links to the instructions and the form for submitting an IRB/IEC registration can be found on OHRP's website, https://www.hhs.gov/ohrp/register-irbs-and-obtain-fwas/forms/irb-registration-form/index.html.

[18] 21 C.F.R. § 56.106(c); 45 C.F.R. § 46.505(a).

[19] 21 C.F.R. § 56.106(e); 45 C.F.R. § 46.505(b), (d).

[20] OHRP, *Assurance Process Frequently Asked Questions*, https://www.hhs.gov/ohrp/register-irbs-and-obtain-fwas/fwas/assurance-process-faq/index.html. The 2018 Common Rule removed the option for institutions with an active FWA to "check the box." The 2018 Common Rule states that "institutions could, if they so desire, continue for purposes of their own internal rules to voluntarily extend the regulations to all research conducted by the institution, but this voluntary extension will no longer be part of the assurance process and such research will not be subject to OHRP oversight." 82 Fed. Reg. 7149 at 7181 (Jan. 19, 2017).

[21] OHRP, *IRB and FWA Database*, https://ohrp.cit.nih.gov/search/search.aspx?styp=bsc.

or expertise. This information is simply used to enable OHRP and FDA to determine the level of activity of an IRB, to assign its quality improvement, educational, and compliance oversight resources based on an IRB's activity level.[22] In fact, FDA conducts on-site IRB inspections to assess whether an IRB's operations comply with FDA regulatory provisions.[23] These inspections may be scheduled or may be unscheduled and are typically performed by FDA personnel from the District Office closest to the IRB.[24]

4.4 IRB Membership

Both OHRP and FDA regulations require that each IRB have at least five members with varying backgrounds to promote complete and adequate review of research activities commonly conducted at the institution.[25] The membership is expected to be diverse to foster a comprehensive approach to safeguarding the rights and welfare of subjects, including both scientific and non-scientific members, institution-affiliated members, and members not affiliated with the institution, who may be from the local community (*e.g.*, lawyers, lay members, physicians, nurses, social workers, members of the clergy, etc.).[26] IRB members are expected to be familiar with specific local conditions affecting the conduct of the research and the protection of the human subjects, so IRBs (particularly those conducting non-local review) need to be knowledgeable about the community from which the subjects are drawn to have the tools necessary to review for subject protection and the appropriate consent process for the subject population involved.[27]

IRBs may appoint alternate members as long as the IRB has written procedures describing their appointment and function; *ad hoc* substitutes are not permissible.[28] Alternate members are listed on the roster of IRB members submitted to OHRP with IRB registration. Formally appointed alternate members may substitute for absent IRB members, provided the alternate's qualifications are comparable to the absent member's qualifications and the alternate has access to the same materials.[29] An alternate member's presence and the absence of the member for whom the alternate is substituting should be noted in the minutes; if both are present, only one can vote.[30]

---

[22] 74 Fed. Reg. 2358 (Jan. 15, 2009).

[23] FDA, *Information Sheet Guidance for IRBs, Clinical Investigators, and Sponsors - Institutional Review Board Inspections,* at 2, (Jan. 2006), https://www.fda.gov/downloads/RegulatoryInformation/Guidances/UCM126555.pdf.

[24] *Id.*

[25] 21 C.F.R. § 56.107(a); 45 C.F.R. § 46.107(a).

[26] Wichman, Alison, *Protecting Vulnerable Research Subjects: Practical Realities of Institutional Review Board Review and Approval,* 1 JOURNAL OF HEALTH CARE LAW & POLICY 88 at 91, 92 (1998).

[27] *Id.*; FDA, *Non-Local IRB Review – Information Sheet* (last updated Jan. 25, 2016), https://www.fda.gov/RegulatoryInformation/Guidances/ucm126423.htm (hereafter "FDA Information Sheet Non-Local IRB Review").

[28] FDA Information Sheet FAQ, FAQ 14.

[29] FDA Information Sheet FAQ, FAQ 15.

[30] *Id.*

The IRB must be sufficiently qualified through experience and expertise of its members. The IRB must include individuals knowledgeable about institutional commitments and regulations, applicable law, and standards of professional conduct and practice. Institutions should provide and require initial and on-going training and education for IRB members to ensure their ability to fulfill their roles. If an IRB regularly reviews research that involves a vulnerable category of subjects, such as children, prisoners, pregnant women, or handicapped or mentally disabled persons, it should consider including one or more individuals who are knowledgeable about and experienced in working with these subjects. Regulations require that IRB membership be diverse and balanced to address both community concerns and scientific need for conducting clinical research. The IRB must include at least one member whose primary concerns are in the scientific area and at least one member whose primary concerns are in the nonscientific area.[31] Most IRBs include physicians and Ph.D. level physical or biological scientists.[32] Such members satisfy the requirement for at least one scientist.[33] The FDA believes the intent of the requirement for diversity of disciplines was to include members who had little or no scientific or medical training or experience.[34] Therefore, according to the FDA, nurses, pharmacists, and other biomedical health professionals should not be regarded to have "primary concerns in the non-scientific area."[35] In the past, lawyers, clergy, and ethicists have been cited as examples of persons whose primary concerns would be in non-scientific areas.[36] Some members have training in both scientific and non-scientific disciplines, such as a nurse-attorney.[37] While such members are of great value to an IRB, other members who are unambiguously non-scientific (community or laypersons) should be appointed to satisfy the non-scientific requirement.[38]

The IRB also must include at least one member who is not otherwise affiliated with the institution and who is not part of the immediate family of a person who is affiliated with the institution.[39] The FDA considers the participation of a non-affiliated member an important indicia of diversity and would deem the frequent absence of all non-affiliated members unacceptable.[40]

One member may satisfy more than one of the above requirements.[41] For example, one member could be otherwise unaffiliated with the institution and have a primary concern in a

[31] 21 C.F.R. § 56.107(c); 45 C.F.R. § 46.107(c). The 2018 Common Rule moved this to 45 C.F.R. § 46.107(b).

[32] FDA Information Sheet FAQ, FAQ 17.

[33] *Id.*

[34] *Id.*

[35] *Id.*

[36] *Id.*

[37] *Id.*

[38] *Id.*

[39] 21 C.F.R. § 56.107(d); 45 C.F.R. § 46.107(d). The 2018 Common Rule moved this to 45 C.F.R. § 46.107(c).

[40] FDA Information Sheet FAQ, FAQ 16.

[41] FDA Information Sheet FAQ, FAQ 13.

non-scientific area.[42] This individual would satisfy two of the membership requirements of the regulations.[43] IRBs should strive, however, for a membership that has a diversity of representative capacities and disciplines.[44] Regulations require that, as part of being qualified as an IRB, the IRB must have "... diversity of ... members, including [consideration of] race, gender, and cultural backgrounds and sensitivity to such issues as community attitudes ... ."[45] Nondiscriminatory efforts must be made to ensure that the IRB does not consist entirely of men or entirely of women. In addition, no IRB may consist entirely of one profession.[46]

On occasion, the IRB may invite individuals with competence in special areas to assist in the review of complex issues that require expertise beyond or in addition to that available on the IRB. These individuals may not vote with the IRB, but often serve as consultants to the IRB prior to a decision on whether to approve a clinical research study. IRB policies and procedures should clearly set forth the circumstances of participation for these individuals so that it is well documented in the IRB minutes.

IRB membership structure should also account for situations where a member may have to recuse himself or herself due to a conflict of interest. There is no regulatory provision that restricts a clinical investigator from becoming a member of the IRB. However, the IRB regulations prohibit any member from participating in the IRB's initial or continuing review of any study in which the member has a conflicting interest, except to provide information requested by the IRB.[47] IRBs policies and procedures should define the circumstances that constitute a conflict of interest and therefore require IRB members to recuse themselves from participating in the approval process for a particular study. For example, the IRB member may have a financial interest in the study due to a relationship with the study sponsor. A non-financial conflict of interest may exist if the IRB member has a close relationship with the principal investigator involved in the study or if the IRB member's practice or patients will be potential participants in the study. In either instance, it is important for the IRB to have a process for the member to disclose and address conflicts as they arise. When selecting IRB members, including the IRB chair, the potential for conflicts of interest must be considered.[48] When members frequently have conflicts and must recuse themselves from deliberation and voting, their contributions

---

[42] *Id.*

[43] *Id.*

[44] *Id.*

[45] 21 C.F.R. § 56.107(a); 45 C.F.R. § 46.107(a).

[46] 21 C.F.R. § 56.107(b); 45 C.F.R. § 46.107(b). The 2018 Common Rule removed the requirement in 45 C.F.R. § 46.107(b) that IRBs consists of both genders and varying professions. However, these requirements are inherent in the remaining language of section 46.107 requiring diversity in gender and backgrounds for IRB members.

[47] 21 C.F.R. § 56.107(e); 45 C.F.R. § 46.107(e). The 2018 Common Rule moved this requirement to 45 C.F.R. § 46.107(d).

[48] FDA Information Sheet FAQ, FAQ 12.

to the IRB review process may be diminished and could hinder the review procedure.[49] Even greater disruptions may result if this person is the IRB chair.[50]

4.5 IRB Policies and Procedures

One of the most critical operational components of an IRB involves the development of robust policies and procedures. IRB written procedures must be designed in a manner that provides the IRB members, the IRB chair, and the IRB administrative staff with an understanding of how to carry out their duties consistently and effectively in ways that ensure that the rights and welfare of subjects are protected, and that the IRB operates in compliance with the regulations.[51] When preparing IRB written procedures, IRBs should identify who carries out specific duties by reference to position title (*e.g.*, IRB Administrator) rather than by employee name to avoid the need to update written procedures if an employee's duties change or there are changes in IRB staff.[52] Federal regulations require that institutions make certain assurances for research supported by federal funding.[53] The regulations also require that IRBs draft certain written procedures that address the following:[54]

- conducting initial and continuing review of research and reporting findings and actions to the investigator and the institution;
- determining which projects require review more often than annually and which projects need verification from sources other than the investigators that no material changes have occurred since previous IRB review;
- ensuring prompt reporting to the IRB of proposed changes in a research activity, and ensuring that such changes in approved research, during the period for which IRB approval has already been given, may not be initiated without IRB review and approval except when necessary to eliminate apparent immediate hazards to the subject; **and**
- ensuring prompt reporting to the IRB, appropriate institutional officials, OHRP if federally funded, and the department or agency head of (i) any unanticipated problems involving risks to subjects or others or any serious or continuing noncompliance with this policy or the requirements or determinations of the IRB; and (ii) any suspension or termination of IRB approval.

---

[49] *Id.*

[50] *Id.*

[51] OHRP/FDA, *Institutional Review Board (IRB) Written Procedures: Guidance for Institutions and IRBs* (May 2018), https://www.fda.gov/downloads/RegulatoryInformation/Guidances/UCM512761.pdf (hereafter "Written Procedures").

[52] *Id.*

[53] 45 C.F.R. § 46.103.

[54] 21 C.F.R. § 56.108; 45 C.F.R. § 46.103,108. The 2018 Common Rule moved the requirements for certain written procedures from 45 C.F.R. § 46.103 to 45 C.F.R. § 46.108.

OHRP and FDA have noted during IRB audits that IRB written procedures do not provide sufficient detail for staff and investigators to operationalize the procedures. IRBs should take care to draft policies and procedures that are meaningful to the IRB's needs and are not a mere restatement of the federal regulations.[55] In the combined guidance, OHRP and FDA include a Written Procedures Checklist for IRBs to engage in a thorough examination of existing policies and areas for improvements.[56] The checklist asks a series of questions to assist in determining whether the IRB has addressed certain regulatory requirements within its policies and procedures. IRBs may utilize this checklist for conducting internal audits, for compliance reviews, and for determining additional policies that may be required for effective operations.

IRBs should share their written policies and procedures with those seeking approval to perform clinical research. Investigators, in turn, should utilize the policies and procedures as a guiding tool for meeting IRB deadlines for initial review and understanding the continuing review process and expectations for reporting deviations, amendments, and adverse events. Investigators should understand that IRBs rely on the policies as the source to suspend, terminate, or otherwise restrict clinical research activities.

4.6 IRB Member Compensation

Many IRB members volunteer their time and do not receive any payment for their services to the IRB. Some are institutional employees who are being compensated for their time related to IRB meetings and activities as part of their job duties. However, the current rules governing IRBs do not preclude an institution from separately paying its IRB members.[57] FDA cautions that payment should not be related to or dependent upon a favorable decision.[58]

In the past, most research was conducted at academic institutions. These institutions did not compensate IRB members, who were mostly faculty and administrators who considered their IRB service as a component of their overall academic responsibilities.[59] As the amount of research performed in privately owned research institutions, through contract research organizations, or at other health care institutions, has increased, the number of IRB members receiving payment for their services has increased.[60] An institution may pay a consulting fee to the IRB Chairman and reimburse IRB members for travel and expenses, such as parking and provide meals during the meeting.[61] However, paying substantial fees or salaries to IRB members may create an implied obligation on the part of these members to approve research

---

[55] Written Procedures.

[56] *Id.*

[57] FDA Information Sheet FAQ, FAQ 8.

[58] *Id.*

[59] *See* Ryan, Mary Kay, RESEARCH INVOLVING MEDICAL DEVICES IN HUMAN SUBJECT RESEARCH: A HANDBOOK FOR INSTITUTIONAL REVIEW BOARDS, 107 (Robert A. Greenwald, *et al.*, eds., 1982).

[60] *See* Burke, Kelly, *Loose-fitting Genes: The Inadequacies in Federal Regulation of Institutional Review Boards*, 3 B.U.J. SEL. & TECH. L., 10, 39 (Spring 1997).

[61] *Id.*

that is financially advantageous for the institution, regardless of whether it is beneficial to human subjects.[62] IRB members should never be compensated in a manner that is related to or dependent upon a favorable decision.

Note that institutions that choose to compensate physician members for their IRB work should also consider the federal physician self-referral statute, known as Stark, and the Anti-Kickback Statute implications of such arrangements. Other federal laws, state law, and professional association agreements may also restrict the ability of physician members to obtain compensation. It is recommended that any compensation arrangement for a physician member include the advice of counsel.

4.7 Quorum

IRB approval of research is achieved by a majority vote of those IRB members present during the meeting.[63] IRB minutes for each meeting should document all voting and non-voting individuals present during the meeting. A quorum is the minimum number and type of IRB members who must be present at a convened meeting for the IRB to conduct business.[64] Except when an expedited review procedure is used, research must be reviewed at a convened meeting at which a majority of the members of the IRB are present (either in person, or by video, web, or telephonically, if allowed by the IRB's procedures), including at least one member whose primary concerns are in a nonscientific area.[65] It is necessary to maintain a quorum in order to hold a vote. When the use of video, web or telephone conferencing is utilized, it must be verified that all members have the ability to participate in the discussion and that all votes are counted.[66] IRB members may choose to abstain from voting on a particular matter. A member who abstains from voting is still counted toward the quorum, making an abstention essentially a "no" vote. Where a member recuses himself or herself, the member cannot be counted toward the quorum. Should the quorum fail during the meeting (*i.e.*, by loss of a majority through recusal of members with conflicting interests or early departures, or by absence of all nonscientific members), the IRB may not take further actions or votes unless the quorum can be restored.[67]

4.8 IRB Records

IRBs are required to maintain detailed records of (i) all research proposals including scientific evaluations, if required or provided, approved consent forms, progress reports submitted

[62] *Id.*

[63] 21 C.F.R. § 56.108(c); 45 C.F.R. § 46.108(b).

[64] OHRP/FDA, *Minutes of Institutional Review Board (IRB) Meetings - Guidance for Institutions and IRBs*, § III.A (Sept. 2017), https://www.hhs.gov/ohrp/minutes-institutional-review-board-irb-meetings-guidance-institutions-and-irbs.html-0 (hereafter "Minutes Guidance").

[65] 21 C.F.R. § 56.108(c); 45 C.F.R. § 46.108(b).

[66] Minutes Guidance, § III.A.

[67] *Id.*

by investigators, and reports of subject injuries; (ii) minutes, including a record of attendance, votes, rationale for required changes or disapprovals, summary of controverted issues and their resolutions, etc.; (iii) record of continuing review activities; (iv) correspondence with researchers; (v) list of IRB members with details of qualifications; (vi) written procedures of the IRB; and (vii) record of significant new findings provided to subjects. All required records must be kept for a minimum of three years after the completion of the research and must be available for inspection by the responsible governmental agency (*e.g.*, OHRP or FDA).[68] Further, federal regulations require that IRBs determine a timeline for which protocols require continuing review based on the risks associated with the study. For studies requiring continuing review, this review must occur at least annually, but the IRB may choose to conduct such review more frequently based upon the degree of risk.[69] OHRP recommends that the minutes of IRB meetings clearly reflect these determinations regarding risk and approval period (review interval).[70]

IRB minutes should contain enough detail to show the actions taken by the IRB during the course of the meeting. OHRP and FDA interpret "actions taken by the IRB" (also called "IRB actions") to refer to any vote taken by the IRB related to a proposed research activity. The minutes must provide a summary of all research activities reviewed by the IRB at the meeting, the members present during the IRB vote on a particular research study, and the vote outcome, including votes for, against, and abstentions. The minutes should serve as a central repository for IRB decisions on proposed research activities.

Generally in its policies and procedures, an IRB sets forth the required documents that must be submitted for the various types of review. For an initial review, the IRB should consider, at a minimum, the following:

- IRB's Initial Review Submission Form
- Protocol
- Current professional license for Principal Investigator, showing the expiration date (medical staff membership may suffice)
- Curriculum Vitae (CV) for Principal Investigator and each Sub-Investigator
- Consent form
- Other materials to be provided to the subjects that are not included in the protocol, such as advertisements, questionnaires, subject diaries, etc.
- Investigator's Drug Brochure, if applicable
- Documentation from sponsor or FDA

[68] 21 C.F.R. § 56.115; 45 C.F.R. § 46.115.

[69] 21 C.F.R. § 56.109; 45 C.F.R. § 46.109. Under the 2018 Common Rule, continuing review is not required for research studies under expedited categories, studies that require limited IRB review, or studies which have progressed to only (1) data analysis and/or (2) accessing data from procedures involved in clinical care.

[70] Minutes Guidance, § III.B; *see also* OHRP Continuing Review Guidance (2010), https://www.hhs.gov/ohrp/regulations-and-policy/guidance/guidance-on-continuing-review-2010/index.html#section-g1.

- FDA letter granting the Investigational Device Exemption (IDE), if applicable

These materials should be provided to the IRB members prior to the meeting to discuss the clinical research.

The FDA also recommends IRBs' records include data relating to subjects who withdraw from trials or who are withdrawn from the trial by their legally authorized representative or the clinical trial investigator.[71] Maintenance of these records is consistent with the underlying FDA regulations, and it reflects the FDA's view of ethical and quality standards in clinical research.[72] The FDA believes that removal of data collected on subjects who subsequently withdraw from a trial would undermine the scientific and ethical integrity of the research, placing other current and future subjects and, ultimately, users of an approved product at unreasonable risk.[73]

On occasion, IRBs may be required to furnish records related to a particular clinical research study. IRB records have been the subject of discovery requests by both federal and state courts. In some instances, a sponsor may request access to an IRB's records. While sponsors are required to assure the FDA that a study will be conducted in compliance with the informed consent and IRB regulation, they are not obligated to determine IRB compliance with those regulations. The investigator's provision of any IRB correspondence to the sponsors provides adequate assurance that the IRB is functioning according to the regulations.[74] The sponsor (or anyone) may also request the IRB's Establishment Inspection Report summarizing its most recent FDA inspection.[75] IRBs and institutions should establish a written policy on which, if any, IRB records will be provided to sponsors and other parties. In some instances, IRBs and investigators may rely upon Certificates of Confidentiality (Certificates) to restrict disclosure of certain information obtained for NIH-funded research studies. Recent NIH guidance states that research covered by the NIH policy, NIH-funded research where identifiable, sensitive information is collected or used, will automatically be issued a Certificate to protect the privacy of human subjects.[76]

4.9 Non-Local IRB Reviews

Most institutions that conduct research maintain at least one IRB, but research may also be conducted by investigators unaffiliated with an institution with an IRB. Federal regulations permit an institution to arrange for an outside (non-local) IRB to be responsible for initial and continuing review of clinical studies conducted at the non-IRB institution. This outside IRB

[71] FDA, Office of the Commissioner, Good Clinical Practice Program, *Guidance for Sponsors, Clinical Investigators, and IRBs – Data Retention When Subjects Withdraw from FDA-Regulated Clinical Trials* (October 2008), http://www.fda.gov/downloads/RegulatoryInformation/Guidances/UCM126489.pdf.

[72] *Id.*

[73] *Id.*

[74] FDA, *Sponsor – Investigator - IRB Interrelationship – Information Sheet* (last updated Jan. 25, 2016), https://www.fda.gov/RegulatoryInformation/Guidances/ucm126425.htm.

[75] *Id.*

[76] NIH, *Notice of Changes to NIH Policy for Issuing Certificates of Confidentiality* (effective Oct. 1, 2017), https://grants.nih.gov/grants/guide/notice-files/NOT-OD-17-109.html.

may be: (i) an independent IRB; (ii) a regional IRB; (iii) a national IRB; (iv) a multi-institutional IRB; or (v) the IRB of another institution.

Most local institutional IRBs have jurisdiction over all studies conducted within their respective institution. However, a non-local IRB may become the IRB of record for those studies upon written agreement with the institution or the in-house IRB. For large multi-center research studies, industry researchers and pharmaceutical entities often rely on a consolidated approach for oversight of a research protocol. This practice is more common in circumstances where a single IRB of record has the responsibility for overseeing all clinical research sites participating in a multisite study. In past, these IRBs have been known in the industry as "Independent IRBs." In 2016, the National Institutes of Health moved toward adopting this practice by issuing a formal policy regarding the use of single IRBs (sIRBs) for NIH-funded research.[77]

Non-local IRBs may face special challenges in meeting some IRB requirements due to the lack of physical proximity to the research activities. Consequently, non-local IRBs may need to visit the study site, contact sponsors' research monitors for information on site visits, or have a consultant from the relevant community advise the IRB on local attitudes and mores.

When non-local IRB review takes place, the reviewing IRB must document its role and responsibility. An IRB may review outside studies on an individual basis when the minutes clearly show the members are aware of where the study is to be conducted and when the IRB possesses appropriate knowledge about the study site(s); but if such reviews are expected to occur with any frequency, the IRB's policies should authorize such reviews and the process should be described in the IRB's written procedures. Additionally, a written agreement should be executed between the institution conducting the research (*e.g.*, private practitioner's office, clinic, etc.) and the IRB or its institution confirming the authority of the IRB to oversee the study.[78] This process should be similar to that described below for Cooperative Research.

4.10 Cooperative Research

A number of studies involve more than one institution, referred to as cooperative research studies. One institution involved in the study may have primary responsibility for conducting the study and coordinating IRB review with other institutions' IRBs, or an entity that does not actually conduct the study or even have an IRB may coordinate the study among the participating institutions. In either event, in the interest of avoiding duplication of effort, the institutions may enter into joint review arrangements in which they rely upon another qualified IRB's initial and ongoing review either for a particular study, a designated category of studies, or even

[77] NIH, *Final NIH Policy on the Use of a Single Institutional Review Board for Multi-Site Research* (June 21, 1016), https://grants.nih.gov/grants/guide/notice-files/NOT-OD-16-094.html.

[78] FDA Information Sheet Non-Local IRB Review.

all studies. The use of a single IRB for research funded by Common Rule agencies generally will be required effective January 20, 2020.[79]

In delegating to another IRB, the delegating institution is agreeing to abide by the reviewing IRB's decisions but remains responsible for ensuring research conducted within its facilities complies with the IRB's decisions. The reviewing IRB should consider factors such as the delegating institution's facilities and capabilities, measures taken by the delegating institution to ensure compliance with the IRB's decisions, and attitudes in the delegating institution's local community, and the reviewing IRB should communicate its determinations to the investigator and delegating institution at each location for which the IRB has assumed responsibility.[80]

Any delegation by an institution to another institution's IRB must be documented, with copies maintained by both the delegating institution and the reviewing IRB. If the research is subject to HHS regulations, the FWA Terms of Assurance require such documentation. The arrangements or agreements may be subject to approval by HHS through OHRP and should be executed in accordance with OHRP's instructions.[81] OHRP provides a sample IRB/Independent Ethics Committee (IEC) Authorization Agreement that may be used to document reliance on the IRB/IEC of another institution.[82] Where one institution relies on an IRB for review of clinical research matters, the authorization agreement serves as the parties' memorialization of the relationship. The agreement may cover specific types of protocols or a research program. Individuals with authority on behalf of the institution should complete the agreement. It is important to note that the initial review and continuing oversight of the reviewing IRB must comply with the terms of the OHRP-approved Assurance and all applicable regulations.

---

[79] 21 C.F.R. § 56.114; 45 C.F.R. § 46.114. The 2018 Common Rule compliance date for 45 C.F.R. § 46.114 is January 20, 2020.

[80] FDA, *Cooperative Research — Information Sheet* (last updated Jan. 25, 2016), https://www.fda.gov/RegulatoryInformation/Guidances/ucm126422.htm.

[81] *Id.*

[82] A sample Institutional Review Board (IRB) Authorization Agreement can be found on the OHRP website at https://www.hhs.gov/ohrp/register-irbs-and-obtain-fwas/forms/irb-authorization-agreement/index.html.

Chapter 5
The IRB Review Process

Sarah E. Swank

Kate Bowen

Lynn E. Smith

Introduction

UNDER FEDERAL REGULATIONS, an IRB must review all non-exempt research activities prior to commencement and either approve, require modification to (to secure approval), or disapprove the proposed research activities.[1] The IRB must also continually review the research protocols to ensure they are in compliance with federal regulations and may suspend or terminate its approval of the research if there has been unanticipated serious harm to human subjects or if the researcher fails to abide by the IRB's requirements and federal regulations.[2]

The IRB review process was designed to foster open discussion and debate at convened meetings of the full IRB membership. While some IRBs choose to provide every IRB member copies of all study materials, it is not required, as long as each member is provided with sufficient information to be able to actively and constructively participate. There are several methods of IRB review, which are discussed in detail below.

5.1 Criteria for Approval of Research

To approve research, an IRB should determine that all of the following conditions are satisfied:

- Risks to human subjects are minimized by using procedures that are consistent with sound research design and that do not unnecessarily expose subjects to risk and, whenever appropriate, by using procedures already being performed on the subjects for diagnostic or treatment purposes;
- Risks are reasonable in relation to anticipated benefits, if any, to human subjects and the importance of the knowledge that may reasonably be expected to result;[3]

---

[1] 45 C.F.R. § 46.109(a); 21 C.F.R. § 56.109(a).

[2] 45 C.F.R. § 46.113; 21 C.F.R. § 56.113; *see also* David J. Powell, *Using The False Claims Act as a Basis for Institutional Review Board Liability*, 69 UNIVERSITY OF CHICAGO LAW REVIEW 1402 (Summer 2002).

[3] One IRB was ultimately disqualified due, in part, to its failure to include an individual with the professional competence necessary to determine whether the risks to subjects were reasonable in relation to the anticipated ben-

- Selection of human subjects is equitable taking into account the purposes of the research and the setting in which the research will be conducted;
- Informed consent will be sought from each prospective subject or the subject's legally authorized representative, unless appropriately waived;
- Informed consent will be appropriately documented, or appropriately waived;
- When appropriate, the research plan makes adequate provision for monitoring the data collected to ensure the safety of human subjects;
- When appropriate, there are adequate provisions to protect the privacy of human subjects and to maintain the confidentiality of data; and
- Where some or all of the human subjects are likely to be vulnerable to coercion or undue influence, such as children, prisoners, individuals with impaired decision-making capacity, or economically or educationally disadvantaged persons, additional safeguards have been included in the study to protect the rights and welfare of those subjects.[4]

Under the 2018 Common Rule, certain research may qualify for limited IRB review under the exempt category of storage or maintenance of information or specimens for secondary research, for which only broad consent is required. In those instances, the IRB is not required to make the above determinations, but instead must ensure the following occur in accordance with the applicable regulations:

- Broad consent for storage, maintenance, and secondary research use of identifiable private information or identifiable biospecimens is obtained,
- Broad consent is appropriately documented or waiver of documentation is appropriate; and
- If there is a change made for research purposes in the way the identifiable private information or identifiable biospecimens are stored or maintained, there are adequate provisions to protect the privacy of subjects and to maintain the confidentiality of data.[5]

5.2 Initial Review

In conducting the initial review of proposed research, IRBs must obtain information in sufficient detail to make the determinations discussed above in **Section 5.1**. Review mate-

---

efits to subjects and importance of the knowledge that may be expected to result. *See* U.S. Food & Drug Admin., Warning Letter to Texas Applied Biomedical Services Research Review Committee IRB (Sept. 24, 2012); U.S. Food & Drug Admin., Notice of Opportunity for Hearing to Texas Applied Biomedical Services Research Review Committee IRB (Sept. 16, 2014); *see also* U.S. Food & Drug Admin., Warning Letter to Burzynski Research Institute Institutional Review Board (Sept. 23, 2013) [hereafter *BRI Warning Letter*].

[4] 45 C.F.R. § 46.111; 21 C.F.R. § 56.111. The FDA adds that research involving children must comply with 21 C.F.R Part 50 Subpart D. HHS also has regulations governing research with children at 45 C.F.R. § 46.401 *et seq*.

[5] *See* 83 Fed. Reg. 2885, 7197, to be codified at 45 C.F.R. §46.111(a)(8).

rials should include the full protocol, a proposed informed consent form, the investigator's brochure (if one exists), and any recruitment materials, including advertisements intended to be seen or heard by potential human subjects. Furthermore, for HHS-supported multi-center clinical trials, the IRB should receive a copy of the complete HHS-approved sample informed consent document and the complete HHS-approved protocol, if they exist.[6] IRBs may require additional documentation, such as an IRB-developed form to facilitate consistent summaries of protocols.

Unless a primary reviewer system (described in **Section 5.2.1**, below) is used, all members should receive a copy of the complete documentation. These materials should be received by the IRB members sufficiently in advance of the meeting date to allow review of the material.

5.2.1 Primary Reviewer System

If the IRB uses a primary reviewer system, a single reviewer is assigned to do a pre-meeting in-depth review of all pertinent documents listed in **Section 5.2** above and summarize the information at the IRB meeting. All other IRB members should receive, at a minimum, a copy of the consent documents, a summary of the protocol in sufficient detail to enable the member to determine the criteria for approval mentioned above are satisfied, as well as the appropriateness of the study-specific statements in the consent documents and recruitment materials. In addition, the complete documentation should be available to all IRB members for their review, both before and at the IRB meeting.

5.2.2 Pre-meeting Review by In-House Counsel

Many institutions have discovered that it is beneficial to have in-house counsel review all informed consent forms, amendments, and other documents in advance of the scheduled IRB meetings. Pre-review allows in-house counsel to discuss requested clarifications and proposed revisions with the principal investigator and/or study coordinator. To the extent documents can be provided to in-house counsel at the same time or prior to the time that they are delivered to the IRB, the pre-review process may allow for revised documents to be presented at the scheduled meetings. This expedites the review process and time required for the IRB meeting. It is important that all comments and drafts generated be provided to the IRB office to ensure a complete file related to the review.

5.3 Expedited Review

An expedited review procedure consists of initial or continuing review by the IRB chair or by one or more experienced reviewers designated by the chair from among members of the IRB.[7] It may be used for research involving no more than minimal risk or minor changes in

[6] *See* 45 C.F.R. § 46.115(a)(1); 21 C.F.R. 56.115(a)(1); FDA, *Institutional Review Boards Frequently Asked Questions – Information sheet*, #32, https://www.fda.gov/RegulatoryInformation/Guidances/ucm126420.htm.

[7] 45 C.F.R. § 46.110(b); 21 C.F.R. § 56.110.

currently approved research, including but not limited to a list of research categories identified by FDA and HHS.[8] Minimal risks are those ordinarily encountered in daily life or during routine physical or psychological exams or tests, such as non-invasive prospective collection of biospecimens, data collection, and survey research.[9]

Under the 2018 Common Rule, an IRB may use the expedited review procedure to review the following:

- Some or all of the research appearing on the list described in regulations, unless the reviewer determines that the study involves more than minimal risk;
- Minor changes in previously approved research during the period for which approval is authorized; or
- Research for which limited IRB review is a condition of exemption.[10]

Expedited review may not be used to grant "provisional approval" of single patient protocols (also known as expanded access programs) pending full board review at a convened meeting.[11] HHS may restrict, suspend, terminate, or choose not to authorize an institution's or IRB's use of the expedited review procedure.[12]

The reviewer(s) may exercise all the authorities of the IRB *except* disapproval. Research may only be disapproved following review by the full IRB. The IRB is required to adopt a method of keeping all members advised of research that has been approved by expedited review. Many IRBs accomplish this by adding to the full IRB's agenda a list of all research that was approved by the expedited procedure since the last meeting of the convened IRB.

5.4 Continuing Review

Effective periodic review by IRBs during the actual course of a research study is essential to the protection of human subjects and is required even if no subjects have been enrolled. The purpose of continuing review is to allow the IRB to consider any changes in the research or research-related events and to ensure appropriate subject protection is in place throughout the study's duration. The regulations regarding continuing review require an IRB to develop and follow written procedures for:

- Conducting continuing review of greater than minimal risk research by the convened IRB at intervals appropriate to the degree of risk as determined by the IRB,

---

[8] 21 C.F.R. § 56.110(a); 45 C.F.R. § 46.110(a). The HHS list is available at https://www.hhs.gov/ohrp/sites/default/files/ohrp/sachrp/mtgings/2013%20March%20Mtg/expeditedreviewcategories.pdf. The FDA list is published at 63 Fed. Reg. 60353 (Nov. 9, 1998) and is available at http://frwebgate.access.gpo.gov/cgi-bin/getdoc.cgi?dbname=1998_register&docid=98-29748-filed.pdf.

[9] 45 C.F.R. § 46.102(j); 21 C.F.R. § 56.102(i).

[10] *See* 83 Fed. Reg. 2885, 7207 (adding the third criterion), to be codified at 45 C.F.R. § 46.110(b).

[11] *BRI Warning Letter*.

[12] 45 C.F.R. § 46.110(d).

but not less than once per year (except as described below), and reporting actions to the investigator and the institution;

- Determining which studies need verification from sources, other than the investigator, that no material changes in the research have occurred since the previous IRB review;
- Ensuring that changes in approved research are promptly reported to, and approved by, the IRB and that changes are not initiated prior to the IRB approval, except to eliminate apparent immediate hazards to the subjects; and
- Suspending or terminating approval of research that is not being conducted in accordance with the IRB's requirements.[13]

Under the 2018 Common Rule, the continued review obligations were revised to ensure that the IRB's time is efficiently used. Unless the IRB determines otherwise, continuing review is not required if:

- The research is eligible for expedited review,
- The research is reviewed by the IRB in accordance with the limited IRB review procedure described in certain exempt categories, or
- The research has progressed to the point that it involves data analysis (including analysis of identifiable information or identifiable biospecimens) or access to follow-up clinical data from procedures that subjects would undergo as part of clinical care.[14]

If the IRB chooses to conduct continuing review in these situations, the rationale for doing so must be documented.[15]

During the continuing review process, IRBs are responsible for reviewing the same criteria for initial review as outlined above in **Section 5.1**. The continuing review regulations outline minimum requirements, but they do not dictate the continuing review framework. Therefore, IRBs may impose greater and more detailed standards of protection for human subjects than those specified by the regulations and develop procedures appropriate to its needs. OHRP and FDA provide guidance on meaningful continuing review.[16] For example, under the 2018 Common Rule, the IRB has authority to observe or have a third party observe the consent process and the research.[17]

---

[13] 21 C.F.R. §§ 56.108(a), 56.109(f), 56.113; 45 C.F.R. §§ 46.109(e), 46.113.

[14] 82 Fed. Reg. 7149, 7205 (Jan. 19, 2017), to be codified at 45 C.F.R. § 46.109(e), (f)(1).

[15] *Id.*, to be codified at 45 C.F.R. § 46.115(a)(3).

[16] FDA, *Guidance for IRBs, Clinical Investigators, and Sponsors: IRB Continuing Review after Clinical Investigation Approval* (Feb. 2012), https://www.fda.gov/downloads/RegulatoryInformation/Guidances/UCM294558.pdf [hereafter *2012 FDA Continuing Review Guidance*]; OHRP, *Continuing Review Guidance (2010)* (Nov. 10, 2010), https://www.hhs.gov/ohrp/regulations-and-policy/guidance/guidance-on-continuing-review-2010/index.html [hereafter *2010 OHRP Continuing Review Guidance*].

[17] *See* 83 Fed. Reg. 2885, 7264, to be codified at 45 C.F.R. § 46.109(g).

The clock for continuing review starts on the date of approval, whether or not human subjects have been enrolled. The regulations make no provision for any grace period extending the conduct of research beyond the expiration date of IRB approval. Thus, it is important that timely notice be provided to the principal investigator of upcoming continuing review to enable the investigator to provide a progress report prior to the expiration date. A sample Continuing Review Notice Letter and continuing review information sheet are attached as **Exhibits 5.4.1** and **5.4.2**. If the IRB does not re-approve the research by the specified expiration date, human subject accrual should be suspended pending re-approval by the IRB. Continuation of research interventions or interactions of already enrolled human subjects should continue only when the IRB finds that it is in the best interest of the human subjects to do so. If IRB approval of a study lapses, the IRB should document the reason for the lapse and steps taken to prevent future lapses. If the lapse was due to a failure on the part of the investigator to provide required information to the IRB, the IRB should determine whether a pattern of non-compliance exists and, if so, take appropriate corrective action.

The continuing review process should focus on changes in the research as well as the progress of the entire study. Continuing review records should contain information such as the number of subjects enrolled and withdrawn, their experiences (benefits and adverse reactions), reasons for withdrawals, results and risk-benefits assessment to date, the investigators' brochure and any new information since the IRB's last review, particularly any that may affect subjects' willingness to continue participation, such as recalls or withdrawal or suspension from marketing in any country.[18] The IRB should also review the current protocol and consent documents to ensure they are still accurate and complete and, if applicable, a summary of the amendments to date. Much of the relevant information is reflected in sponsors' annual FDA progress reports. Sponsors of device studies are required to provide those reports to each reviewing IRB,[19] and IRBs that review drug studies may also ask sponsors for their progress reports.

5.5 Adverse Events and Unanticipated Problems

IRBs are required to have written procedures for ensuring (directly or through other parties such as sponsors) prompt reporting to institutional and government officials when "unanticipated problems involving risks to subjects or others" occur.[20] However, neither HHS nor FDA regulations define or use the term "adverse event." The phrase "unanticipated problem involving risks to subjects or others" is found, but also not defined, in HHS and FDA regulations.

[18] *2012 FDA Continuing Review Guidance.*

[19] 21 C.F.R. 812.150(b)(5).

[20] 45 C.F.R. § 46.108(a)(4)(i); 21 C.F.R. § 56.108(b). Note that regulatory language refers to the occurrence of "risks," which may not involve actual harm; *see also* OHRP, *Federalwide Assurance (FWA) for the Protection of Human Subjects,* term #4(a)1, https://www.hhs.gov/ohrp/register-irbs-and-obtain-fwas/fwas/fwa-protection-of-human-subjecct/index.html.

OHRP considers unanticipated problems, in general, to include those events that (i) are not expected given the nature of the research procedures and the subject population being studied; (ii) are related or possibly related to participation in the research, and (iii) suggest that the research places subjects or others at a greater risk of harm (including economic or social harm as well as physical or psychological harm) related to the research than was previously known or recognized. Unanticipated problems are reportable. Adverse events may also be unanticipated problems and thus reportable, but unanticipated problems are not limited to adverse events.[21]

Adverse events, in general, can be divided into the following three categories:

- Adverse events that are serious, unexpected, and related or possibly related to participation in the research. In general, OHRP considers this category to be the most important group of adverse events that represents unanticipated problems. OHRP notes that IRBs must have authority to suspend or terminate approval of research that, among other things, has been associated with unexpected serious harm to subjects.
- Serious adverse events that are expected in some subjects, but are determined to be occurring at a significantly higher frequency or severity than expected.
- Other unexpected adverse events, regardless of severity, that may alter the IRB's analysis of the risk versus potential benefit of the research *and*, as a result, warrant consideration of substantive changes in the research protocol or informed consent process/document.

FDA guidance on reporting of adverse events attempts to define unanticipated problems in terms of adverse events and similar terms used in the FDA regulations. This guidance states that reportable unanticipated problems include:

- single occurrence of a serious, unexpected event that is uncommonly and strongly associated with drug exposure;
- a single occurrence or a small number of occurrences of a serious, unexpected event not commonly associated with drug exposure but uncommon in the study population;
- multiple occurrences of an adverse event that based on aggregate analysis is determined to be an unanticipated problem;
- an adverse event described in the investigator's brochure, protocol, or informed consent documents, but which occurs at specificity or severity that is inconsistent with prior observations;

[21] OHRP, *Unanticipated Problems Involving Risks & Adverse Events Guidance (2007)* (Jan. 15, 2007), https://www.hhs.gov/ohrp/regulations-and-policy/guidance/reviewing-unanticipated-problems/index.html (stating that "...harm to a subject need not occur for an event to be an unanticipated problem.") [hereafter *2007 OHRP Guidance on Unanticipated Problems*].

- a serious adverse event described in the investigator's brochure, protocol or informed consent documents, but which is occurring at a significantly increased frequency; or
- any other adverse event or safety finding that would cause the sponsor to modify the investigator's brochure, protocol, or informed consent documents.[22]

Adverse event reports are generally filed with the IRB when an event is deemed to be serious, such as one that, among other things: (i) results in death; (ii) is life-threatening event; (iii) results in hospitalization (including extension of a planned hospital stay); (iii) results in persistent or significant disability or incapacity; (iv) results in a congenital anomaly/birth defect (adverse pregnancy outcome following exposure to study procedures prior to conception or during pregnancy); or (vi) may result in harm and may require medical or surgical intervention to prevent one of the preceding outcomes.[23]

In multi-center clinical trials, IRBs routinely receive a large volume of reports of individual adverse events experienced by subjects enrolled at sites other than the site(s) over which the IRB has jurisdiction. OHRP refers to these events as external adverse events.[24] Although not required by HHS regulations, the sponsors or coordinating centers of multi-center clinical trials frequently distribute reports of external adverse events to all principal investigators at all study sites; these reports often represent the majority of adverse event reports submitted by investigators to IRBs.

Internal adverse events are those adverse events experienced by subjects enrolled at the site(s) under the IRB's jurisdiction for either multi-center or single-center research projects. In the case of an internal adverse event, the principal investigator typically becomes aware of the adverse event directly from the subject, another collaborating local investigator, or the subject's health care provider.

When adverse events are reported to the IRB, the IRB must then determine if they are unanticipated problems, and require reporting, and if so, whether this reporting is being done through other processes, such as via a sponsor, or whether reporting must be done by the IRB. There may also be occurrences within the study which are not adverse events but which present risk to subjects or others. These occurrences should also be analyzed to determine if they are reportable unanticipated problems.

5.6 IRB Suspension or Termination

Both FDA and HHS regulations provide that an IRB shall have the authority to "suspend or terminate approval of" research that is not being conducted in accordance with the IRB's

---

[22] FDA, *Guidance for Clinical Investigators, Sponsors, and IRBs: Adverse Event Reporting to IRBs – Improving Human Subject Protection* (Jan. 2009), *available at* http://www.fda.gov/downloads/RegulatoryInformation/Guidances/UCM126572.pdf.

[23] *2007 OHRP Guidance on Unanticipated Problems*; *see also* 21 C.F.R. § 312.32(a).

[24] *2007 OHRP Guidance on Unanticipated Problems.*

requirements or that has been associated with unexpected serious harm to subjects.[25] The regulations further provide that any suspension or termination of approval shall include a statement of the reasons for the IRB's action and shall be reported promptly to the investigator, appropriate institutional officials, and the department or agency head.[26]

The IRB should have written procedures on study suspension or termination to ensure protection of subjects' rights and welfare, subjects are not put at risk and subjects receive appropriate care while the IRB and investigator are resolving any remaining issues.[27] This may include decisions as to whether subjects will continue to receive the investigational item, be transferred to another participating investigator or site or obtain care from a provider that does not participate in the trial. In the event subjects continue to receive the investigational item, the IRB should also consider how data will continue to be collected and reported to the IRB.

[25] 45 C.F.R. § 46.113; 21 C.F.R. § 56.113.

[26] 45 C.F.R. §§ 46.113, 46.103(b)(5); 21 C.F.R. §§ 56.113, 56.108(b). Terms of FWA include reporting to "any applicable regulatory body, and OHRP."

[27] *2012 FDA Continuing Review Guidance.*

Chapter 6

Roles and Responsibilities of Investigators

Beverly H. Lorell

Igor Gorlach

Introduction

The Common Rule does not discuss the roles and responsibilities of investigators in human subjects research. However, the FDA's regulations governing investigational new drug (IND) applications and investigational device exemptions (IDE) both enumerate multiple investigator responsibilities, as well as potential penalties for non-compliance with these responsibilities. This chapter summarizes each of the investigator responsibilities identified in the FDA's regulations and guidance.

6.1 Responsibilities of an Investigator in FDA-Regulated Clinical Trials

Under the FDA's regulations, an "investigator" is "an individual who actually conducts a clinical investigation, i.e., under whose immediate direction the test article is administered or dispensed to, or used involving, a subject, or, in the event of an investigation conducted by a team of individuals, is the responsible leader of that team."[1] While the specific responsibilities of investigators in drug[2] trials are somewhat different from responsibilities of investigators in medical device trials, the general responsibilities are essentially the same: an investigator is responsible for ensuring that an investigation is conducted according to the signed investigator statement, the investigational plan, and applicable regulations; for protecting the rights, safety, and welfare of subjects under the investigator's care; and for the control of the drug or device under investigation.[3]

---

[1] 21 C.F.R. § 812.3; *see also* 21 C.F.R. § 312.3 (using virtually identical definition for drugs and biological products). "Investigator means an individual who actually conducts a clinical investigation (i.e., under whose immediate direction the drug is administered or dispensed to a subject). In the event an investigation is conducted by a team of individuals, the investigator is the responsible leader of the team."

[2] As used in this chapter, the term "drugs" includes biological products subject to 21 C.F.R. pt. 312.

[3] *See* 21 C.F.R. pt. 312 ("Investigational New Drug Application") and 21 C.F.R. pt. 812 (Investigational Device Exemptions).

21 C.F.R. § 312.60 provides as follows:

> An investigator is responsible for ensuring that an investigation is conducted according to the signed investigator statement, the investigational plan, and applicable regulations; for protecting the rights, safety, and welfare of subjects under the investigator's care; and for the control of drugs under investigation. An investigator shall, in accordance with the

6.1.1 Statement of Investigator

An investigator must submit to the study sponsor a signed "statement of investigator," further describing and acknowledging intent to comply with the commitments of the investigator. The statement of the investigator for device studies must include three commitments:[4]

> (1) *Conduct the investigation in accordance with the agreement, the investigational plan, this part and other applicable FDA regulations, and conditions of approval imposed by the reviewing IRB or FDA;*
>
> (2) *supervise all testing of the device involving human subjects; and*
>
> (3) *ensure that the requirements for obtaining informed consent are met.*

For drug investigations, an investigator must use Form FDA 1572 (Statement of Investigator) and agree to the following commitments:[5]

> (1) *I agree to conduct the study(ies) in accordance with the relevant, current protocol(s) and will only make changes in a protocol after notifying the sponsor, except when necessary to protect the safety, rights, or welfare of subjects.*
>
> (2) *I agree to personally conduct or supervise the described investigation(s).*
>
> (3) *I agree to inform any patients, or any persons used as controls, that the drugs are being used for investigational purposes, and I will ensure that the requirements relating to obtaining informed consent in 21 C.F.R. Part 50 and institutional review board (IRB) review and approval in 21 C.F.R. Part 56 are met.*
>
> (4) *I agree to report to the sponsor adverse experiences that occur in the course of the investigation(s) in accordance with 21 C.F.R. § 312.64. I have read and understand the information in the investigator's brochure, including the potential risks and side effects of the drug.*
>
> (5) *I agree to ensure that all associates, colleagues, and employees assisting in the conduct of the study(ies) are informed about their obligations in meeting the above commitments.*

> provisions of part 50 of this chapter, obtain the informed consent of each human subject to whom the drug is administered, except as provided in §§ 50.23 or 50.24 of this chapter.

21 C.F.R. § 812.100 provides as follows:

> An investigator is responsible for ensuring that an investigation is conducted according to the signed agreement, the investigational plan and applicable FDA regulations, for protecting the rights, safety, and welfare of subjects under the investigator's care, and for the control of devices under investigation. An investigator also is responsible for ensuring that informed consent is obtained in accordance with part 50 of this chapter.

[4] 21 C.F.R. § 812.43(c).

[5] 21 C.F.R. § 312.53(c). The two commitments that are not identified in the regulations as required components of the statement are marked with an "*".

(6) *I agree to maintain adequate and accurate records in accordance with 21 C.F.R. § 312.62 and to make those records available for inspection in accordance with 21 C.F.R. § 312.68.**

(7) *I will ensure that an IRB that complies with the requirements of 21 C.F.R. Part 56 will be responsible for the initial and continuing review and approval of the clinical investigation. I also agree to promptly report to the IRB all changes in the research activity and all unanticipated problems involving risks to human subjects or others. Additionally, I will not make any changes in the research without IRB approval, except where necessary to eliminate apparent immediate hazards to human subjects.**

(8) *I agree to comply with all other requirements regarding the obligations of clinical investigators and all other pertinent requirements in 21 C.F.R. Part 312.*

6.1.2 Investigator Responsibilities

6.1.2.1 Conduct Study in Accordance with Protocol

An investigator must agree to conduct the study in accordance with the relevant, current protocol(s), and to only make changes in a protocol after notifying the sponsor, except when necessary to protect the safety, rights, or welfare of subjects.[6] Adherence to the protocol is a broad responsibility that affects both the conduct of the study and the protection of the rights, safety, and welfare of study subjects. The protocol includes, among other specifications, the specific aims of the study, criteria for inclusion and exclusion of subjects, actions and timing of events regarding administration of the investigational product and follow-up, definitions of specific safety events, and if applicable, procedures for conducting the study in a blinded manner. To successfully comply with investigator responsibility, investigators must ensure that all of the individuals on the study team are familiar with the protocol or at least with the parts of the protocol that are most relevant to each individual's task. Members of the study team should also be informed of any updates to the protocol.

The protocol must be adhered to even where other legal requirements or other applicable requirements (*e.g.*, requirements established by a facility) are less strict. For example, a protocol may specify that a clinician performing a procedure must be trained in a specific subspecialty, even though such training is not a prerequisite to perform the procedure under the applicable laws and other applicable requirements. In such case, a deviation from the protocol, even if compliant with other legal requirements and standards, is not permissible.[7]

---

[6] *See* 21 C.F.R. §§ 312.60, 812.100, 812.43.

[7] FDA, GUIDANCE FOR INDUSTRY: INVESTIGATOR RESPONSIBILITIES – PROTECTING THE RIGHTS, SAFETY, AND WELFARE OF STUDY SUBJECTS (Oct. 2009), at p. 3, *available at* https://www.fda.gov/downloads/Drugs/.../Guidances/UCM187772.pdf. [hereafter *FDA Guidance for Protecting, Rights, Safety, and Welfare of Study Subjects*].

In drug investigations, an investigator may not make changes in the research without the IRB's approval, except as necessary to eliminate an immediate hazard to human subjects.[8] Upon making a change in the research, an investigator must promptly report to the IRB such change.[9] In device investigations, prior to deviating from the investigational plan, an investigator must acquire prior approval from the sponsor, and—if the deviation may affect the scientific soundness of the plan or the rights, safety, or welfare of human subjects—from the FDA and the IRB.[10] The investigator may, however, deviate from the investigational plan without prior approval if the deviation is to protect the life or physical well-being of a subject in an emergency.[11] An investigator must notify the IRB of such deviation as soon as possible, but no later than five working days after the emergency occurred.[12]

6.1.2.2 Personally Supervise the Investigation and Ensure that Study Staff are Informed about Investigator Commitments

Investigators conducting investigations of drugs must personally conduct or supervise the investigation.[13] Investigators conducting investigations of devices must supervise all testing of the device involving human subjects.[14] These broad requirements are appropriately coupled with the suggestion that the investigator be given adequate resources.[15] The supervision responsibility has generated some uncertainty, possibly because investigations vary in the type of tasks that are delegated, the qualifications of the individuals to whom tasks are delegated, and the type of supervision provided by investigators over other members of the study team at the site.

Generally, the delegation of study-related tasks is permissible so long as the investigator provides adequate supervision.[16] The FDA determines whether supervision is adequate based on four criteria.[17] First, the delegatee must be appropriately qualified by education, training, competence, and experience (and state licensure where relevant) to perform the task. Qualification concerns primarily arise in connection with clinical or medical tasks, which often require medical training, licensing, or certification. The investigator should maintain a list that documents qualified study personnel to whom significant trial-related duties were delegated. In its guidance, the FDA offers examples of tasks that have been inappropriately delegated: screening evaluations (including obtaining medical histories and assessment of inclusion/exclusion

---

[8] 21 C.F.R. § 312.66.

[9] *Id.*

[10] 21 C.F.R. § 812.150(a)(4).

[11] *Id.*

[12] *Id.*

[13] 21 C.F.R. § 312.53(c)(1)(vi)(c).

[14] 21 C.F.R. § 812.43(c)(4)(ii).

[15] ICH, GOOD CLINICAL PRACTICE (July 1996), at p. 14, *available at* https://ec.europa.eu/health/sites/health/files/files/eudralex/vol-10/3cc1aen_en.pdf [hereafter *ICH Good Clinical Practice*].

[16] *FDA Guidance for Protecting, Rights, Safety, and Welfare of Study Subjects.*

[17] *See id.* at 2-7.

criteria), physical examinations, evaluation of adverse events, assessments of primary study endpoints, and obtaining informed consent.

Second, an investigator must ensure that all study staff (including staff hired after the study has commenced) receive adequate training. Staff should be familiar with the purpose of the study, the details of the protocol, the attributes of the investigational product needed to perform their assigned tasks, and the standards and regulatory requirements for the conduct of trials and the protection of human subjects. The investigator should inform staff of any pertinent changes during the trial and provide additional training as appropriate. Finally, the investigator should ensure that staff receives all training that is offered by the sponsor in connection with the conduct of the study.

Third, an investigator must provide adequate supervision and involvement in the ongoing conduct of the study. There must be a single supervising investigator (and not merely a subinvestigator) for each study site; and any subinvestigators must report directly to the investigator. The investigator's supervision should be appropriate to the staff, nature of the trial, and the subject population. In its guidance, the FDA identifies the following as factors that may affect an investigator's ability to provide adequate supervision: inexperienced study staff, demanding workload for study staff, complex trials, large number of subjects, subject population that is seriously ill, conducting multiple studies concurrently, conducting a study from an off-site location, and conducting a study at multiple sites under the oversight of a single investigator, particularly where those sites are not in close proximity. To ensure appropriate supervision, the investigator should develop a *supervision and oversight plan* that includes meetings with staff, meetings with sponsor's monitors, and procedures for the following: correcting and documenting problems; documenting or reviewing the performance of delegated tasks; ensuring that the consent process is compliant with regulatory requirements; ensuring that source data are accurate, contemporaneous, and original; ensuring that information in source documents is captured on case report forms; dealing with data queries and discrepancies; ensuring study staff comply with protocol and adverse event assessment/reporting requirements; and addressing medical and ethical issues in a timely manner.

Fourth, the investigator must provide adequate supervision or oversight of any third parties involved in the conduct of a study, to the extent reasonably possible. This criterion is relevant when the sponsor retains a site management organization (SMO), and as a result, the SMO's personnel or forms are used. An investigator remains responsible for supervising the study tasks performed by staff, even if the staff is not employed by the investigator. If a crucial aspect of a study is performed by a third party (*e.g.*, radiologic assessment) and is not under the direct control of the clinical investigator, the sponsor is responsible for ensuring the party performing the task is competent to fulfill, and does fulfill, its responsibilities under the study. If the investigator retains the services of a facility to perform study assessments, the investigator must take steps to ensure that the facility is adequate (*e.g.*, licensed and certified), and may also institute procedures to ensure the integrity of data and records obtained. The investigator must evaluate, to the extent possible considering the study design, whether results appear reasonable and document the evaluation. If an investigator is assisted by a field clinical engineer (*e.g.*, device sponsor employee), such field clinical engineer may introduce bias, and therefore must be supervised by the investigator. If the field engineer has face-to-face contact with a subject or is involved in activities that directly affect the subject, those activities must be described in the informed consent.

6.1.2.3 Comply with Informed Consent and IRB Review Requirements

An investigator must inform subjects in the investigation, as well as subjects who participate as controls, that the product that is being tested is being used for investigational purposes, and ensure that the informed consent requirements at 21 C.F.R. Part 50 are met.[18] The informed consent process and the related HIPAA requirements are further discussed in **Chapters 9 and 10** of this primer. An investigator must also generally ensure that the investigation is in compliance with IRB approval and initial and continuing review requirements set forth at 21 C.F.R. Part 56.[19] The IRB review and approval process is discussed further in **Chapter 5** of this primer. Importantly, although the IRB must comply with all requirements for informed consent in 21 C.F.R. Part 50, an IRB may require additional components of the informed consent process and written informed consent document.

6.1.2.4 Report Adverse Events and Unanticipated Adverse Device Effects

With respect to investigations of drugs, an investigator must "immediately report to the sponsor any serious adverse event,[20] whether or not considered drug-related, including those listed in the protocol or investigator brochure, and must include an assessment of whether there is a reasonable possibility that the drug caused the event."[21] An investigator must record nonserious adverse events and report them to the sponsor according to the timetable for reporting specified in the protocol.[22] An investigator must also report to the IRB all unanticipated

---

[18] 21 C.F.R. §§ 312.60, 812.100; *ICH Good Clinical Practice*.

[19] 21 C.F.R. §§ 312.60, 812.110.

[20] Under 21 C.F.R. § 312.32, "adverse event" is defined as "any untoward medical occurrence associated with the use of a drug in humans, whether or not considered drug related;" and "serious adverse event" is defined as follows:

> An adverse event or suspected adverse reaction is considered "serious" if, in the view of either the investigator or sponsor, it results in any of the following outcomes: Death, a life-threatening adverse event, inpatient hospitalization or prolongation of existing hospitalization, a persistent or significant incapacity or substantial disruption of the ability to conduct normal life functions, or a congenital anomaly/birth defect. Important medical events that may not result in death, be life-threatening, or require hospitalization may be considered serious when, based upon appropriate medical judgment, they may jeopardize the patient or subject and may require medical or surgical intervention to prevent one of the outcomes listed in this definition. Examples of such medical events include allergic bronchospasm requiring intensive treatment in an emergency room or at home, blood dyscrasias or convulsions that do not result in inpatient hospitalization, or the development of drug dependency or drug abuse.

[21] 21 C.F.R. § 312.64(b).

[22] *Id.*

problems involving risk to human subjects or others.[23] In guidance, the FDA instructs that an adverse effect observed during the conduct of a study should be considered an unanticipated problem involving risk to human subjects and reported to the IRB "only if it were unexpected, serious, and would have implications for the conduct of the study (*e.g.*, requiring a significant and usually safety-related change in the protocol, such as revising inclusion/exclusion criteria or including a new monitoring requirement, informed consent, or investigator's brochure)."[24]

As a related responsibility, an investigator in a drug investigation must acknowledge that he/she read and understood the investigator's brochure, including the potential risks and side effects of the drug.[25] An investigator's brochure is a compilation of the clinical and nonclinical data on the investigational product that are relevant to the study of the product in human subjects, the purpose of which is to provide information to facilitate the understanding of the rationale for, and compliance with, key features of the protocol.[26] This commitment is particularly important for investigators whose involvement in the investigation is limited. The commitment further helps to ensure that all of the investigators who participate in the investigation are familiar with the information in the investigator's brochure.

As for device investigations, an investigator must submit to the sponsor and the reviewing IRB a report of any unanticipated adverse device effect[27] occurring during an investigation as soon as possible, but no later than within 10 working days of learning of such effect.[28]

6.1.2.5 Maintain and Make Available Adequate Records

An investigator must maintain adequate and accurate records and make those records available for inspection by the FDA.[29] Investigators of drugs and devices are required to maintain records pertaining to (i) disposition of drugs or devices, as applicable (*e.g.*, dates, quantity, and use by subjects) and (ii) case histories (*i.e.*, relevant information on each individual, including consent forms and medical record information that is the primary source data for entries that must be submitted to the sponsor).[30] In addition, investigators in device investigations must

[23] 21 C.F.R. § 312.66.

[24] FDA, GUIDANCE FOR CLINICAL INVESTIGATORS, SPONSORS, AND IRBS: ADVERSE EVENT REPORTING TO IRBS – IMPROVING HUMAN SUBJECT PROTECTION (Jan. 2009), at p. 3, *available at* https://www.fda.gov/downloads/RegulatoryInformation/Guidances/UCM126572.pdf.

[25] Form FDA 1572 (2/16), p. 2, *available at* https://www.fda.gov/downloads/AboutFDA/ReportsManualsForms/Forms/UCM074728.pdf.

[26] *ICH Good Clinical Practice,* at 42-43.

[27] Under 21 C.F.R. § 812.3(s), an "unanticipated adverse device effect" means:

> any serious adverse effect on health or safety or any life-threatening problem or death caused by, or associated with, a device, if that effect, problem, or death was not previously identified in nature, severity, or degree of incidence in the investigational plan or application (including a supplementary plan or application), or any other unanticipated serious problem associated with a device that relates to the rights, safety, or welfare of subjects.

[28] 21 C.F.R. § 812.150(a)(1).

[29] 21 C.F.R. §§ 312.62, 312.68, 812.140(a), 812.145.

[30] 21 C.F.R. §§ 312.62, 812.140(a).

maintain (iii) correspondence with other investigators, an IRB, the sponsor, a monitor, or the FDA, (iv) the protocol, including documentation of deviations from the protocol, and (v) other records determined to be required by the FDA.[31]

In drug investigations, investigators must retain study records for two years following the date a marketing application is approved for the drug or two years after the investigation is discontinued and the FDA is notified.[32] For investigational device studies, records must be retained for two years after the latter of (i) the date on which the investigation is terminated or completed, or (ii) the date after which the records are no longer required for supporting a premarket application or a notice of completion of a product development protocol.[33]

The investigator must, upon request, allow the FDA to review and copy records pertaining to the investigation.[34] The FDA's inspections of investigators (and inspections of IRBs and sponsors) are conducted under the FDA's Bioresearch Monitoring Program (BIMO) for the purpose of ensuring the protection of human subjects and the integrity of the clinical data, and field investigators must comply with the *FDA Compliance Program Guidance Manual*.[35] The investigator is not required to identify subjects unless the FDA has reason to believe that the records do not represent actual case studies or do not represent actual results obtained.[36]

6.1.2.6 Protect the Rights, Safety, and Welfare of Study Subjects

The FDA's regulations provide that an investigator is responsible for protecting the rights, safety, and welfare of subjects under their care during a clinical trial.[37] The FDA's guidance distills this broadly-worded regulatory commitment into three components.[38] First, the investigator should provide reasonable medical care for study subjects for medical problems arising during participation in the trial that are, or could be, related to the study intervention.[39] If the investigator does not possess the expertise to provide needed medical care, the investigator must ensure that the subject is able to obtain the necessary care from a qualified practitioner. The care provided to a subject, whether by the investigator or another practitioner, should be provided until any emergent condition related to the study intervention is resolved, even if the follow-up period extends beyond the end of the study at the investigative site. In addition, if medical care is needed for conditions or illnesses unrelated to the study intervention, which are

---

[31] 21 C.F.R. § 812.140(a).

[32] 21 C.F.R. § 312.62(c).

[33] 21 C.F.R. § 812.140(d).

[34] 21 C.F.R. §§ 312.68, 812.145(b)-(c).

[35] FDA, COMPLIANCE PROGRAM GUIDANCE MANUAL FOR FDA STAFF (Dec. 8, 2008), *available at* https://www.fda.gov/ICECI/EnforcementActions/BioresearchMonitoring/ucm133562.htm.

[36] *Id.*

[37] 21 C.F.R. §§ 312.60, 812.100.

[38] Unless noted otherwise, the discussion in this section of an investigator's responsibilities with respect to protecting the rights, safety, and welfare of study subjects is based on FDA's guidance document *FDA Guidance for Protecting, Rights, Safety, and Welfare of Study Subjects.*

[39] *ICH Good Clinical Practice,* at 14-15.

readily apparent or identified through screening procedures and eligibility criteria, the investigator must inform the subject and advise the subject to seek appropriate care.

Second, the investigator should be available to subjects during the conduct of the trial for medical care related to participation in the study. For example, if a study drug has potentially fatal toxicity risks, the investigator, or specifically designated subinvestigators, should be readily available by phone or other electronic communication 24 hours a day and in reasonably close proximity to the study subjects. Subjects should be given the adequate information to contact the investigator (*e.g.*, phone number). If the investigator is not available, the responsibility for medical care should be delegated to a specific qualified physician. The investigator should make adequate provision for any necessary medical care that the investigator is not qualified to provide.

Finally, the investigator must ensure adherence to the protocol so that study subjects are not exposed to unreasonable risks. While investigators are generally responsible for the study's adherence to the protocol, certain non-adherence may be also considered failure to protect the rights, safety, and welfare of subjects. For example, failure to perform safety assessments intended to detect drug toxicity or adverse events following administration of a medical device within protocol-specified time frames may be considered failure to protect the rights, safety, and welfare of the enrolled subject.

6.1.2.7 Maintain Control of Investigational Product

An investigator must maintain control of the drug or device under investigation.[40] In investigations involving drugs, an investigator may administer the investigational drug only to subjects under the investigator's personal supervision or under the supervision of a subinvestigator responsible to the investigator, and may not supply the investigational drug to any person not authorized to receive it.[41] An investigator is responsible for the return or disposition of the investigational drug or device upon the completion or termination of a clinical investigation or the investigator's part of an investigation, or at the sponsor's request.[42]

6.1.2.8 Furnish Investigator Reports Pertaining to Study Progress, Completion, and Financial Interest

An investigator must furnish to the sponsor certain reports pertaining to study progress, completion of investigator participation or of the investigation, and financial disclosures.[43] These reports regarding study progress and financial disclosures must be submitted by the investigator in addition to the other reports that must be submitted by the investigator, as discussed elsewhere in this chapter (*e.g.*, reports pertaining to adverse events, informed con-

[40] 21 C.F.R. §§ 312.60, 312.61, 812.100; *ICH Good Clinical Practice,* at 16.

[41] 21 C.F.R. § 312.61.

[42] 21 C.F.R. §§ 312.62(a), 812.110(e).

[43] 21 C.F.R. §§ 312.64, 812.150(a); 21 C.F.R. pt. 54.

sent, IRB review, and deviations from the protocol or investigational plan). Progress reports are intended to assist the sponsor in submitting its annual reports to the FDA, which include information such as list of subjects who died during participation in the investigation, and a list of the preclinical studies completed and a summary of findings.[44] Final reports are provided by the investigator at the completion of the investigator's participation in the investigation or the completion of the investigation.[45]

Financial disclosure reports described at 21 C.F.R. Part 54 contain information about financial interest arrangements with the sponsor involving each clinical investigator who was not an employee of a sponsor of the clinical study, including such investigator's spouse and each dependent child.[46] Disclosable financial interests and arrangements include (i) any compensation made to the investigator by any sponsor of a study in which the value of compensation could be affected by study outcome, (ii) a proprietary interest in the tested product, (iii) any equity interest in any sponsor of the covered clinical study, (iv) any equity interest in any sponsor of the covered study if the sponsor is a publicly held company and the interest exceeds $50,000 in value, and (v) significant payments (*i.e.*, over $25,000) of other sorts made by the sponsor to the investigator or the investigator's institution during the time the investigator is carrying out the study and for one year after completion.[47] This financial information is submitted to the FDA at the same time the sponsor submits a marketing application for the investigational product to the agency.

6.1.3 FDA Inspections of Clinical Investigators

The FDA regularly conducts inspections and for-cause audits to determine whether clinical investigators fulfill their responsibilities and comply with the applicable regulatory requirements. The FDA's inspections of investigators (and inspections of IRBs and sponsors) are conducted under the FDA's BIMO program for the purpose of ensuring the protection of human subjects and the integrity of the clinical data. Field investigators must comply with the *FDA Compliance Program Guidance Manual*.[48] Such inspections and audits involve an on-site inspection designed to document how the study was actually conducted at the clinical investigator's site. The inspector conducts the inspection by inspecting records and talking to individuals involved in the conduct of the clinical investigation.

[44] 21 C.F.R. §§ 312.64(a), 812.150(a)(3), 312.33.

[45] 21 C.F.R. §§ 312.64(c), 812.150(a)(6).

[46] 21 C.F.R. §§ 54.2, 54.4; FDA, GUIDANCE FOR CLINICAL INVESTIGATORS, INDUSTRY, AND FDA STAFF: FINANCIAL DISCLOSURE BY CLINICAL INVESTIGATORS (Feb. 2013), *available at* https://www.fda.gov/downloads/RegulatoryInformation/Guidances/UCM341008.pdf.

[47] 21 C.F.R. §§ 54.2, 54.4.

[48] FDA, COMPLIANCE PROGRAM GUIDANCE MANUAL FOR FDA STAFF (Dec. 8, 2008), *available at* https://www.fda.gov/ICECI/EnforcementActions/BioresearchMonitoring/ucm133562.htm.

Inspectors seek to ascertain whether the investigator complied with the applicable requirements by inquiring the following:[49]

(1) who performed various aspects of the protocol for the study (e.g., who verified inclusion and exclusion criteria, who obtained informed consent, who collected adverse event data);

(2) whether the IRB approved the protocol, informed consent form, and any amendments to the protocol prior to implementation;

(3) whether the clinical investigator and study staff adhered to the sponsor's protocol and investigational plan and whether protocol deviations were documented and reported appropriately;

(4) whether informed consent documents were signed by the subject or the subjects' legally authorized representative prior to entry in the study (i.e., performance of any study related procedures);

(5) whether authority to conduct aspects of the study was delegated, and if so, how the conduct of the study was supervised by the clinical investigator;

(6) where specific aspects of the investigation were performed;

(7) how the study data were obtained and where the study data were recorded;

(8) accountability for the investigational product, including shipping records and disposition of unused investigational product;

(9) whether the clinical investigator disclosed information regarding his financial interests to the sponsor and/or interests of any subinvestigator(s), spouse(s), and dependent children;

(10) the monitor's communications with the clinical investigator;

(11) the monitor's evaluations of the progress of the investigation; and

(12) corrective actions in response to previous FDA inspections, if any, and regulatory correspondence or sponsor and/or monitor correspondence.

The inspector may also review the study data (by comparing the original medical record source data with the data filed with the sponsor), including review of the subjects' written or electronic

---

[49] FDA, INFORMATION SHEET GUIDANCE FOR IRBS, CLINICAL INVESTIGATORS, AND SPONSORS: FDA INSPECTIONS OF CLINICAL INVESTIGATORS (June 2010), at p. 4, *available at* https://www.fda.gov/downloads/RegulatoryInformation/Guidances/UCM126553.pdf.

medical records to verify subject eligibility, adherence to protocol, and accuracy of data submitted to the sponsor in comparison with the original source data.[50]

At the end of an inspection, the FDA conducts an exit interview, and the findings are discussed with the investigator. Following the inspection, the FDA inspector prepares an Establishment Inspection Report for the appropriate FDA Center, which classifies the inspection report as (i) No Action Indicated (NAI); (ii) Voluntary Action Indicated (VAI), or (iii) Official Action Indicated (OAI), which means that regulatory and/or administrative/civil/criminal actions will be recommended. For year 2016, FDA BIMO inspection metrics reported that 755 inspections were conducted of investigators participating in clinical trials of drugs or medical devices. Of these inspections, approximately 2% were classified as "Official Action Indicated."[51] According to the FDA, the following regulatory deficiencies were most commonly found during inspections of clinical investigators: (i) failure to follow the investigational plan or regulations, or both; (ii) protocol deviations; (iii) inadequate recordkeeping; (iv) inadequate human subjects protection, including informed consent issues and failure to report adverse events; (iv) inadequate accountability for the investigational product; (v) inadequate communication with IRB; and (vi) misrepresentation of the investigational product as safe and effective.[52]

Upon reviewing the Report, the FDA Center may send the investigator one of four types of letters: (i) a letter of general compliance, stating observed basic compliance with pertinent regulations (if no deficiencies are found, the FDA may opt to not send any letter); (ii) an informational or untitled letter, stating that certain deviations were observed and should be responded to in writing by the clinical investigator; or (iii) a warning letter, stating that serious deviations from regulatory requirements were observed and must be promptly corrected to avoid an enforcement action. In rare instances, among other potential administrative actions, the FDA may issue a "Notice of Initiation of Disqualification Proceedings and Opportunity to Explain" (NIDPOE), which initiates a process to disqualify the clinical investigator from receiving investigational new drugs or devices because the investigator has repeatedly or deliberately failed to comply with applicable regulatory requirements or submitted false information to the FDA or the sponsor in any required report.[53]

The results of the inspection are shared with the FDA division assigned to review the marketing submission, and are considered by the division in reviewing the marketing submis-

---

[50] *Id.*

[51] FDA, BIORESEARCH MONITORING (BIMO) METRICS – FY'16, *available at* https://www.fda.gov/downloads/ScienceResearch/SpecialTopics/RunningClinicalTrials/UCM561049.pdf.

[52] *Id.*

[53] *Id.* at 7-8. The disqualification process is governed by 21 C.F.R. §§ 312.70 (drugs) and 812.119 (devices). Upon the receipt of a NIDPOE, the investigator may request an informal conference at the FDA Center. The investigator may opt to enter into a consent agreement (typically limiting or barring the investigator's use of investigational products) instead of contesting the allegations set forth in the NIDPOE. The investigator is also given the opportunity for an informal regulatory hearing under 21 C.F.R. pt. 16.

sion.[54] The FDA may choose to reject data from an investigator's site based on the results of an inspection.

6.2 Pre-2018 Common Rule: SACHRP Committee Recommendations

The roles and responsibilities of investigators in human subjects research are not discussed directly in the Pre-2018 Common Rule. The HHS Office for Human Research Protections (OHRP) has, however, received numerous recommendations to amend the Common Rule to address investigator responsibilities. Despite these recommendations, extensive amendment to the 2018 Common Rule still does not address investigator responsibilities.[55]

In a 2011 report, the Presidential Commission for the Study of Bioethical Issues recommended that the pre-2018 Common Rule "be revised to include a section directly addressing the responsibilities of investigators," stating that the revision would bring the Common Rule into harmony with the FDA regulations and international standards, as well as contribute to building a stronger culture of responsibility among investigators.[56] Two years later, in 2013, HHS Secretary's Advisory Committee on Human Research Protections (SACHRP) also recommended the addition of regulations to the Common Rule to address investigator responsibilities, referencing the 2011 report of the Presidential Commission.[57] SACHRP's recommendation letter to the HHS Secretary was accompanied with a more granular proposal in the form of draft regulatory language for inclusion in the 2018 Common Rule (45 C.F.R. Part 46).

SACHRP's draft regulations are generally similar to the FDA's regulations. SACHRP proposed defining "investigator" as "any individual responsible for the conduct of research involving human subjects, either for the study as a whole or for an individual site. If the research is conducted by a team at a study site, the investigator is the responsible leader of the team." SACHRP's draft regulations identify the following responsibilities for investigators: (i) ensuring that the research is conducted according to sound research design and methods, the protocol, applicable terms of grant, contract, or funding agreements, and applicable laws and regulations; and (ii) ensuring that members of the research team are appropriately qualified, trained, and supervised. The draft regulations also establish that investigators must possess the appropriate education, training, and experience, and must possess the required time and resources to properly conduct and supervise the research. Finally, the draft regulations require

---

[54] FDA, Information Sheet Guidance for IRBs, Clinical Investigators, and Sponsors: FDA Inspections of Clinical Investigators (June 2010), at p. 8, *available at* https://www.fda.gov/downloads/RegulatoryInformation/Guidances/UCM126553.pdf.

[55] Federal Policy for the Protection of Human Subjects, Final Rule, 82 Fed. Reg. 7149-7274 (Jan. 19, 2017). Effective date delayed in 83 Fed. Reg. 2885-2894 (Jan. 22, 2018), and again in 83 Fed. Reg. 28497 (Jun. 19, 2018).

[56] Presidential Comm'n for the Study of Bioethical Issues, Moral Science: Protecting Participants in Human Subjects Research (2011), *available at* https://bioethicsarchive.georgetown.edu/pcsbi/sites/default/files/Moral%20Science%20June%202012.pdf.

[57] U.S. Dep't of Health & Human Servs., January 10, 2013 SACHRP Letter to the HHS Secretary (Jan. 10, 2013), *available at* https://www.hhs.gov/ohrp/sachrp-committee/recommendations/2013-january-10-letter/index.html.

investigators to store, protect, and ensure accuracy and completeness of data, maintain records appropriate to research and permit access to such records, and submit reports to the IRB.

Chapter 7
Children in Research

Gelvina Rodriguez Stevenson

Leah A. Voigt

Introduction

INCLUDING CHILDREN IN CLINICAL RESEARCH serves at least two important scientific aims. First, and perhaps foremost, certain interventions target childhood diseases and conditions, and children are therefore the primary participants in research studies. Second, children may be just one segment of the population for whom a drug, device, or other intervention holds promise. Because of age and other physical characteristics of children, however, treatments that can benefit adults may be harmful to children, and the results of research involving adults cannot easily be extrapolated to this younger population. Understanding the full scope of the benefits and risks of a new clinical intervention may therefore require the inclusion of children in the research process.

From a legal standpoint, involving children in research raises a unique set of concerns, based both in state and federal law and regulation. Because children do not typically have legal authority to make their own medical decisions, parents, guardians, and other legal surrogates are responsible for deciding whether children and infants will participate in research studies. In addition, children are considered vulnerable subjects accorded special protections for their participation. IRBs and legal counsel must understand this unique set of obligations and regulatory requirements with respect to the participation of children in research.

It is important to point out that federal regulations distinguish neonates from other infants and children. Research involving newborn infants, or "neonates," is addressed separately in Subpart B of HHS Regulations, while Subpart D pertains to children and infants more broadly. This chapter focuses solely on Subpart D of HHS regulations.[1] The 2018 Common Rule revisions discussed in **Chapter 1** did not include amendments to Subpart D. However, some of the 2018 Common Rule revisions modify the way in which the IRB reviews research involving children, as described in greater detail below.

---

[1] The FDA also has parallel regulations governing research with children, found at 21 C.F.R. Part 50, Subpart D. These regulations are cited herein, and if a study falls under FDA jurisdiction, the FDA regulations should be consulted.

7.1 Who are "Children"?

HHS regulations define "children" as "persons who have not attained the legal age for consent to treatments or procedures involved in the research, under the applicable law of the jurisdiction in which the research will be conducted."[2] The definition of "children also depends on state laws pertaining to medical decision-making and informed consent. These laws typically define when an individual reaches the legal age of majority, or, in other words, when the individual is no longer considered a "minor." A minor lacks the legal capacity to make decisions concerning his or her own medical treatment. Thus, state laws define who may make those decisions—often, it is a parent, a guardian, or another caregiver.

In some limited circumstances, minors may make their own treatment decisions. A minor individual who is "emancipated," as defined by state law, may make his or her own medical decisions, and, in the case of an emergency, a minor's consent to treatment may be implied. State laws may also allow minors to make their own treatment decisions with respect to sexually transmitted diseases, pregnancy-related services, mental health, and substance abuse.

When a proposed research study involves children, HHS regulations impose additional requirements on an IRB. For instance, the regulations may require the IRB to include in its membership, or encourage it to obtain as consultants, individuals who are knowledgeable about working with children. Subpart D also directs an IRB to take note of special considerations pertaining to the risks and benefits of the proposed research.[3]

7.2 IRB Membership

When an IRB reviews a research proposal involving children, HHS encourages the IRB to include in its membership individuals who are knowledgeable and experienced in working with this vulnerable population.[4] For example, an IRB may include a teacher, child psychologist, or pediatrician if the IRB regularly reviews research with children as subjects. If the IRB does not regularly review research involving children, it may invite an individual with this special competence to assist in reviewing specific pediatric research proposals.[5]

7.3 Categories of Allowable Research in Children

IRBs may approve research involving children when the research fits into one of three categories under Subpart D. These categories are distinguished by the level of risk, the potential

---

[2] 45 C.F.R. § 46.402(a); FDA regulations vary slightly, defining a child as one not having attained the legal age for consent to treatment or procedures involving clinical investigations under applicable law of the jurisdiction where the clinical investigation will be conducted. 21 C.F.R. § 50.3(o).

[3] *Special Protections for Children as Research Subjects*, OFFICE FOR HUMAN RESEARCH PROTECTIONS, *available at* https://www.hhs.gov/ohrp/regulations-and-policy/guidance/special-protections-for-children/index.html; *see also Research with Children FAQs*, OFFICE FOR HUMAN RESEARCH PROTECTIONS, *available at* https://www.hhs.gov/ohrp/regulations-and-policy/guidance/faq/children-research/index.html.

[4] 45 C.F.R. § 46.107(a); 21 C.F.R. § 56.107(a).

[5] 45 C.F.R. § 46.107(f); 21 C.F.R. § 56.107(f).

for direct benefit, and the potential to yield "generalizable" knowledge about the condition at issue.[6]

The first category permits research with children when the proposed research does not pose a greater than minimal risk to the child.[7] "Minimal risk" means that "the probability and magnitude of harm or discomfort anticipated with the research is not greater than the harm or discomfort ordinarily encountered in daily life or during routine physical or psychological examinations or tests."[8] Minimal risk, as used in Subpart D, should be interpreted as the type of risk encountered by average, healthy children during daily life or during routine physical or psychological examinations or tests.[9]

The HHS Secretary's Advisory Committee on Human Research Protections (SACHRP) has made several recommendations regarding the interpretation of minimal risk.[10] SACHRP recommended that the baseline standard for determining minimal risk be the level of risk posed to children living in a safe environment and should not be higher for children living in less safe environments.[11] The committee also recommended that the evaluation of minimal risk should be indexed against the risk posed to other children of the same age and developmental status as the subject population.[12]

The second category of allowable research with children involves a greater than minimal risk if the proposed research also has the potential for providing direct benefit to the child.[13] The anticipated benefit to risk relationship must be at least as favorable as that presented by available alternative approaches.[14] In other words, the extent of the risk must be proportional to the probability and magnitude of benefit.[15]

The third category of allowable research with children (i) poses a minor increase over minimal risk but provides no prospect of direct benefit; (ii) results in an experience similar to those normally associated with the child's actual or expected medical, dental, psychological, social, or educational situation; and (iii) is likely to yield knowledge that is vital to understanding or ameliorating the condition at issue.[16] A "minor increase over minimal risk" is not defined

[6] 45 C.F.R. §§ 403–406; 21 C.F.R. §§ 50.50–50.53.

[7] 45 C.F.R. § 46.404; 21 C.F.R. § 50.51.

[8] 45 C.F.R. § 46.102(j); 21 C.F.R. § 50.3(k); 21 C.F.R. § 56.102(i).

[9] *July 28, 2005 SACHRP Chair Letter to HHS Secretary Regarding Recommendations*, HHS.gov (July 28, 2005), *available at* https://www.hhs.gov/ohrp/sachrp-committee/recommendations/2005-july-28-letter/index.html [hereafter *Letter to HHS Secretary*].

[10] *Id.* at Appendix B in *Letter to HHS Secretary*. These recommendations were made by the Subcommittee on Research Involving Children (SRIC) and were approved by SACHRP.

[11] *Id.*

[12] *Id.*

[13] 45 C.F.R. § 46.405; 21 C.F.R. § 50.52.

[14] 45 C.F.R. § 46.405(b); 21 C.F.R. § 50.52(b).

[15] *Letter to HHS Secretary*, *supra* note 9.

[16] 45 C.F.R. § 46.406; 21 C.F.R. § 50.53.

in the regulations; however, SACHRP has recommended that transient or reversible harm be included in this risk category. An extremely small probability of experiencing severe pain, discomfort, stress, or other harm, should also be included in this category.[17]

If the proposed research does not fit into one of these categories, the IRB may submit the proposal to the Office for Human Research Protections (OHRP) for approval. OHRP will approve the research if it presents "a reasonable opportunity to further the understanding, prevention, or alleviation of a serious problem affecting the health or welfare of children."[18] Through OHRP, HHS may approve the research if the following conditions are met: HHS consults with a panel of experts and allows public comment; HHS finds that the research falls into one of the three allowable categories or if HHS agrees with the IRB's analysis regarding importance; if the research will be conducted in accordance with ethical principles; and if consent and/or assent will be obtained in accordance with Subpart D.[19]

All four categories of research require parental or guardian consent and assent of the child to participate in a study.[20]

7.4 Expedited Review and Exempt Research

For research involving children, the same expedited review procedure for research involving adults is utilized; however, the categories for exempt research are slightly different when children are the subjects of the research. Exemption from the Pre-2018 Common Rule requirements regarding educational tests does not apply to research involving children when information recorded by the investigator can be readily ascertained.

The category for exempt research involving educational tests, survey or interview procedures, or observations of public behavior applies to research involving children in a more limited manner than when involving adults.[21] For example, the pre-2018 Common Rule provides that research involving educational tests is exempt from the Rule's requirements if the information is recorded by the investigator in a manner such that the identity of the subjects cannot be readily ascertained; however research that involves children is exempt only if the investigator is *not* participating in the research activity being observed.[22] Similarly, while the pre-2018 Common Rule exempts research involving educational tests when any disclosure of subjects' responses outside of the research would not reasonably place the subjects at risk of criminal or civil liability, or be damaging to the subjects' financial standing, employability, educational advancement, or reputation, this exemption applies to research involving children

---

[17] *Letter to HHS Secretary*, *supra* note 9.

[18] 45 C.F.R. § 46.407(a); 21 C.F.R. § 50.54(a).

[19] 45 C.F.R. § 46.407(b); 21 C.F.R. § 50.54(b).

[20] 45 C.F.R. § 404-408; 21 C.F.R. § 50.51-55.

[21] 45 C.F.R. § 46.104(b)(3).

[22] *Id.*

only if the investigator does not participate in any research activity being observed.[23] By way of example, an investigator does not participate in the research activity being observed when he or she only observes children's interactions on a playground but does not rearrange equipment, add objects to the playground, or videotape the interactions.

7.5 Parental Permission and Assent of the Child

There are two components of the informed consent process when research involves children: the permission of the parent and the assent of the child. Permission is the agreement of a parent or guardian to the participation of his or her child or ward in research.[24] Assent refers to the child's affirmative agreement to participate in research.[25]

The IRB is responsible for determining whether adequate provisions exist for obtaining and documenting the permission of the parent consistent with the requirements set forth in **Chapter 9** for informed consent. Where research is approved under § 46.404 or 46.405 of Subpart D, the permission of one parent is acceptable. When research is approved under § 46.406 or 46.407, the permission of both parents is required unless one parent is deceased, unknown, incompetent, not reasonably available, or when one parent has legal responsibility for the care and custody of the child.[26] In these circumstances, investigators should maintain documentation of the reason why the second parent's permission was not obtained. This is further discussed in **Section 9.4**.

In certain circumstances the parental permission requirement may be waived by the IRB under HHS regulations. The options for waiver or alteration of informed consent apply to research involving children. In addition, if an IRB determines that a research study is designed for conditions or for a subject population for which parental permission is not a reasonable requirement, the IRB may waive the parental permission requirement under HHS regulations.[27] The IRB must ensure that the waiver is in compliance with other applicable laws, including state and local laws. The IRB also must substitute an appropriate procedure for protecting the subjects. In determining an appropriate procedure, the IRB should consider the risks, anticipated benefits, and the subjects' age, maturity, and condition. An example may include research involving older adolescents and treatment for which they may consent, under applicable state law, on their own behalf (*e.g.*, treatment for sexually transmitted diseases or drug abuse).

An IRB must ensure that adequate provisions are made to obtain the assent of the children when the IRB determines they are capable of assenting. The IRB must take into account the age, maturity, and psychological state of the children involved. An assent form for younger children (ages 7 through 11) should include simple language that explains what the study is

---

[23] *Id.*

[24] 45 C.F.R. § 46.402(c); 21 C.F.R. § 50.3(r).

[25] 45 C.F.R. § 46.402(b); 21 C.F.R. § 50.3(n).

[26] 45 C.F.R. § 46.408(b). FDA has parallel provisions, at 21 C.F.R. § 50.55.

[27] 45 C.F.R. § 46.408(c).

about, the procedures, the risks, the potential benefits, a statement that they do not have to participate, an invitation to ask questions, and the names and phone numbers of whom to contact with questions. For older children (ages 12 through 17), the IRB may utilize the parental permission form for the assent of the child. State and local laws may have variations on when and how assent is to be obtained. IRBs may establish guidelines, but should not establish rigid rules based solely on age. Determinations of appropriate assent must also include considerations of maturity and psychological state of the children.[28] When assent is required, the IRB must determine whether and how assent must be documented.[29]

If an IRB determines that some or all of the children cannot reasonably consent, or the intervention involved in the research is only available in the research context and holds out the prospect of direct benefit that is important to the health and well-being of the child, assent is not necessary.[30] Assent may also be waived by the IRB is accordance with requirements set forth in **Chapter 9** (**Section 9.4**).

7.6 Wards

Children who are wards of the state or any other agency, institution or entity can be included in research approved under §§ 46.404 or 46.405. The IRB must ensure there is an appropriate process in place for obtaining permission from the guardian and assent from the child. Wards may also be included in research approved under §§ 46.406 or 46.407 only if the research is (i) related to their status as wards or (ii) conducted in schools, camps, hospitals, institutions, or similar settings in which the majority of children involved as subjects are not wards. In these latter circumstances, the IRB must appoint an advocate for each child who is a ward, in addition to any other person acting on behalf of the child as a guardian. One advocate may be provided for multiple wards. The advocate shall have the background and experience to act in the best interest of the child throughout the duration of the research and shall be independent of the researchers.[31] IRBs working regularly with children who are wards should have procedures in place to ensure that these additional requirements are met.

For a child in foster care, determining who has legal authority to consent to the child's participation in research will likely be a fact-specific analysis, based on state law and the terms of the foster care arrangement. An IRB considering research that may include children in foster care should consult legal counsel to determine whether these children can be enrolled in the research, under what circumstances and, importantly, who can make the decision to participate on behalf of the children under foster care.

---

[28] 45 C.F.R. § 46.408(a); 21 C.F.R. § 50.55(b).

[29] 45 C.F.R. § 46.408(e); 21 C.F.R. § 50.55(g).

[30] 45 C.F.R. § 46.408(a); 21 C.F.R. § 50.55(c).

[31] 45 C.F.R. § 46.409; 21 C.F.R. § 50.56.

Chapter 8
Special Categories of Review

Alice K. Marcee

Introduction

There are several situations regarding FDA-regulated items that involve special consideration. As discussed in **Chapter 3**, an FDA-regulated product, including a drug, biological product, or medical device for human use, must receive FDA approval before it is introduced or delivered into interstate commerce and marketed for a specific use. The FDA's approval process generally involves use of such investigational FDA-regulated products, as "test articles," in clinical trials, and includes requirements for the prospective approval and continued oversight of the clinical trial by the IRB, the submission of scientific data to support the approval of the test article, and the completion of the clinical trial. The timeframe for completing clinical trials averages six to seven years.[1]

Certain situations may justify access to a test article outside of the clinical trial approval process; however, the IRB continues to play its critical role in approving and monitoring outside this standard process. This chapter addresses the use of test articles outside of a clinical trial that may, for example, include situations involving a serious or life-threatening disease or condition for which there is no available standard of care therapy or diagnostic method under the expanded access program, or allowing access to medical devices for rare diseases or conditions that are classified by the FDA as humanitarian use devices. Right-to-try laws involve similar use of unapproved therapies, but without IRB involvement. This chapter also includes a discussion of off-label use of approved FDA-regulated products. Health care institutions would be wise to consider policies or guidelines regarding this practice to differentiate off-label use from research.

8.1 Expanded Access for Treatment Use

Expanded access to test articles for treatment uses, commonly referred to as "compassionate use," is the practice of using an investigational drug, biologic, or medical device outside of a clinical trial to treat a patient with a serious or immediately life-threatening disease or condition for which no acceptable treatment alternative is available. It generally allows access for patients who do not meet the requirements for inclusion in a clinical investigation or where

[1] *Biopharmaceutical Research & Development: The Process Behind New Medicines*, PhRMA (Aug. 20, 2015), *available at* http://phrma-docs.phrma.org/sites/default/files/pdf/rd_brochure_022307.pdf.

there is no active investigation, but for whom the treating physician believes the drug, biologic, or medical device may provide a benefit in treating and/or diagnosing their disease or condition. FDA approval and—unless an exception applies—IRB approval are required for expanded access. Informed consent requirements also must be met. The FDA uses its regulatory discretion in determining whether such use should occur.[2] The FDA has provided guidance addressing all expanded access uses, including emergency uses.[3]

For all individual expanded access uses, the following criteria must be met: (i) the patient to be treated has a serious or immediately life-threatening disease or condition and no comparable or satisfactory alternative is available; (ii) the probable risk from use of the investigational product is not greater than the probable risk from the disease or condition; (iii) the FDA determines that there is sufficient evidence of the safety and effectiveness of the investigational product to support the proposed use; (iv) the FDA determines that expanded access to the investigational product for the specific disease or condition will not interfere with the initiation, conduct, or completion of any clinical trials to support marketing approval, or compromise the development of the investigational product in the context of the specific disease or condition; (v) appropriate application is submitted; and (vi) the patient is unable to obtain the investigational product under an existing Investigational New Drug application (IND) or in a clinical trial.[4] Meeting these criteria, obtaining patient informed consent, and pending prospective IRB approval—except for emergency use and where waivable[5]—are required for all expanded access uses.

The three different patient categories of expanded access to investigational drugs or biologics include (i) individual patients,[6] (ii) intermediate-size patient populations,[7] and (iii) larger

---

[2] 21 C.F.R. § 312.305; 21 C.F.R. § 812.36; Investigational New Drugs: FDA Has Taken Steps to Improve the Expanded Access Program but Should Further Clarify How Adverse Events Data Are Used, GAO-17-564 (July 11, 2017), *available at* https://www.gao.gov/assets/690/685729.pdf.

[3] Expanded Access (Compassionate Use), FDA, *available at* https://www.fda.gov/NewsEvents/PublicHealthFocus/ExpandedAccessCompassionateUse/default.htm.

[4] *Id.*; 21 C.F.R. § 312.305.

[5] Information Sheet Guidance for Sponsors, Clinical Investigators, and IRBs: Waiver of IRB Requirements for Drug and Biological Product Studies, FDA (updated Oct. 2017), *available at* https://www.fda.gov/downloads/regulatoryinformation/guidances/ucm126500.pdf. Waiver of full IRB review at a convened IRB meeting for individual patient expanded access INDs using Form FDA 3926 is appropriate when the requesting physician obtains concurrence by the IRB chair or another designated IRB member before the treatment use begins. The FDA has indicated that this same modified IRB procedure would be used for continuing review or for changes/amendments. Physicians submitting Form FDA 1571 for individual patient expanded access may submit an application for waiver of full IRB review.

[6] 21 C.F.R. § 312.310; Individual Patient Expanded Access Applications: Form FDA 3926: Guidance for Industry, FDA (updated Oct. 2017), *available at* https://www.fda.gov/downloads/Drugs/GuidanceComplianceRegulatoryInformation/Guidances/UCM432717.pdf. The 21st Century Cures Act (Pub. L. 114-255, Dec. 13, 2016) required certain drug manufacturers or distributors to make publicly available, such as on their websites, their policies for expanded access; *see also* Reagan-Udall Foundation for the Food and Drug Administration at www.reaganudall.org for an individual patient expanded access navigator.

[7] 21 C.F.R. § 312.315.

populations under a treatment protocol or treatment IND.[8] In addition, there are two different categories of expanded access to investigational devices: (i) compassionate use (individual patient/small group access),[9] and (ii) treatment use (larger populations, but limited number of study sites and enrollment).[10] The FDA has guidance on expanded access for medical devices[11] and has developed a training slide deck regarding use of unapproved medical devices.[12]

8.1.1 Right-to-Try

On May 30, 2018, the federal Right to Try Act (the Act) was signed into law.[13] The Act amends the federal Food, Drug, and Cosmetic Act and allows patients to directly request access to investigational drugs as long as the patient is an "eligible patient" and the investigational drug is an "eligible investigation drug." An eligible patient is a patient who (i) is diagnosed with a life-threatening disease or condition, (ii) has exhausted approved treatment options and is unable to participate in a clinical trial involving the eligible investigational drug, as certified by a physician, and (iii) has provided the treating physician written informed consent.[14] The physician that certifies that the patient has exhausted all other avenues for treatment must be in good standing with the physician's licensing body and not be directly compensated by the investigational drug manufacturer for this certification.[15]

An eligible investigational drug, an investigational drug that has not been approved or licensed by the FDA for any use, is subject to and covered by an IND with the FDA, and has completed a Phase 1 clinical trial.[16] The investigational drug must be undergoing active development or production by the manufacturer and under no clinical holds. Finally, the clinical trials for this investigational drug must intend to serve as the basis for a claim of effectiveness that will support a request to the FDA for approval of this drug.[17] In addition, the clinical trial investigations for the investigational drug cannot be unduly prolonged in order to be in compliance with the Act.[18] Information will be provided to the FDA regarding uses of the

---

[8] 21 C.F.R. § 312.320.

[9] The physician desiring expanded access should contact the device sponsor for permission to use the device under expanded access. If the sponsor agrees to the use, the sponsor submits an investigational device exemption (IDE) supplement requesting approval of a protocol deviation in order to treat a patient (*see* 21 C.F.R. § 812.35(a)).

[10] 21 C.F.R. § 812.36.

[11] Expanded Access for Medical Devices, FDA, *available at* https://www.fda.gov/medicaldevices/deviceregulationandguidance/howtomarketyourdevice/investigationaldeviceexemptionide/ucm051345.htm.

[12] Emergency Uses and Compassionate Use of Unapproved Devices, FDA, *available at* https://www.fda.gov/downloads/Training/CDRHLearn/UCM180888.pdf.

[13] Right to Try Act (Pub. L. 115-176 (May 30, 2018)).

[14] 21 U.S.C. § 360bbb-0a (a)(1).

[15] *Id.*

[16] 21 U.S.C. § 360bbb-0a (a)(2).

[17] *Id.*

[18] Exemptions under the Act are available as long as the sponsor does not unduly prolong an investigation after finding that the results of the investigation appear to establish sufficient data to support a marketing appli-

investigational drugs under the Act and some information will be posted on the FDA website; however, use of clinical outcomes in the FDA review process is limited.[19]

Of great interest is this Act's exemption from IRB approval and oversight of a patient taking an investigational drug as long as the eligibility of the patient and the investigational drug are met.[20] This exemption from IRB approval, and related oversight and requirements for informed consent, is contingent on compliance with drug labeling, promotion, and charging limitations. While the Act requires patients to provide their physicians with written informed consent, the Act exempts meeting the informed consent requirements or elements found under 21 C.F.R. Part 50, Protection of Human Subjects. As long as compliance is maintained, the oversight for patient safety under this Act appears to be left to the sponsor, manufacturer, prescriber, or dispenser.

A sponsor or manufacturer will not be liable for providing an experimental drug in compliance with the Act; all others will not be liable for providing an experimental drug in compliance with the Act unless their acts constitute reckless or willful misconduct, gross negligence, or an intentional tort under any applicable state law. There is no liability for any party for not providing access to an investigational drug under the Act. The patient's right to otherwise bring a private action under any state or federal product liability, tort, consumer protection, or warranty law is not barred, however.[21] The FDA is tasked with implementing the Act for patients "in a way that seeks to protect their autonomy, their safety, and the safety of others following in their paths."[22]

On the surface, this Act appears to have created an additional access point to investigational drugs—albeit drugs with limited FDA review for safety and effectiveness, having only completed Phase 1 safety testing with 20 to 100 subjects, for patients with serious or immediately life-threatening diseases or conditions for which no acceptable treatment alternative is available. However, there is no requirement to provide patients access to eligible investigational drugs under the Act. Patients can make requests, but they have no right to access to these investigational drugs.

In addition, 41 states have passed right-to-try laws, which were not specifically preempted by the Act. These state laws have a similar intent but the provisions vary, with some providing more limitations of investigational drug access, and some expanding the provisions to include access to medical devices. The interaction of these laws will develop over time.

---

cation, in addition to other applicable compliance requirements. *See* 21 U.S.C. §360bbb-0a(b), referencing 21 C.F.R. §312.7(c).

[19] 21 U.S.C. §360bbb-0a (c).

[20] Exemption from IRB approval and oversight are available as long as all requirements of the Act are met. *See* 21 U.S.C. §360bbb-0a(b), referencing 21 C.F.R. Parts 50, 56.

[21] *See* 21 U.S.C. §360bbb-0a, *citing* Pub.L. 115-176, §2(b) (May 30, 2018).

[22] FDA, Statement from FDA Commissioner Scott Gottlieb, M.D., on the signing of the Right to Try Act (May 30, 2018), *available at* https://www.fda.gov/newsevents/newsroom/pressannouncements/ucm609258.htm.

8.2 Expanded Access for Emergency Use

"Emergency use" is a specific subset of expanded access and is defined as the use of a test article for a patient in a life-threatening situation in which no standard acceptable treatment is available, and in which there is not sufficient time to obtain IRB approval.[23] "Life-threatening," for the purposes of section 56.102(d), includes the scope of both life-threatening and severely debilitating, as defined below:[24]

- Life-threatening means diseases or conditions where the likelihood of death is high unless the course of the disease is interrupted and diseases or conditions with potentially fatal outcomes, where the end point of clinical trial analysis is survival. The criteria for life-threatening do not require the condition to be immediately life-threatening or to immediately result in death. Rather, the subjects must be in a life-threatening situation requiring intervention before review at a convened meeting of the IRB is feasible.
- Severely debilitating means diseases or conditions that cause major irreversible morbidity. Examples of severely debilitating conditions include blindness, loss of arm, leg, hand or foot, loss of hearing, paralysis, or stroke.

The emergency use of an unapproved investigational drug or biologic requires an IND.[25] If the intended patient does not meet the criteria of an existing study protocol, or if an approved study protocol does not exist, the usual procedure is to contact the manufacturer and determine if the drug can be made available for the emergency use under the company's IND. The need for an investigational drug may arise in an emergency situation that does not allow time for submission of an IND. In such a case, the FDA may authorize shipment of the investigational drug or device for a specialized use in advance of the IND submission. Requests for such authorization for drugs and biologics may be made by telephone or other communication means.[26] An expanded access submission must be made within 15 days of the FDA's authorization of use.[27] A similar process is applicable to the use of investigational devices in emergency situations.[28]

Emergency use of a test article is exempt from prospective IRB review requirements, provided that such emergency use is reported to the IRB within five working days and any subsequent use of the test article at the institution is subject to IRB review.[29] Although FDA

[23] 21 C.F.R. § 56.102(d).

[24] Emergency Use of an Investigational Drug or Biologic–Information Sheet, FDA, *available at* https://www.fda.gov/RegulatoryInformation/Guidances/ucm126491.htm.

[25] *Id.*, an Investigational New Drug application is needed to use an unapproved investigational drug or biologic in a research trial; *see* 21 C.F.R. Part 312.

[26] 21 C.F.R. § 312.310(d).

[27] *Id.*

[28] Expanded Access for Medical Devices, FDA, *available at* https://www.fda.gov/medicaldevices/deviceregulationandguidance/howtomarketyourdevice/investigationaldeviceexemptionide/ucm051345.htm; *see also* Emergency Use and Compassionate Use of Unapproved Devices, FDA, *available at* https://www.fda.gov/downloads/Training/CDRHLearn/UCM180888.pdf.

[29] 21 C.F.R. § 56.104(c).

regulations require that any subsequent use of the investigational product at the institution have prospective IRB review and approval, FDA acknowledges that it would be inappropriate to deny emergency treatment to a second individual if the only obstacle is that the IRB has not had sufficient time to convene a meeting to review the issue.

Institutional procedures may require that the IRB be notified prior to an emergency use; however, this notification should not be construed as an IRB approval. Notification should be used by the IRB to initiate tracking to ensure that the investigator files a report within the five day time-frame required by 21 C.F.R. § 56.104(c). The FDA regulations do not provide for expedited IRB approval in emergency situations. An IRB must either convene and give "full board" approval of the emergency use or, if the conditions of 21 C.F.R. § 56.102(d) are met and it is not possible to convene a quorum within the time available, the use may proceed without any IRB approval.

Some manufacturers will agree to allow the use of the test article but require "an IRB approval letter" before the test article will be shipped. If it is not possible to convene a quorum of the IRB within the time available, some IRBs have sent to the sponsor a written statement that the IRB is aware of the proposed use and considers the use to meet the requirements of 21 C.F.R. § 56.104(c). Although this is not an IRB approval, the acknowledgment letter has been acceptable to manufacturers and they have allowed the shipment to proceed.

Informed consent requirements must still be met for emergency use.

8.3 Humanitarian Use Devices

A Humanitarian Use Device (HUD) is a medical device intended to benefit patients in the treatment or diagnosis of a disease or condition that affects or is manifested in no more than 8,000 individuals in the United States per year.[30] Such rare diseases or conditions create challenges to gathering scientific evidence to support safety and effectiveness in a timely manner, and thereby limit access to treatment or diagnostics. Once the medical device is designated by the FDA as a HUD, the next step is the completion of a Humanitarian Device Exemption (HDE). The HDE is an application that is similar to a premarket approval (PMA) application, but is exempt from the effectiveness requirements of a PMA, and instead establishes a threshold of "probable benefit."[31] FDA approval of an HDE authorizes marketing of a HUD, subject to certain restrictions. The purpose of this alternative pathway is to encourage the discovery and use of devices to benefit patients suffering from rare diseases or conditions.[32]

[30] The 21st Century Cures Act (Pub. L. 114-255 (Dec. 13, 2016)) increased the population from fewer than 4,000 to no more than 8,000 individuals; *see* 21 C.F.R. §§ 814.3(n), 814.100(a),(b).

[31] 21 C.F.R. § 814.104.

[32] 21 C.F.R. § 814.100(a), (b); Getting a Humanitarian Use Device to Market, *available at* https://www.fda.gov/medicaldevices/deviceregulationandguidance/howtomarketyourdevice/premarketsubmissions/humanitarianddeviceexemption/ucm563286.htm.

The HUD is not considered "investigational," nor is use of the device considered "research" as long as the use of a HUD is not in a clinical investigation (*i.e.*, collection of safety and effectiveness data) and use is for its HDE-approved purpose. The federal statute and implementing regulations do, however, require IRB review and approval before a HUD is used, except in emergency situations in which the physician determines that approval cannot be obtained in time to prevent serious harm or death to the patient.[33] The IRB is responsible for the initial, as well as continuing, review of the HUD. For initial review, the IRB is required to perform a full board review. For continuing review, the IRB may use the expedited review process, unless the IRB determines that a full board review should be performed. The IRB of record will receive copies of the medical device reports sent to the FDA where a death or serious injury was caused by, or may have been caused by, the HUD.[34]

The IRB does not need to review and approve each individual use of a HUD. As long as the HUD is used within the FDA-approved indication, the IRB may approve the use of the device without further restrictions, or, if it so desires, the IRB can require approval of the device on a case-by-case basis.

The HUD regulations do not require informed consent because an approved HDE provides for marketing approval and the use of the HUD does not constitute research or an investigation that would normally require specific informed consent. Guidance issued by the FDA does state, however, that there is nothing in the federal regulations that prohibits an institution from requiring prospective informed consent.[35] It states that most HDE holders have developed patient information packets that include information to assist a patient in making an informed decision about the use of the device. The FDA guidance also indicates that such patient information packets contain a discussion of the potential risks and benefits of the device, as well as any procedures associated with the use of the HUD. Lastly, the guidance reflects that the patient information packets generally contain a statement that the device is a humanitarian use device for which effectiveness for the labeled indication has not been demonstrated, which must be included in the labeling of the HUD. It is up to the individual IRB to determine whether specific informed consent should be obtained. At a minimum, it is recommended that patients receive a copy of the HDE holder's patient information packet.

[33] 21C.F.R. § 814.124(a). Within five days after use in an emergency situation, written notification to the chair of the IRB must be provided, including identification of the patient, the date of device use, and the reason for such use—notification is not IRB approval.

[34] 21 C.F.R. § 814.126(a).

[35] Information Sheet Guidance for IRBs, Clinical Investigators, and Sponsors, Frequently Asked Questions About Medical Devices, FDA (Jan. 2006), *available at* https://www.fda.gov/downloads/RegulatoryInformation/Guidances/UCM127067.pdf; Humanitarian Device Exemption (HDE) Regulation: Questions and Answers, Draft Guidance for HDE Holders, Institutional Review Boards (IRBs), Clinical Investigators, and Food and Drug Administration Staff, FDA (July 8, 2010), *available at* https://www.fda.gov/downloads/MedicalDevices/DeviceRegulationandGuidance/GuidanceDocuments/ucm110203.pdf (update for compliance with the 21st Century Cures Act is pending.); Humanitarian Device Exemption (HDE) Program: Guidance for Industry and Food and Drug Administration Staff, FDA (June 13, 2018) (when final, this guidance will supersede the guidance issued July 8, 2010), *available at* https://www.fda.gov/downloads/MedicalDevices/DeviceRegulationandGuidance/GuidanceDocuments/UCM389275.pdf.

Counsel may be called upon to assist the IRB in determining whether an informed consent should be drafted for a HUD. Thus, it is important for counsel to understand the HUD requirements. A general HUD Information Sheet is attached as **Exhibit 8.3**.

8.4 Off-Label Uses

The term "off-label" refers to the medical practice of prescribing FDA-approved drugs, biologics, or medical devices for uses that are not identified in the approved labeling, and it reflects the fact that any lawfully marketed drug, biologic, or medical device approved by the FDA for a given use may be prescribed for any use that a physician believes will best serve the patient. Off-label use occurs when a physician prescribes a drug or biologic or uses a medical device outside the scope of the FDA-approved labeling. While FDA approval means that the drug, biologic, or medical device may be sold or marketed in a certain way, the FDA does not dictate to physicians how they can use approved drugs, biologics, or medical devices.[36]

A physician using his/her best medical judgment may make a decision to prescribe or administer a legally marketed drug, biologic, or medical device for an unindicated or off-label use to a patient for the treatment of the patient's particular condition or disease. From a legal and ethical standpoint, off-label use represents a delicate balance between the regulatory objective of protecting patients from unsafe or ineffective drugs, biologics, and medical devices on the one hand, and, on the other hand, the prerogative of physicians to use their professional judgment in treating patients.

Off-label uses for patient treatment may not fall within the definition of research, or even be considered investigational or experimental. The off-label use of a drug, biologic, or medical device does not require an IND or IDE or require review by an IRB if that use is solely for the "practice of medicine."[37] Health care institutions should, however, have policies and procedures that define research and the procedures where research is involved, as well as guidelines for off-label and investigational uses of drugs, biologics, and medical devices. In appropriate circumstances, health care institutions may desire to have the physician utilize an informed consent for an off-label use. A sample consent for off-label use is included at **Exhibit 8.4**. An institution may also require an innovative off-label use to be done within a research protocol.

---

[36] 21 C.F.R. § 312.2(d); 21 U.S.C. § 396.

[37] "Off-Label" and Investigational Use of Marketed Drugs, Biologics and Medical Devices—Information Sheet, FDA, *available at* https://www.fda.gov/RegulatoryInformation/Guidances/ucm126486.htm.

Chapter 9

Understanding Research Informed Consent

Laura M. Odwazny

Haley N. Bavasi

Introduction

Informed consent is both a legal standard for medical care and a regulatory requirement for research. Unless the general requirements for written informed consent are waived or altered, each human subject must be provided with and sign an informed consent document before being enrolled in a research study. The process of educating research subjects begins during the initial recruitment contact and continues throughout the duration of their research participation. When counsel is reviewing a proposed informed consent form for a research study, it is often helpful to utilize a checklist that itemizes the specific elements required by the federal regulations (and applicable state laws and institutional policies) to ensure that the proposed consent addresses all of the necessary elements. Many Institutional Review Boards (IRBs) have created an informed consent checklist for use in its review process. In addition, the Food and Drug Administration (FDA) published draft guidance expanding on informed consent in July 2014,[1] and the Office for Human Research Protections (OHRP) website contains an informed consent checklist, tips, and FAQs.[2] Sample informed consent checklists are attached as **Exhibit 9.0.1:** Sample Informed Consent Checklist, pre-2018 Common Rule and FDA; **Exhibit 9.0.2:** Sample Study-Specific Informed Consent Checklist, 2018 Common Rule; and **Exhibit 9.0.3:** Sample Broad consent Checklist, 2018 Common Rule.

The FDA informed consent requirements set forth at 21 C.F.R. Part 50 and the pre-2018 Common Rule, as codified at Subpart A of 45 C.F.R. Part 46 for the Department of Health and Human Services (HHS), are largely congruent in the basic requirements, though there are some differences due to different regulatory scope. Where a research study is governed by both the FDA and the Common Rule, the requirements of both sets of regulations must be met. This chapter will discuss both the FDA and Common Rule requirements, with an emphasis on recent legal developments and their impact on the federal informed consent requirements for research.

---

[1] FDA, Informed Consent Information Sheet: Guidance for IRBs, Clinical Investigators, and Sponsors, Draft Guidance (July 2014) (hereafter FDA Draft Guidance July 2014), *available at https://www.hhs.gov/sites/default/files/hipaa-future-research-authorization-guidance-06122018%20v2.pdf.*

[2] *See* Ofc. for Human Research Protections (OHRP), Informed Consent, *available at* https://www.hhs.gov/ohrp/regulations-and-policy/guidance/informed-consent/index.html.

9.1 Recent Legal Developments

Revisions to the Common Rule. A revision to the pre-2018 Common Rule was published on January 19, 2017 (2018 Common Rule). The 2018 Common Rule initially was scheduled to become effective on January 19, 2018; however, on January 22, 2018, the 2018 Common Rule departments and agencies published an interim final rule delaying the effective date and general compliance date of the revised rule for six months, until July 19, 2018. Then, on April 20, 2018, they published a notice of proposed rulemaking seeking comment on a further six month delay of the general compliance date of the revised rule, until January 21, 2019, during which period regulated entities could implement certain burden-reducing provisions of the 2018 Common Rule requirements.[3] In June 2018, a final rule implemented that proposed delay.[4]

The 2018 Common Rule significantly changes the regulatory requirements for informed consent. It is important to note that, for human subjects research initiated prior to January 21, 2019, the 2018 Common Rule contains a transition provision that would allow research institutions to choose either (i) to continue to conduct such ongoing research in compliance with the pre-2018 Common Rule requirements for the lifetime of the study, or (ii) to conduct such research in compliance with the 2018 Common Rule requirements, as of January 21, 2019.[5] Given that some ongoing research may continue to be conducted in compliance with the pre-2018 Common Rule for the lifetime of the study—which, for certain longitudinal studies, could be 80 or more years, or the lifetime of the study subjects—counsel must be knowledgeable about both the informed consent requirements of the pre-2018 Common Rule, as well as the changed regulatory structure of the 2018 Common Rule.

The 2018 Common Rule made substantial changes to the requirements for how informed consent is obtained, including adding: revised or new definitions; additional elements of consent; a new regulatory allowance for subjects to provide "broad consent" to the storage, maintenance, and secondary research use of identifiable biospecimens or identifiable private information; revised criteria for waiver of consent; and a public posting requirement for clinical trial informed consent forms.[6] These new regulatory requirements are addressed in the pertinent sections of this chapter.

---

[3] 83 Fed. Reg. 17595 (Apr. 20, 2018). The compliance date regarding cooperative research and use of a single IRB remains January 20, 2020, 82 Fed. Reg. 7149, 7265 (Jan. 19, 2017) (to be codified at 45 C.F.R. §___.114(b)).

[4] 83 Fed. Reg. 28497 (June 19, 2018).

[5] 82 Fed. Reg. 7149 at 7259 (Jan. 19, 2017) (to be codified at 45 C.F.R. §____.101(l)).

[6] As of the date of this publication, FDA regulations do not incorporate the 2018 Common Rule's changes to the regulatory requirements relevant to informed consent. However, Section 2023 of the 21st Century Cures Act (P.L. No. 114-255 (Dec. 13, 2016)) directs HHS and FDA to harmonize differences between the Common Rule and FDA Human Subjects Regulations. Further, the preamble to the 2018 Common Rule states that "Finally, it is important to note that, to the extent appropriate, the intent is to eventually amend the other subparts of the HHS human subjects protection regulations in 45 C.F.R. Part 46 (Subparts B, C, D, and E), and consider the need for updates to FDA regulations . . . ." 82 Fed. Reg. 7149 at 7151 (Jan. 19, 2017).

According to the interim final rule published January 22, 2018, regulated entities must continue to comply with the requirements of the pre-2018 Common Rule until the general compliance date which has since been delayed to January 21, 2019.[7] Note that the provisions of the 2018 Common Rule that do not conflict with the requirements of the pre-2018 Common Rule may be implemented at any time by institutions. Many of these provisions relate to informed consent; for example, institutions may redraft their informed consent templates according to the new formatting requirements of the 2018 Common Rule, and include the new required elements of consent. However, prior to the general compliance date, regulated entities must still meet the requirements of the pre-2018 Common Rule and, unless following the June 19, 2018 rules for transitioning research discussed in footnote 4 above, cannot implement any provisions of the 2018 Common Rule that conflict with the requirements of the pre-2018 Common Rule—for example, the exception from the informed consent requirements for certain pre-research activities. These referenced provisions are discussed subsequently in this chapter.

Newborn Screening Saves Lives Reauthorization Act of 2014. The Newborn Screening Saves Lives Reauthorization Act of 2014 (Pub. L. 113–240), enacted in December 2014, included certain provisions that serve to apply the existing Common Rule (*i.e.*, the pre-2018 Rule) informed consent requirements to research using newborn dried blood spots that is funded by HHS pursuant to the federal Public Health Service Act (PHS Act). The Newborn Screening Saves Lives Reauthorization Act deems such research to be considered research with human subjects, even if the newborn dried blood spots are nonidentified, and provides that the provisions allowing an IRB to waive informed consent for certain research studies cannot be applied to such research. The overall effect is to require that the pre-2018 Rule's informed consent requirements be met for all PHS Act-funded research that uses newborn dried blood spots.

The Newborn Screening Saves Lives Reauthorization Act provides that the requirements of the statute with respect to the pre-2018 Rule's regulation of research using nonidentified blood spots will no longer be applicable as of the date the updates to the pre-2018 Common Rule (the 2018 Common Rule) are "promulgated." The specific language of the statute appears to indicate that, for ongoing research using nonidentified newborn dried blood spots to which the pre-2018 Common Rule applies by virtue of the statute, the research will no longer will be regulated as human subjects research as of the date of promulgation of the 2018 Common Rule. The statute's language also appears to indicate that research using nonidentified newborn dried blood spots that is initiated after the date of promulgation of the 2018 Common Rule, no matter when the blood spots were collected, will not be regulated as human subjects research. The preamble to the 2018 Common Rule states that the changes made by the Newborn Screening Saves Lives Reauthorization Act will no longer apply after the effective date of the 2018 Common Rule, July 19, 2018.

---

[7] 83 Fed. Reg. 2885 at 2886 (Jan. 22, 2018). *See also* 82 Fed. Reg. 7149 at 7259 (Jan. 19, 2017) (to be codified at 45 C.F.R. §____.101(l)); 83 Fed. Reg. 28497 (June 19, 2018).

Certificates of Confidentiality. The 21st Century Cures Act (Pub. L. 114-255) (Cures Act), enacted in December 2016, meaningfully altered the way a Certificate of Confidentiality (CoC) is conceptualized and applied. The National Institutes of Health (NIH) incorporated the changes made by the Cures Act in a revised CoC policy, effective October 1, 2017.[8] Pursuant to the Cures Act and NIH policy, the CoC disclosure requirements prohibit disclosure of the name of research subjects or any identifiable research information, document, or biospecimen to anyone not connected with the research except under very specific circumstances as detailed in NIH's CoC policy. CoCs are issued automatically for any NIH-funded project using identifiable, sensitive information that is ongoing on or after December 13, 2016. In addition, previously-issued CoCs have been converted to CoCs that apply according to the Cures Act requirements for CoCs and the revised NIH policy.

If an investigator obtains informed consent for research covered by a CoC, NIH expects that the investigator will inform subjects about the CoC protections and any exceptions to those protections. NIH provides suggested informed consent language on its website,[9] which should be edited as necessary for the study population:

> This research is covered by a Certificate of Confidentiality from the National Institutes of Health. The researchers with this Certificate may not disclose or use information, documents, or biospecimens that may identify you in any federal, state, or local civil, criminal, administrative, legislative, or other action, suit, or proceeding, or be used as evidence, for example, if there is a court subpoena, unless you have consented for this use. Information, documents, or biospecimens protected by this Certificate cannot be disclosed to anyone else who is not connected with the research except, if there is a federal, state, or local law that requires disclosure (such as to report child abuse or communicable diseases but not for federal, state, or local civil, criminal, administrative, legislative, or other proceedings, see below); if you have consented to the disclosure, including for your medical treatment; or if it is used for other scientific research, as allowed by federal regulations protecting research subjects.
>
> **[INCLUDE IF APPLICABLE:]** The Certificate cannot be used to refuse a request for information from personnel of the United States federal or state government agency sponsoring the project that is needed for auditing or program evaluation by [*THE AGENCY*] which is funding this project or for information that must be disclosed in order to meet the requirements of the federal Food and Drug Administration (FDA). You should understand that a Certificate of Confidentiality does not prevent you from voluntarily releasing information about yourself or your involvement in this research. If you want your research information released to an insurer, medical care provider, or

---

[8] *See* Nat'l Inst. of Health, NOT-OD-17-109, Notice of Changes to NIH Policy for Issuing Certificates of Confidentiality (Sept. 7, 2017), *available at* https://grants.nih.gov/grants/guide/notice-files/NOT-OD-17-109.html.

[9] *See* Nat'l Inst. of Health, Suggested Consent Language Describing CoC Protections, *available at* https://humansubjects.nih.gov/coc/suggested-consent-language.

any other person not connected with the research, you must provide consent to allow the researchers to release it.

[INCLUDE IF APPLICABLE (if researcher intends to disclose information covered by a Certificate, such as potential child abuse, or intent to hurt self or others in response to specific federal, state, or local laws).] The Certificate of Confidentiality will not be used to prevent disclosure as required by federal, state, or local law of *[list what will be reported, such as child abuse and neglect, or harm to self or others]*.

[INCLUDE IF APPLICABLE (if researcher intends to disclose information covered by a Certificate, with the consent of research participants).] The Certificate of Confidentiality will not be used to prevent disclosure for any purpose you have consented to in this informed consent document *[restate what will be disclosed, such as including research data in the medical record]*.

9.2 Overarching Requirements for Obtaining Informed Consent

The introductory language in the FDA and the Common Rule informed consent provisions (both pre-2018 and 2018 versions) contain several general requirements for how informed consent must be obtained. Both FDA regulations and the Common Rule require legally effective informed consent to (i) be obtained from the subject or the subject's legally authorized representative; (ii) be in language understandable to the subject or representative; and (iii) be obtained under circumstances that provide the subject with the opportunity to consider whether or not to participate.[10] The regulations or accompanying guidance impose three particular requirements that merit additional discussion:

Coercion or Undue Influence. Both FDA regulations and the Common Rule require that informed consent be obtained in circumstances that minimize the possibility of coercion or undue influence.[11] Coercion occurs when an overt or implicit threat of harm is intentionally presented by one person to another in order to obtain compliance, *e.g.*, an investigator might tell prospective subjects that they will lose access to health services if they do not agree to participate in the study. In contrast, undue influence can occur through an offer of excessive or inappropriate reward in order to obtain agreement; or can be presented by a situation in which prospective subjects are encouraged to act against their interests (which otherwise they would not choose to do). Undue influence need not be an excessive monetary reward, but may be more subtle. For example, patients might feel pressure to participate in research at the request of their personal physician, or, in the case of students, if their professor is the investigator. Context is therefore highly relevant, and it is difficult for an IRB to draw bright lines as to what is undue influence.

---

[10] 45 C.F.R. § 46.116; 82 Fed. Reg. 7149 at 7265 (Jan. 19, 2017) (to be codified at 45 C.F.R §___,116(a)); 21 C.F.R. § 50.20.

[11] *Id. See also* OHRP, Informed Consent FAQs, What does it mean to minimize the possibility of coercion or undue influence?, *available at* https://www.hhs.gov/ohrp/regulations-and-policy/guidance/faq/informed-consent/index.html; FDA Draft Guidance July 2014, at Section III.A.2.

In addition, IRBs also must give special consideration to additional safeguards for subjects who may be more vulnerable to coercion or undue influence. The pre-2018 Common Rule provides the following categories of subjects as examples of populations who may be more vulnerable to coercion or undue influence: children, prisoners, pregnant women, mentally disabled persons, or economically disadvantaged persons.[12] The 2018 Common Rule has modified this list, eliminating the reference to pregnant women as a vulnerable population, and referring to individuals with impaired decision-making capacity rather than "mentally disabled persons."[13]

While IRBs may find it difficult to determine whether the level of monetary or non-monetary compensation provided to research subjects is ethically or regulatorily appropriate, compensation for research participation is not *per se* coercive or a form of undue influence, and providing reasonable compensation to research subjects is not uncommon. Participating in a clinical research trial can be time consuming and otherwise burdensome for subjects, and compensating them for that time and inconvenience is acceptable. This is distinguishable from compensation that would be so significant to the participants as to influence their determination to voluntarily consent to participate. Similarly, it is important that a non-monetary incentive is not of such significant value that it interferes with the participant's ability to make a reasoned and informed determination as to whether to participate in the research. This topic is further discussed in **Chapter 11**, *Payment to Research Subjects*.[14]

Exculpatory Language. Both FDA regulations and the Common Rule require that informed consent not include exculpatory language through which the subject is made to waive or appear to waive any legal rights, or which releases, or appears to release, the investigator, sponsor or institution from responsibility for malpractice, negligence, blame, fault, or guilt.[15] For example, if an informed consent document contains language through which a subject waives the right to be compensated for injuries caused by research participation, this statement is exculpatory language and the IRB should not approve the informed consent document as drafted. FDA and OHRP draft guidance also clarifies that waiver by an individual to compensation for use of the subject's biospecimens is not "exculpatory" as long as the waiver does not have the general effect of freeing or appearing to free an individual or an entity from responsibility for

[12] 45 C.F.R. § 46.111(a)(3).

[13] 82 Fed. Reg. 7149 at 7264 (Jan. 19, 2017) (to be codified at 45 C.F.R. §__.111(a)(3)).

[14] *See* OHRP, Informed Consent FAQs, When does compensating subjects undermine informed consent or parental permission?, *available at* https://www.hhs.gov/ohrp/regulations-and-policy/guidance/faq/informed-consent/index.html; *see also* FDA, Payment and Reimbursement to Research Subjects–Information Sheet (Jan. 25, 2018), *available at* https://www.fda.gov/RegulatoryInformation/Guidances/ucm126429.htm.

[15] 45 C.F.R. § 46.116; 82 Fed. Reg. 7149 at 7265 (Jan. 19, 2017) (to be codified at 45 C.F.R. §___.116(a)); 21 C.F.R. § 50.20. *See also* FDA and OHRP, Guidance on Exculpatory Language in Informed Consent, Draft Guidance (Aug. 19, 2011), *available at* https://www.fda.gov/downloads/RegulatoryInformation/Guidances/UCM271036.pdf; 76 Fed. Reg. 55390 (Sept. 7, 2011). A prior final guidance is found at OHRP, Exculpatory Language in Informed Consent (1996), *available at* https://www.hhs.gov/ohrp/regulations-and-policy/guidance/exculpatory-language-in-informed-consent-documents/index.html. There is some reference to exculpatory language in FDA, A Guide to Informed Consent—Information Sheet, *available at* https://www.fda.gov/RegulatoryInformation/Guidances/ucm126431.htm.

malpractice or negligence, or from blame, fault, or guilt. This joint FDA and OHRP guidance is not yet final

Financial Relationships and Interests. Both FDA and HHS guidance state that investigators and IRBs should consider whether certain financial relationships or interests could have a potential effect on the rights and welfare of human subjects, and if so, what actions could be undertaken to protect those subjects.[16] For example, a question to consider is whether individuals involved in the study (*e.g.*, principal investigators) or institutions (such as those where the study site is located) receive compensation that may be affected by or tied to the study outcome. Depending on the potential financial interest or relationship, an IRB may decide that an appropriate safeguard is to provide information disclosing such financial relationships or interests directly to subjects.

Added by the 2018 Common Rule:

The 2018 Common Rule includes two changes designed to enhance the presentation of information to subjects and facilitate more understandable consent forms. First, the 2018 Common Rule requires that a prospective subject or the legally authorized representative be provided with the information that a reasonable person would consider important in order to make an informed decision about whether to participate in the research study, as well as an opportunity to discuss that information.[17] Second, except in the case of broad consent, informed consent must begin with a concise and focused presentation of the key information in a way that facilitates comprehension, and must as a whole provide information in sufficient detail relating to the research and be organized and presented in a way that does not merely provide lists of isolated facts, all in a manner that is most likely to assist a prospective subject or a legally authorized representative in understanding the reasons why one may or may not want to participate in the research.[18]

9.3 Elements of Informed Consent

9.3.1 Basic Elements of Informed Consent–HHS and FDA

The following information must be provided to each subject:

- A statement that the clinical study involves research, an explanation of the purposes of the research and the expected duration of the subject's participation, a

[16] *See* OHRP, Financial Conflict of Interest: HHS Guidance (2004), *available at* https://www.hhs.gov/ohrp/regulations-and-policy/guidance/financial-conflict-of-interest/index.html; FDA, Informed Consent Information Sheet, Guidance for IRBs, Clinical Investigators, and Sponsors, Draft Guidance, Section IV.B.2., Financial Relationships and Interests (July 2014), *available at* https://www.fda.gov/RegulatoryInformation/Guidances/ucm404975.htm#financialrelationships.

[17] 82 Fed. Reg. 7149 at 7265 (Jan. 19, 2017) (to be codified at 45 C.F.R. §__.116(a)(4)).

[18] 82 Fed. Reg. 7149 at 7265, 7266 (Jan. 19, 2017) (to be codified at 45 C.F.R. §__.116(a)(5)(i)-(ii). Note that FDA regulations do not presently contain these additional requirements to obtain informed consent as of the date of this publication.

description of the procedures to be followed, and identification of any procedures that are experimental;

- A description of any reasonably foreseeable risks and discomforts to the subject;
- A description of any benefits to the subject or others that may reasonably be expected from the research;
- A disclosure of appropriate alternative procedures or courses of treatment, if any, that might be advantageous for the subject;
- A statement describing the extent, if any, to which confidentiality of records identifying the subject will be maintained, and noting the possibility that the FDA may inspect the records, if applicable;[19]
- For research involving more than minimal risk, an explanation as to whether any compensation and an explanation as to whether any medical treatments are available if injury occurs and, if so, what they consist of, or where further information may be obtained;
- An explanation as to whom to contact for answers to pertinent questions about the research and the research subject's rights, and whom to contact in the event of a research-related injury to the subject; ***and***
- A statement that participation is voluntary, refusal to participate will involve no penalty or loss of benefits to which the subject is otherwise entitled, and the subject may discontinue participation at any time without penalty or loss of benefits to which the subject is otherwise entitled.[20]

Added by the 2018 Common Rule:

- One of the following statements about any research that involves the collection of identifiable private information or identifiable biospecimens:
  - A statement that identifiers might be removed from the identifiable private information or identifiable biospecimens and that, after such removal, the information or biospecimens could be used for future research studies or distributed to another investigator for future research studies without obtaining additional informed consent from the subject or the legally authorized representative (if such a transfer is a possibility); ***or***
  - A statement that the subject's information or biospecimens collected as part of the research, even if identifiers are removed, will not be used or distributed for future research studies.[21]

[19] Note the specific requirement of possible disclosure to FDA is not required under 45 C.F.R. § 46.116(b).

[20] 45 C.F.R. § 46.116 (a); 82 Fed. Reg. 7149 at 7266 (Jan. 19, 2017) (to be codified at 45 C.F.R. § __.116(b)(1)–(8)); 21 C.F.R. § 50.25(a).

[21] 82 Fed. Reg. 7149 at 7266 (Jan. 19, 2017) (to be codified at 45 C.F.R. § __.116(b)(9)).

9.3.2 Additional Elements of Informed Consent–HHS and FDA

When appropriate, one or more of the following elements of information must be provided to each subject:

- A statement that the particular treatment or procedure may involve risks to the subject (or to the embryo or fetus, if the subject is or may become pregnant) that are currently unforeseeable;
- Anticipated circumstances under which the subject's participation may be terminated by the investigator without regard to the subject's or the legally authorized representative's consent;
- Any additional costs to the subject that may result from participation in the research;
- The consequences of a subject's decision to withdraw from the research and procedures for orderly termination of participation by the subject;
- A statement that significant new findings developed during the course of the research that may relate to the subject's willingness to continue participation will be provided to the subject; ***and***
- The approximate number of subjects involved in the study.[22]

Added by the 2018 Common Rule:

- A statement that the subject's biospecimens (even if identifiers are removed) may be used for commercial profit, and whether the subject will or will not share in this commercial profit;
- A statement regarding whether clinically relevant research results, including individual research results, will be disclosed to subjects, and if so, under what conditions; ***and***
- For research involving biospecimens, whether the research will (if known) or might include whole genome sequencing (*i.e.*, sequencing of a human germline or somatic specimen with the intent to generate the genome or exome sequence of that specimen).[23]

9.3.3 An Additional Element of Informed Consent for Certain FDA-Regulated Studies

- For clinical trials that will be posted on the website www.ClinicalTrials.gov,[24] the following statement must be provided to each subject of such trial in the informed consent document:

---

22 45 C.F.R. § 46.116(b); 82 Fed. Reg. 7149 at 7266 (Jan. 19, 2017) (to be codified at 45 C.F.R. §__.116(c)(1)–(6)); 21 C.F.R. § 50.25(b).

23 82 Fed. Reg. 7149 at 7266 (Jan. 19, 2017) (to be codified at 45 C.F.R. §__.116(c)(7)–(9)).

24 Clinical trials subject to this requirement are defined in 42 U.S.C. § 282(j)(1)(A).

"A description of this clinical trial will be available on http://www.ClinicalTrials.gov, as required by U.S. law. This Web site will not include information that can identify you. At most, the Web site will include a summary of the results. You can search this Web site at any time."[25]

Added by the 2018 Common Rule:

9.3.4 Broad Consent

The 2018 Common Rule includes an option to obtain a subject's broad consent for the storage, maintenance, and secondary research use of identifiable private information or identifiable biospecimens. Broad consent is available only for *secondary research use*, meaning that the identifiable private information or identifiable biospecimens were collected for a study other than the proposed research or for a non-research purpose.[26]

Required elements of broad consent are:

- A description of any reasonably foreseeable risks or discomforts to the subject;
- A description of any benefits to the subject or to others that may reasonably be expected from the research;
- A statement describing the extent, if any, to which confidentiality of records identifying the subject will be maintained;
- A statement that participation is voluntary, refusal to participate will involve no penalty or loss of benefits to which the subject is otherwise entitled, and the subject may discontinue participation at any time without penalty or loss of benefits to which the subject is otherwise entitled;
- For research involving biospecimens, a statement that the subject's biospecimens (even if identifiers are removed) may be used for commercial profit and whether the subject will or will not share in this commercial profit;
- For research involving biospecimens, whether the research will (if known) or might include whole genome sequencing (*i.e.*, sequencing of a human germline or somatic specimen with the intent to generate the genome or exome sequence of that specimen);
- A general description of the types of research that may be conducted with the identifiable private information or identifiable biospecimens, which description must include sufficient information such that a reasonable person would expect that the broad consent would permit the types of research conducted;
- A description of the identifiable private information or identifiable biospecimens that might be used in research, whether sharing of identifiable private informa-

[25] 21 C.F.R. § 50.25(c).

[26] 82 Fed. Reg. 7149 at 7266 (Jan. 19, 2017) (to be codified at 45 C.F.R. §__.116(d)).

tion or identifiable biospecimens might occur, and the types of institutions or researchers that might conduct research with the identifiable private information or identifiable biospecimens;

- A description of the period of time that the identifiable private information or identifiable biospecimens may be stored and maintained (which period of time could be indefinite), and a description of the period of time that the identifiable private information or identifiable biospecimens may be used for research purposes (which period of time could be indefinite);
- Unless the subject or legally authorized representative will be provided details about specific research studies, a statement that they will not be informed of the details of any specific research studies that might be conducted using the subject's identifiable private information or identifiable biospecimens, including the purposes of the research, and that they might have chosen not to consent to some of those specific research studies;
- Unless it is known that clinically relevant research results, including individual research results, will be disclosed to the subject in all circumstances, a statement that such results may not be disclosed to the subject; ***and***
- An explanation of whom to contact for answers to questions about the subject's rights and about storage and use of the subject's identifiable private information or identifiable biospecimens, and whom to contact in the event of a research-related harm.[27]

Sample Informed Consent Forms are attached as **Exhibit 9.3.1:** Sample Informed Consent, Pre-2018 Common Rule and FDA; **Exhibit 9.3.2:** Sample Study-Specific Informed Consent, 2018 Common Rule; and **Exhibit 9.3.3:** Sample Broad Consent, 2018 Common Rule.

9.4 Who Can Consent

Ensuring that subjects have the capacity to consent is an area where legal counsel can play a critical role. In addition to federal regulations, state laws vary and can be important in determining whether a subject has properly consented to the research, including whether an appropriate legally authorized representative or guardian has provided effective consent on behalf of certain subjects where they cannot provide their own.

9.4.1 Subjects with Diminished Decision-making Capacity

FDA and OHRP guidance advise that when a subject's consent capacity is sufficiently impaired such that the subject is unable to provide legally effective informed consent, the sub-

[27] 82 Fed. Reg. 7149 at 7266–7267 (Jan. 19, 2017) (to be codified at 45 C.F.R. §__.116(d)(1)–(7)). The HHS Office for Civil Rights (OCR), in its June 2018 guidance on HIPAA and individual authorizations (published in response to a 21st Century Cures Act mandate) provides additional information on OCR's views regarding the circumstances in which an authorization for uses and disclosures of PHI for future research contains a sufficient description of the purpose of the use or disclosure being authorized, *available at* https://www.hhs.gov/sites/default/files/hipaa-future-research-authorization-guidance-06122018%20v2.pdf. *See* **Chapter 10**, *HIPAA Compliance in Clinical Trials,* for further discussion of the HIPAA requirements.

ject may not be enrolled unless the subject's legally authorized representative consents on the subject's behalf. Some subjects may have a partial impairment that requires modification to the consent form and/or process but still enables them to consent on their own behalf. Diminished decision-making capacity may arise as a result of trauma, intellectual disability, age, and some forms of mental illness or dementia, whether temporary, progressive, or permanent. While the regulations are silent on specific consent procedures for individuals with impaired decision-making capacity, they expressly state that additional safeguards must be included to protect the rights and welfare of subjects that are likely to be vulnerable to coercion or undue influence, which includes "mentally disabled persons" or, under the 2018 Common Rule, "individuals with impaired decision-making capacity."[28]

IRBs and investigators should consider carefully whether the inclusion of subjects who lack decision-making capacity is ethical and scientifically necessary.[29]

9.4.2 Additional HHS and FDA Protections for Children and Other Persons in Protected Classes Involved as Subjects in Research[30]

Some of the Common Rule departments and agencies have published agency-specific regulations that provide additional protections to certain populations involved as subjects in research conducted or supported by the federal department or agency. When pertinent, these protections apply in addition to the requirements of the Common Rule. HHS has published additional protections for research conducted or supported by HHS that involves children, 45 C.F.R. §§ 46.401 to 46.409 (Subpart D); pregnant women, fetuses, or neonates, 45 C.F.R. §§ 46.201 to 46.207 (Subpart B); and prisoners, 45 C.F.R. §§ 46.301 to 46.306 (Subpart C). FDA has published regulations providing additional protections to children who are subjects of FDA-regulated clinical investigations subject to 21 C.F.R. Part 50, 21 C.F.R. §§ 50.50-50.56 (Subpart D).

Children. Under FDA and HHS regulations, "children" are individuals who have not attained the legal age for consent to treatments or procedures involved in the research under the applicable law of the jurisdiction in which the research will be conducted.[31] The legal age is often 18 years, but may vary by state, and state law also may address certain circumstances in which a person younger than the legal age of adulthood is legally authorized to consent to medical procedures or treatments. If the proposed research activity consists of such medical procedures or treatments, the IRB should generally treat the subjects as adults for purposes of

---

[28] 45 C.F.R. § 46.111(b); 82 Fed. Reg. 7149 at 7264 (Jan. 19, 2017) (to be codified at 45 C.F.R. §____.111(a) (changing the language to "individuals with impaired decision-making capacity)); 21 C.F.R. §§ 56.111(b). *See also* OHRP, Informed Consent FAQs, What should be considered in seeking informed consent from individuals with diminished decision-making capacity?, *available at* https://www.hhs.gov/ohrp/regulations-and-policy/guidance/faq/informed-consent/index.html; FDA Draft Guidance July 2014, at 35.

[29] FDA Draft Guidance July 2014, at 35.

[30] The HHS regulations at 45 C.F.R. Part 46, Subparts B, C and D were not revised with the overall revisions to the Common Rule.

[31] 45 C.F.R. § 46.402(a); 21 C.F.R. § 50.3(o).

research, unless other research-specific state laws would restrict this interpretation. In addition, emancipated minors may be legally able to consent to research.[32] See **Chapter 7**, *Children in Research* for further discussion.

When consent on behalf of a child is required, the permission of the parent, either biological or adoptive, must be sought. The IRB may find that the permission of only **one** parent is sufficient for research that does not involve more than minimal risk,[33] or for research involving more than minimal risk, but presenting the prospect of direct benefit to the child.[34] However, unless one parent is deceased, unknown, incompetent, not reasonably available, or when only one parent has legal responsibility for the care and custody of the child, **both parents must give their permission** when (i) the research involves greater than minimal risk and no prospect of direct benefit to individual subjects,[35] or (ii) the research is not otherwise approvable but presents an opportunity to understand, prevent, or alleviate a serious problem affecting the health or welfare of children.[36]

Note that in addition to biological and adoptive parents, a child's legal guardian may also provide permission for the child to participate in research. HHS and FDA regulations define a "guardian" as an individual who is authorized under applicable state or local law to consent on behalf of a child to general medical care, as discussed further below in **Section 9.4.3**.[37] In addition, even in the absence of a legal guardian, HHS regulations permit an IRB to waive parental permission and find an appropriate substitute mechanism after making certain documented findings; for example, such a procedure may be used in the case of neglected or abused children, and may include additional protections, such as appointing a child advocate.[38]

Even where children are not able to provide legally effective informed consent, they may be able to give their "assent." Assent means a child's affirmative agreement to participate in research. Mere failure to object does not, absent affirmative agreement, constitute assent.[39] The IRB must determine whether adequate measures have been taken to obtain assent from those child-subjects who could provide it; or, determine that the intervention or procedure involved in the research holds out a prospect of direct benefit that is important to the health or well-being of the child, and is available only in the context of the research, in which case the assent of the

[32] *Id. See also* OHRP, Vulnerable Populations, Special Protections for Children as Research Subjects, *available at* https://www.hhs.gov/ohrp/regulations-and-policy/guidance/special-protections-for-children/index.html.

[33] 45 C.F.R. § 46.404; 21 C.F.R. § 50.51.

[34] 45 C.F.R. § 46.405; 21 C.F.R. § 50.52.

[35] 45 C.F.R. § 46.406; 21 C.F.R. § 50.53.

[36] 45 C.F.R. §§ 46.407, 46.408(b); 21 C.F.R. §§ 50.54, 50.55(e). *See also* 45 C.F.R. § 46.408(c) regarding waiver of parental consent under HHS regulations.

[37] 45 C.F.R. § 46.402(e); 21 C.F.R § 50.3 (s).

[38] 45 C.F.R. § 46.116; 45 C.F.R. § 46.408(c).

[39] 45 C.F.R. §§ 46.402(b) and 46.408(a); 21 C.F.R. §§ 50.3(n) and 50.55.

child is not a necessary condition for proceeding with the research.[40] The IRB may still waive the requirement to obtain assent from those children who could provide it if certain requirements are met.[41]

IRBs should consider whether to require the assent of children before they are enrolled in a research study.[42] For research involving children, IRBs may require that two consent documents be developed, one for obtaining parental permission and another which outlines the study in simplified language for obtaining the assent of children who are capable of understanding the relevant concepts.

Pregnant Women, Fetuses, and Neonates. Subpart B of 45 C.F.R. Part 46 provides additional requirements for informed consent for research in which pregnant women, fetuses, or and/or neonates are subjects.

Where required by the Common Rule informed consent provisions, the consent of only the pregnant woman is required if the research holds out (i) the prospect of direct benefit to the pregnant woman, (ii) the prospect of a direct benefit both to the pregnant woman and the fetus, or (iii) no prospect of benefit for the woman nor the fetus, but where the risk to the fetus is not greater than minimal and the purpose of the research is the development of important biomedical knowledge that cannot be obtained by any other means.[43]

By contrast, the consent of both the pregnant woman and the father is required if the research holds out the prospect of direct benefit solely to the fetus. However, the father's consent is not required if he is unable to consent because of unavailability, incompetence, or temporary incapacity, or if the pregnancy resulted from rape or incest.[44]

The pregnant woman and, if applicable, the father, must be fully informed regarding the reasonably foreseeable impact of the research on the fetus or neonate.[45]

Subpart B contains separate requirements for informed consent regarding neonates of uncertain viability and nonviable neonates involved in research. In each case, the individual(s)

[40] 45 C.F.R. § 46.408(a); 21 C.F.R. § 50.55(d); OHRP, Research with Children FAQs, When does child assent have to be obtained for research and can it be waived?, *available at* https://www.hhs.gov/ohrp/regulations-and-policy/guidance/faq/children-research/index.html; *see also* FDA, Additional Protections for Children (last updated March 29, 2018), *available at* https://www.fda.gov/ScienceResearch/SpecialTopics/RunningClinicalTrials/ucm119111.htm.

[41] 45 C.F.R. § 46.116; 45 C.F.R. § 46.408(a); 21 C.F.R. § 50.55(d). *See* OHRP, Vulnerable Populations, Special Protections for Children as Research Subjects, *available at* https://www.hhs.gov/ohrp/regulations-and-policy/guidance/special-protections-for-children/index.html.

[42] ICH, Integrated Addendum to ICH E6(R1): Guideline to Good Clinical Practice E6(R2), Section 4.8.12 (Nov. 9, 2016), "...the [child] should be informed about the trial to the extent compatible with the [child]'s understanding and, if capable, the [child] should assent, sign and personally date the written informed consent," *available at* http://www.ich.org/fileadmin/Public_Web_Site/ICH_Products/Guidelines/Efficacy/E6/E6_R2__Step_4_2016_1109.pdf; *see also* 78 Fed. Reg. 12937 at 12944.

[43] 45 C.F.R. § 46.204(d).

[44] 45 C.F.R. § 46.204(e).

[45] 45 C.F..R § 46.204(f).

providing consent must be fully informed regarding the reasonably foreseeable impact of the research on a neonate that is nonviable or of uncertain viability.

For neonates of uncertain viability, the legally effective informed consent of either parent of the neonate is required to be obtained. If, however, neither parent is able to consent because of unavailability, incompetence, or temporary incapacity, the legally effective informed consent of either parent's legally authorized representative may be obtained in place of the parents. The consent of the father or his legally authorized representative need not be obtained if the pregnancy resulted from rape or incest.[46]

For nonviable neonates, the legally effective informed consent of both parents of the neonate is required to be obtained, and the waiver and alteration provisions set forth in 45 C.F.R. § 46.116(c) and (d) do not apply. If, however, either parent is unable to consent because of unavailability, incompetence, or temporary incapacity, the informed consent of one parent of a nonviable neonate will be sufficient, except that the consent of the father need not be obtained if the pregnancy resulted from rape or incest. Note that the consent of a legally authorized representative of either or both of the parents of a nonviable neonate does not meet the regulatory requirements under Subpart B.[47]

FDA informed consent regulations do not contain specific requirements for research involving pregnant women and fetuses that are comparable to Subpart B of the HHS human subjects regulations, although FDA recommends that the Subpart B requirements be met for FDA-regulated clinical research. FDA recently has taken steps to aid the FDA-regulated community in assessing the appropriate inclusion of pregnant women as research subjects. In April 2018, FDA published draft guidance for industry entitled *Pregnant Women: Scientific and Ethical Considerations for Inclusion in Clinical Trials*."[48] While the draft guidance primarily addresses general scientific and ethical considerations involved with the inclusion of pregnant women in clinical trials, the draft guidance also provides FDA's views on two specific informed consent considerations. First, FDA recommends that if pregnant women are being enrolled in clinical trials, the informed consent should disclose whether trial data will be assessed in a way (*e.g.*, real-time data analysis and feedback) that can potentially benefit the subject during the course of the trial. Second, regarding women who are not pregnant upon enrollment, but who become pregnant during clinical trial participation, FDA recommends that the trial should be unblinded; the risks and benefits of continuing trial participation versus withdrawal should be reviewed with the pregnant woman; and the pregnant woman should undergo a second informed consent process that reflects these additional risk-benefit considerations. (As of the date of this publication, the FDA guidance is still in draft form.)

---

[46] 45 C.F.R. § 46.205(b).

[47] 45 C.F.R. § 46.205(c); 45 C.F.R. § 46.116(c) and (d) were moved in the 2018 Common Rule (to be codified at 45 C.F.R. § ___.116(e) and (f).

[48] FDA, Pregnant Women: Scientific and Ethical Considerations for Inclusion in Clinical Trials, Draft Guidance (Apr. 2018), *available at* https://www.fda.gov/downloads/Drugs/GuidanceComplianceRegulatoryInformation/Guidances/ucm603873.pdf.

Prisoners. Subpart C of 45 C.F.R. Part 46 provides additional considerations IRBs must address when research involves prisoners, including providing the information in language understandable by the population; minimizing the potential for undue influence, (*e.g.*, advantages offered that may influence the decision to enroll); ensuring procedures for subject selection is fair to all and without intervention by prison authorities or prisoners, so that it is immune from arbitrary selection of study subjects from the general prison population; and providing effective communication to prisoners of the fact that that their participation will have no effect on their likelihood of parole.[49]

9.4.3 Legally Authorized Representatives

HHS and FDA regulations allow for informed consent to be obtained from a "legally authorized representative" of a subject. A legally authorized representative is defined in FDA regulations and the pre-2018 Common Rule as an individual, or judicial or other body, authorized under applicable law to consent on behalf of a prospective subject to the subject's participation in the procedure(s) involved in the research.[50] In the U.S., applicable state law generally defines who would be considered to be a legally authorized representative. Sources of state law include statutes, regulations, and common law that specifically address consent by someone other than the subject. This could include agents under a power of attorney or legal guardian, although there may be limitations on such persons' powers in the research context. Most states, however, do not specifically address the issue of who may provide consent on behalf of another person in the research context. In these states, OHRP has specified that a law addressing who is authorized to give consent on behalf of another to specific medical procedures, or to general medical treatment, may also serve to authorize an individual to provide surrogate consent to the research participation of another person if there is a reasonable basis for this authority under the state law and the research involves such procedures or treatment.[51] In other states, however, there are no laws permitting a proxy to provide consent for another person in *either* the research or medical treatment context absent a power of attorney, guardianship, or some other specific legal authority. In these states, the lack of legal authority has proven to be a barrier to conducting research involving subjects who cannot consent on their own behalf (*e.g.*, subjects with decisional impairment).

It is recommended that counsel advise investigators, IRB staff, and IRB members as to whether state law authorizes an individual in a particular capacity to serve as a legally authorized representative to consent to a prospective subject's participation in a particular research study.

---

[49] 45 C.F.R. § 46.305(a).

[50] 45 C.F.R. § 46.102(c); 21 C.F.R. § 50.3(l).

[51] OHRP, Informed Consent FAQs, Who can be a legally authorized representative (LAR) for the purpose of providing consent on behalf of a prospective subject?, *available at* https://www.hhs.gov/ohrp/regulations-and-policy/guidance/faq/informed-consent/index.html.

Added by the 2018 Common Rule:

The 2018 Common Rule adds a new sentence to the definition of "legally authorized representative," providing additional flexibility to the term:

> "If there is no applicable law addressing this issue, *legally authorized representative* means an individual recognized by institutional policy as acceptable for providing consent in the non-research context on behalf of the prospective subject to the subject's participation in the procedure(s) involved in the research."[52]

The new definition allows a person to act as a legally authorized representative for purposes of consenting to research where no state law exists to address surrogate consent for research participation, or where no state law allows for surrogate consent without authority under power of attorney, guardianship, or other legal authority. For clarity, the 2018 Common Rule language would not preempt state law on point that would expressly restrict such surrogate consent. The revised definition allows the researchers and IRB to rely on institutional policies for allowing surrogate consent in a non-research context to serve as sufficient authorization for a legally authorized representative in the research context. It is still recommended that counsel be consulted in implementing this basis for consent.

9.5 The Consent Process

Informed consent is more than just a signature on a form; it is a process of information exchange that may include—in addition to the subject reading and signing the informed consent document—subject recruitment materials, verbal instructions, question and answer sessions, and measures of subject understanding. In general, the IRB must review and approve the information provided to subjects, either orally or in writing, during the informed consent process.[53]

The principal investigator is ultimately responsible for ensuring informed consent is obtained from each subject prior to the subject enrolling in the study.[54] While FDA does not require the investigator to personally conduct the consent interview, the investigator remains responsible for the process, even when delegating the task of obtaining informed consent to another individual knowledgeable about the research.[55] The individuals involved in obtaining

[52] 82 Fed. Reg. 7149 at 7260 (Jan. 19, 2017) (to be codified at 45 C.F.R. §__.102(i)).

[53] *See* 45 C.F.R. § 46.109; 82 Fed. Reg. 7149 at 7263 (Jan. 19, 2017) (to be codified at 45 C.F.R. §__.109); 21 C.F.R. § 56.109. Note that OHRP has stated information regarding significant new findings that might affect a subject's willingness to participate may be disclosed to enrolled subjects without undergoing prior review and approval by the IRB (but subsequently providing such information to the IRB) (*see* 45 C.F.R. § 46.116(b)(5); 82 Fed. Reg. 7149 at 7266 (Jan. 19, 2017) (to be codified at 45 C.F.R. § __.116(c)(5), and OHRP, IRB Review of Protocol and Informed Consent Changes in Cooperative Group Protocols (OHRP Memo to the National Cancer Institute, 2008) (Sep. 29, 2008), *available at* https://www.hhs.gov/ohrp/regulations-and-policy/guidance/september-29-2008-letter-to-jeffrey-abrams/index.html.

[54] 45 C.F.R. § 46.116; 82 Fed. Reg. 7149 at 7265 (Jan. 19, 2017) (to be codified at 45 C.F.R. §__.116); 21 C.F.R. § 50.20.

[55] 21 C.F.R. § 312.60; 21 C.F.R. § 812.100; FDA Draft Guidance July 2014, at 25.

consent should be appropriately trained in the ethical principles and regulatory requirements related to conducting human subjects research.[56]

In addition to signing the consent form, the subject or legally authorized representative should enter the date of signature on the consent document, which permits verification that consent was actually obtained before the subject began participation in the study.[57] If consent is obtained the same day that the subject's involvement in the study begins, the subject's medical records/case report form should document that consent was obtained prior to participation in the research.[58] A copy of the consent document must be provided to the subject and the original signed consent document should be retained in the study records.[59] The Common Rule and FDA regulations do not require the subject's copy to be a signed copy, although FDA guidance recommends that a photocopy with signature(s) is preferred.[60]

When written informed consent is required, the use of electronic, including digital, signatures is permitted under FDA regulations, provided execution of the consent form is in compliance with the requirements for Electronic Records and Electronic Signatures.[61] Current combined FDA and OHRP guidance also addresses electronic signatures, permitting them as long as all of the regulatory criteria are met and subjects are provided with an electronic copy of the consent, unless documentation of the consent is waived.[62] The 2018 Common Rule also addresses electronic records by including a definition of "written, or in writing": "*Written,* or *in writing,* for purposes of this part, refers to writing on a tangible medium (*e.g.*, paper) or in an electronic format."[63]

Literacy. A person who speaks and understands English but does not read and write may be enrolled in a study by "making their mark" (*e.g.*, an "X" or a fingerprint) on the consent document when this would constitute a legal signature in accordance with applicable state

---

[56] *Id.* State law should be consulted to determine whether any requirements exist regarding the procedures for obtaining contents of informed consent. *See, e.g.*, *Shinal v. Toms*, 162 A.3d 429 (PA 2017) (finding that a physician cannot delegate responsibilities for obtaining informed consent, including for experimental treatments or procedures under state law); 40 P.S. § 1303.504(a).

[57] *See* FDA Draft Guidance 2014, at 18, *citing* 21 C.F.R. § 50.27(a), an FDA regulation that requires that the consent form to be dated; *see also* OHRP, Informed Consent FAQs, Do signatures on consent forms have to be dated?, *available at* https://www.hhs.gov/ohrp/regulations-and-policy/guidance/faq/informed-consent/index.html.

[58] *See* FDA Draft Guidance 2014, at 18.

[59] 45 C.F.R. § 46.117; 82 Fed. Reg. 7149 at 7267 (Jan. 19, 2017) (to be codified at 45 C.F.R. §__.117); 21 C.F.R. 50.27.

[60] FDA Draft Guidance July 2014, at 18.

[61] 21 C.F.R. Part 11; *see also* FDA Draft Guidance July 2014, at 17.

[62] OHRP, Use of Electronic Informed Consent Questions and Answers, Guidance for Institutional Review Boards, Investigators, and Sponsors (Dec. 2016), *available at* https://www.fda.gov/downloads/drugs/guidances/ucm436811.pdf.

[63] 82 Fed. Reg. 7149 at 7261 (Jan. 19, 2017) (to be codified at 45 C.F.R. §__.102(m)).

or local law.[64] FDA guidance suggests that when orally presenting consent information to a potential subject with lower literacy or numeracy, it is advisable to include the signature of a witness to the oral presentation of the informed consent elements.[65]

Physical Limitations. A potential subject who has physical limitations (*e.g.*, may be physically unable to speak or write or has hearing or vision loss) can enroll in a clinical investigation if competent and able to signal consent when consistent with applicable state law.[66] The consent form should document the method used for communication with the prospective subject and the specific means by which the prospective subject communicated agreement to participate in the study. Consideration may be given as to whether the investigator could use alternative means to assist individuals with physical limitations in the consent process (*e.g.*, making an audio recording of the entire consent form or using a form with enlarged font to assist visually impaired subjects).[67]

9.6 Types of Consent Forms

Sample or draft consent documents may be developed by a sponsor or cooperative study group, but the IRB of record is the final authority on the content of the consent document and other materials used in the consent process that are presented to prospective study subjects.[68] This includes IRB-approved advertisements, recruitment letters, pre-screening phone calls, and study description sheets. When an informed consent form is provided by a sponsor, counsel should coordinate with the institution's study coordinator to request changes to the consent form from the sponsor where necessary so that it is compliant with state and federal law.

Where obtaining informed consent is required, and except when the IRB has approved a waiver of consent documentation, informed consent must be documented by the use of a written consent form approved by the IRB and signed by the subject or the subject's legally authorized representative, as discussed above in **Section 9.5**. The consent document may be either of the following forms:[69]

- A **written consent** document that embodies the elements of informed consent described above. This form may be read to the subject or the subject's legally

[64] FDA, A Guide to Informed Consent—Information Sheet, *available at* https://www.fda.gov/RegulatoryInformation/Guidances/ucm126431.htm; FDA Draft Guidance July 2014, at 34.

[65] FDA, A Guide to Informed Consent—Information Sheet, *available at* https://www.fda.gov/RegulatoryInformation/Guidances/ucm126431.htm; FDA Draft Guidance July 2014, at 34 (referencing the short form consent process described in **Section 9.6**).

[66] FDA Draft Guidance July 2014, at 34.

[67] FDA Draft Guidance July 2014, at 34 and 35.

[68] 45 C.F.R. § 46.109; 82 Fed. Reg. 7149 at 7263 (Jan. 19, 2017) (to be codified at 45 C.F.R. §__.109); 21 C.F.R. § 50.50; 21 C.F.R. § 56.109.

[69] 45 C.F.R. § 46.117; 82 Fed. Reg. 7149 at 7267, 7268 (Jan. 19, 2017) (to be codified at 45 C.F.R. §__.117); 21 C.F.R. § 50.27.

authorized representative, but in any event, the investigator should give either the subject or the representative adequate opportunity to read it before it is signed.

- A **short form written consent** document, stating that the elements of informed consent have been presented orally to the subject or the subject's legally authorized representative. When this method is used, there must be a witness to the oral presentation. Also, the IRB must approve a written summary of what is to be said to the subject or the representative. Only the short form itself is to be signed by the subject or the representative; however, the witness must sign both the short form and a copy of the summary, and the person actually obtaining consent must sign a copy of the summary. A copy of the summary and a copy of the short form must be given to the subject or the representative.

9.7 Language Requirements

The regulations require that information related to informed consent be presented "in language understandable to the subject."[70] FDA draft guidance notes that "understandable" in part means that the information conveyed to subjects must be in a language and at a level that they can comprehend, and points out that (at the time the guidance was published) more than one-third of U.S. adults have basic or below basic health literacy.[71] Technical and medical language should be avoided when possible or translated to "lay" terms for the subject. Institutions often have policies that all patient communications be written to a certain grade level and such policies should be applied to research consent communications with subjects. As discussed in **Section 9.2**, under the 2018 Common Rule, except where broad consent is obtained, the consent also must begin with a concise and focused presentation of the key information about the study that is organized and presented in a way that facilitates comprehension.[72]

In general, subjects who do not speak English should be presented with an informed consent document written in a language understandable to them.[73] OHRP strongly encourages the use of this procedure whenever possible. Alternatively, as described in **Section 9.6**, the regulations permit oral presentation of informed consent information in conjunction with a short form document. When this procedure is used with subjects who do not speak English, (i) the oral presentation and the short form document should be in a language understandable to the subject, (ii) the IRB-approved English language consent document may serve as the summary, and (iii) the witness should be fluent in both English and the language of the subject.[74] When

[70] 45 C.F.R. § 46.116; 82 Fed. Reg. 7149 at 7265 (Jan. 19, 2017) (to be codified at 45 C.F.R. §__.116(a)); 21 C.F.R. § 50.20.

[71] FDA Draft Guidance July 2014, at 5.

[72] 82 Fed. Reg. 7149 at 7265 (Jan. 19, 2017) (to be codified at 45 C.F.R. §__.116).

[73] OHRP, Informed Consent of Subjects Who Do Not Speak English (1995) (Nov. 9, 1995), *available at* https://www.hhs.gov/ohrp/regulations-and-policy/guidance/obtaining-and-documenting-infomed-consent-non-english-speakers/index.html; FDA Draft Guidance July 2014, at 5.

[74] OHRP, Informed Consent of Subjects Who Do Not Speak English (1995) (Nov. 9, 1995), *available at* https://www.hhs.gov/ohrp/regulations-and-policy/guidance/obtaining-and-documenting-infomed-consent-non-

using the short form, a witness to the oral presentation is required and the subject must be given copies of the short form document and the summary.[75] Institutions also must have procedures available to communicate with subjects in a language that they understand throughout the study.

9.8 Exceptions to Informed Consent; Waiver and Alteration of Informed Consent; Waiver of Documentation of Informed Consent

9.8.1 Exceptions to Informed Consent

Emergency Research Protocols. The HHS and FDA regulations both allow an exception to the informed consent requirements for emergency research protocols that meet certain criteria.[76] The FDA regulations outline a detailed procedure for determining that informed consent is not obtainable from human subjects because they are in a "life threatening" situation, available treatments are unproven or unsatisfactory, and, among other factors, the subjects' physical condition precludes obtaining the subjects' consent.[77] The exception from informed consent requirements for emergency research can be implemented under the HHS protection of human subjects regulations pursuant to the terms of an HHS Secretarial waiver.[78]

Individual Emergency Use of a Test Article. In addition, under the FDA regulations, there is an exception to the informed consent requirements for use of a test article for an individual patient who is in a "life threatening" situation, where consent cannot be obtained, and there are no alternative approved or generally recognized methods of therapy that provide an equal or greater likelihood of saving the life of the subject. Specific procedures must to be followed for this exception to obtaining informed consent. This does not address the requirement for IRB review.[79]

Military Use. The FDA permits another exception to obtaining informed consent relating to the administration of an investigational product to members of the armed forces in connection with military operations.[80]

---

english-speakers/index.html; *see also* FDA, A Guide to Informed Consent—Information Sheet, *available at* https://www.fda.gov/RegulatoryInformation/Guidances/ucm126431.htm.

[75] 45 C.F.R. § 46.117(b)(2); 82 Fed. Reg. 7149 at 7268 (Jan. 19, 2017) (to be codified at 45 C.F.R. § __.117(b)(2)); 21 C.F.R. § 50.27(b)(2).

[76] 61 Fed. Reg. 51498 at 51528-51531 (Oct. 2, 1996).

[77] 21 C.F.R. § 50. 24.

[78] 45 C.F.R. § 46.101(i); 82 Fed. Reg. 7149 at 7259 (Jan. 19, 2017) (to be codified at 45 C.F.R. § __.101(i)); OHRP, Informed Consent Requirements in Emergency Research (OPRR Letter 1996) (Oct. 31, 1996), *available at* https://www.hhs.gov/ohrp/regulations-and-policy/guidance/emergency-research-informed-consent-requirements/index.html.

[79] 21 C.F.R. § 50.23.

[80] *Id.*

Added by the 2018 Common Rule:

The 2018 Common Rule adds an exception to informed consent for certain pre-research activities. An IRB may approve a research proposal in which an investigator will obtain information or biospecimens for the purpose of screening, recruiting, or determining the eligibility of prospective subjects without the informed consent of the prospective subject or the subject's legally authorized representative, if either of the following conditions are met:

(1) The investigator will obtain information through oral or written communication with the prospective subject or legally authorized representative, ***or***

(2) The investigator will obtain identifiable private information or identifiable biospecimens by accessing records or stored identifiable biospecimens.[81]

This exception to the general requirement for informed consent is consistent with FDA's application of the FDA informed consent requirements, which do not require informed consent or a waiver of informed consent for such activities, and serves to better harmonize the Common Rule with the FDA informed consent regulations.[82]

9.8.2 Waiver and Alteration of Informed Consent–FDA and HHS

FDA regulations regarding exceptions to the informed consent requirements have traditionally been far more limited than HHS regulations, permitting an exception only in life-threatening situations under certain conditions or when the requirements for emergency research are met. The FDA informed consent regulations do not allow the IRB to approve a general waiver of informed consent or alteration of the informed consent requirements. The

[81] 82 Fed. Reg. 7149 at 7267 (Jan. 19, 2017) (to be codified at 45 C.F.R. §__.116(g)). Similarly, the HIPAA Privacy Rule allows for "preparatory to research" activities, under which provision covered entities may disclose PHI, without authorization, to researchers to aid in study recruitment. The researcher may identify, but not contact, potential study participants if the researcher provides certain representations to the covered entity, and no PHI may leave the covered entity. As per December 2017 guidance developed pursuant to the 21st Century Cures Act, the HHS Office of Civil Rights has allowed that an electronic transmission of PHI is not necessarily considered a "removal" of PHI, and researchers may remotely access PHI provided that reasonable security safeguards are in place and PHI is not copied or retained by the researcher. *See* U.S. Dept. of Health & Human Services., Ofc. for Civil Rights, 21st Century Cures Act Guidance: Remote Access to PHI for Activities Preparatory to Research, *available at* https://www.hhs.gov/sites/default/files/remote-access-research-12-15-17.pdf. If the researcher wishes to contact the prospective subject for such "preparatory to research" activities, the researcher may do so, without authorization, only under limited circumstances: (1) if the researcher is a workforce member of a covered entity, the researcher may contact the prospective subject to seek authorization, or a covered health care provider may discuss research participation with a patient as part of the patient's treatment or health care operations; or a business associate (who may be a researcher) may assist in contacting individuals on behalf of the covered entity to obtain their authorizations, or (2) with documentation that an IRB has partially waived the authorization requirement to disclose PHI to a researcher for recruitment purposes, then the covered entity could disclose to the researcher sufficient PHI necessary for the researcher to contact the prospective subject. *See* U.S. Dept. of Health & Human Services, Health Information Privacy, Research, *available at* https://www.hhs.gov/hipaa/for-professionals/special-topics/research/index.html. *See also* **Chapter 10,** *HIPAA Compliance in Clinical Trials,* for further discussion of the HIPAA requirements.

[82] *See* FDA, Screening Tests Prior to Study Enrollment–Information Sheet, *available at* https://www.fda.gov/RegulatoryInformation/Guidances/ucm126430.htm.

21st Century Cures Act does, however, authorize FDA to create an exception from informed consent requirements when the proposed clinical testing poses no more than minimal risk to the subject and includes appropriate safeguards to protect the rights, safety, and welfare of the subject. Per FDA guidance, FDA does not intend to object to an IRB following the pre-2018 Common Rule regulations regarding waiver and alteration of informed consent (see below in **Section 9.8.3**) until FDA promulgates its own regulations at a later date.[83]

The Common Rule allows an IRB to waive the requirement for informed consent, or approve a waiver or alteration of the required elements of informed consent. Under the pre-2018 Common Rule, an IRB may waive informed consent—or waive or alter the basic and additional elements of consent outlined in **Sections 9.3.1 and 9.3.2**—for some or all subjects if the IRB finds and documents all of the following:

- The research involves no more than minimal risk to the subjects;
- The research could not practicably be carried out without the requested waiver or alteration;
- The waiver or alteration will not adversely affect the rights and welfare of the subjects; ***and***
- Whenever appropriate, the subjects or legally authorized representatives will be provided with additional pertinent information after participation.[84]

The overarching requirements for how informed consent is obtained outlined above in **Section 9.2** cannot be altered or waived if the IRB determines that informed consent must be obtained from subjects, *i.e.*, if the IRB requires that a subject's consent is obtained, these requirements must be met.[85]

For research involving children, the Common Rule allows an IRB to waive parental or guardian permission if the IRB makes and documents the required findings for a general waiver of informed consent.[86] Alternatively, if the IRB determines that a research protocol is designed to study conditions in children or a subject population for which parental or guardian consent is not a reasonable requirement to protect the subjects (*e.g.*, neglected or abused children), the IRB may waive the parental or guardian permission requirements if an appropriate mechanism is in place to protect the children, and provided that the waiver is not inconsistent with

[83] *See* FDA, IRB Waiver or Alteration of Informed Consent for Clinical Investigations Involving No More Than Minimal Risk to Human Subjects, Guidance for Sponsors, Investigators, and Institutional Review Boards (July 2017), *available at* https://www.fda.gov/downloads/RegulatoryInformation/Guidances/UCM566948.pdf.

[84] 45 C.F.R. § 46.116(d).

[85] The waiver provision of the Common Rule refers to the waiver or alteration of the "elements" of consent; 45 C.F.R. § 46.116(d); 82 Fed. Reg. 7149 at 7267 (Jan. 19, 2017) (to be codified at 45 C.F.R. §__.116(f)); 21 C.F.R. § 50.20.

[86] 45 C.F.R. § 46.408(b); 45 C.F.R. §§ 46.116(c) and (d); 82 Fed. Reg. 7149 at 7267 (Jan. 19, 2017) (to be codified at 45 C.F.R. §__.116(e) and (f)).

federal, state, or local law.[87] The FDA regulations do not allow waiver of parental or guardian permission.

Added by the 2018 Common Rule:

The 2018 Common Rule adds an additional criterion for waiver or alteration of informed consent:

- If the research involves using identifiable private information or identifiable biospecimens, the research could not practicably be carried out without using such information or biospecimens in an identifiable format.[88]

The 2018 Common Rule limits the availability of a waiver of consent in certain circumstances in which broad consent was sought. If an individual was asked to provide broad consent for the storage, maintenance, and secondary research use of identifiable private information or identifiable biospecimens and refused to consent, the 2018 Common Rule provides that an IRB cannot waive consent for the storage, maintenance, or secondary research use of the identifiable private information or identifiable biospecimens.[89]

The elements for broad consent cannot be altered or omitted by an IRB. If an investigator chooses to obtain broad consent, the broad consent must be obtained in accordance with all of the regulatory requirements at 82 Fed. Reg. 7149 at 7266, to be codified at §__.116(d).[90]

9.8.3 Waiver of Documentation of Informed Consent

An IRB may waive the requirement for the investigator to obtain a signed consent form for some or all subjects, if it finds:[91]

- For research subject to the Common Rule, that the only record linking the subject and the research would be the consent document, and the principal risk would be potential harm resulting from a breach of confidentiality. Each subject (or legally authorized representative) will be asked whether the subject consents to having documentation linking the subject to the research, and the subject's preference will control; ***or***
- For research subject to the Common Rule or FDA regulation, that the research presents no more than minimal risk of harm to subjects, and involves no procedures for which written consent is normally required outside of the research context.

---

[87] 45 C.F.R. § 46.408(c).

[88] 82 Fed. Reg. 7149 at 7267 (Jan. 19, 2017) (to be codified at 45 C.F.R. § __.116(f)(3)(iii)).

[89] 82 Fed. Reg. 7149 at 7267 (Jan. 19, 2017) (to be codified at 45 C.F.R. § __.116(f)(1)).

[90] 82 Fed. Reg. 7149 at 7267 (Jan. 19, 2017) (to be codified at 45 C.F.R. § __.116 (f)(2)).

[91] 45 C.F.R. § 46.117(c); 82 Fed. Reg. 7149 at 7268 (Jan. 19, 2017) (to be codified at 45 C.F.R. §__.117(c); 21 C.F.R. § 56.109(c).

Added by the 2018 Common Rule:

- For research subject to the Common Rule, if the subjects or legally authorized representatives are members of a distinct cultural group or community in which signing forms is not the norm, that the research presents no more than minimal risk of harm to subjects and provided there is an appropriate alternative mechanism for documenting that informed consent was obtained.[92]

In cases in which the documentation requirement is waived, the IRB may require the investigator to provide subjects with a written statement regarding the research.[93]

9.9 Observation of Research

Federal regulatory agencies do not expect IRBs to routinely observe consent interviews, observe the conduct of the clinical study, or review clinical study records. The Common Rule and FDA regulations do, however, give the IRB the authority to observe, or have a third party observe, the consent process and the research.[94] If the IRB is concerned about the conduct of the clinical study or the process for obtaining consent, the IRB should consider whether, as part of providing adequate oversight of the clinical study, an active audit is warranted.

9.10 IRB Continuing Review

Study protocols often are changed during the course of the study, and such changes may require revision of the informed consent document. Under the pre-2018 Common Rule and FDA regulations, the IRB generally must conduct "continuing review" at least annually throughout the course of the study (note that under the 2018 Common Rule, some categories of research no longer require continuing review). This includes reviewing a copy of the sample informed consent document submitted by the investigator to verify the investigator is using accurate, up-to-date information about the research and that the informed consent document continues to meet the regulatory requirements. OHRP and FDA recommend that IRBs use methods that allow the IRB to readily recognize the most current version of the IRB-approved informed consent document, (*e.g.*, using date stamps, version numbers, or initialing and dating documents to indicate when a version was approved), which the investigator should be using with all new study subjects, as well as, if required by the IRB, re-consenting existing study subjects with the updated consent form. Numbering, dating, or otherwise sequencing the forms helps ensure that only the most current IRB-approved informed consent documents are presented to subjects.[95]

---

[92] 82 Fed. Reg. 7149 at 7268 (Jan. 19, 2017) (to be codified at 45 C.F.R. §__117(c).

[93] 45 C.F.R. § 46.117(c); 21 C.F.R. § 56.109(d).

[94] 45 C.F.R. § 46.109(e); 82 Fed. Reg. 7149 at 7264 (Jan. 19, 2017) (to be codified at 45 C.F.R. §__.109(g); 21 C.F.R. § 56.109(f).

[95] 45 C.F.R. § 46.109(e); 82 Fed. Reg. 7149 at 7264 (Jan. 19, 2017) (to be codified at 45 C.F.R. §__.109(e) (which carves out certain categories of research from the general requirement for annual continuing review); 21 C.F.R. § 56.109(f). *See also* OHRP, Continuing Review Guidance (2010) (Nov. 10, 2010), *available at* https://www.hhs.gov/ohrp/regulations-and-policy/guidance/guidance-on-continuing-review-2010/index.html;

9.11 Informed Consent for Genetic Testing

For studies that involve genetic testing, either in the proposed research or as a secondary use of identifiable private information or identifiable biospecimens, IRBs should be cognizant of additional informed consent requirements. For example, while the Common Rule permits broad or open-ended consent for future research, some jurisdictions require *specific* consent for genetic testing, including a more robust description of the type of testing and future research uses, as well as more stringent requirements with respect to storage and maintenance absent specific consent to the contrary. The Common Rule expressly states it does not preempt any other federal, state, or local law that requires additional information to be disclosed in order for informed consent to be legally effective.[96] When research will be conducted with biospecimens collected from sites outside the U.S., special attention should be paid to international local law that may place additional requirements on the collection and processing of biospecimens for genetic testing purposes.

9.12 Posting of Informed Consent Documents

Added by the 2018 Common Rule:

The 2018 Common Rule requires that, for clinical trials conducted or supported by a Common Rule department or agency, an IRB-approved informed consent form used to enroll subjects must be posted on a publicly available federal website. Either the awardee institution or the Common Rule agency conducting the trial is responsible for posting the consent form. The Common Rule agency conducting or supporting the clinical trial may either permit, or require, that certain information be redacted from the informed consent form before it is posted. For example, confidential commercial information might be redacted from the consent form before it is posted. Legal counsel can play a helpful role in identifying information to be redacted in the informed consent form, and in discussing the proposed redaction with federal department or agency officials.

The informed consent form must be posted after recruitment of subjects for the clinical trial has closed, and no later than 60 days after the last study visit by any subject (as dictated by the clinical trial protocol).[97]

FDA, Guidance for IRBs, Clinical Investigators, and Sponsors–IRB Continuing Review after Clinical Investigation Approval (Feb. 2012), *available at* https://www.fda.gov/downloads/RegulatoryInformation/Guidances/UCM294558.pdf.

[96] 45 C.F.R. § 46.116(e); 82 Fed. Reg. 7149 at 7267 (Jan. 19, 2017) (to be codified at 45 C.F.R. §__116(i)). State law should be consulted for additional requirements regarding genetic testing in the research context. *See, e.g.*, Minn. Stat. § 13.386 (prescribing restrictions on the storage, use and dissemination of genetic information by government and non-government entities), *available at* https://www.revisor.mn.gov/statutes/cite/13.386.

[97] 82 Fed. Reg. 7149 at 7267 (Jan. 19, 2017) (to be codified at 45 C.F.R. §__.116(h)).

Chapter 10

HIPAA Compliance in Clinical Trials

Kimberly H. Gillespie

Melinda G. Murray

Heather L. Fields

Introduction

The Health Insurance Portability and Accountability Act of 1996 (HIPAA) and its implementing regulations, as amended, are referred to herein as the "Privacy Rule."[1] The Privacy Rule[2] provides comprehensive federal protection for the privacy of one's health information. The Privacy Rule defines "research" as "a systematic investigation, including research development, testing and evaluation, designed to develop or contribute to generalizable knowledge,"[3] and it prescribes how a "Covered Entity" (a provider, health plan, or clearinghouse that transmits health information electronically) may make use of protected health information (PHI) and the circumstances under which PHI may be disclosed to others. The U.S. Department of Health and Human Services (HHS) states that disclosure of PHI for research purposes (*e.g.*, clinical trials, etc.) generally is not permitted as part of treatment, payment, or health care operations.[4] This chapter outlines the requirements for a Patient Authorization under the Privacy Rule, and identifies the Privacy Rule provisions that permit use or disclosure of PHI without a Patient Authorization, or with a modified Patient Authorization.

A Covered Entity may use or disclose PHI for research with a Patient Authorization, or if another provision of the Privacy Rule is met, without a Patient Authorization. Patient Authorization under the Privacy Rule is distinct from the concept of informed consent, which is required under the federal regulations for the protection of human subjects.[5] The Privacy Rule does not remove any of the requirements for obtaining informed consent set forth in the other

[1] HHS published the Privacy Rule on Dec. 28, 2000, adopted modifications of the Rule on Aug. 14, 2002, with amendments since that time. Compliance for most Covered Entities was required as of Apr. 14, 2003.

[2] 45 C.F.R. Part 160 and Subparts A and E of Part 164.

[3] 45 C.F.R. § 164.501.

[4] 67 Fed. Reg. 53213 (Aug. 14, 2002).

[5] Federal research regulations have been promulgated by the U.S. Department of Health and Human Services at 45 C.F.R. Part 46 and by the U.S. Food and Drug Administration at 21 C.F.R. Parts 50 and 56.

federal regulations. The Patient Authorization may be combined with the informed consent document, subject to certain additional requirements and considerations.[6]

The Privacy Rule applies to individually identifiable health information created or received and transmitted or maintained in any form by a Covered Entity, *i.e.*, PHI. Researchers themselves are not Covered Entities, unless they are health care providers and engage in any of the covered electronic transactions, and may not be subject to the Privacy Rule. If a researcher is an employee or other workforce member of a Covered Entity, such as a hospital or health insurer, the Covered Entity should consider carefully how the Privacy Rule and the entity's research policies and procedures apply to the researcher's dual role as employee/workforce member and researcher.

Many states have privacy laws that may have additional requirements or limitations that apply to the use of PHI for research. This chapter focuses on the Privacy Rule without consideration to specific state laws.

10.1 Use/Disclosure of PHI for Research

The Privacy Rule permits a Covered Entity to use or disclose PHI for a research study, regardless of the funding source, if the Covered Entity obtains a valid Patient Authorization from the individual whose PHI will be used or disclosed.[7] A Covered Entity may still use or disclose PHI for research when there is no Patient Authorization if the Covered Entity:

- obtains a "waiver" or "alteration" of the Patient Authorization from an Institutional Review Board (IRB) or privacy board;[8] or
- verifies that the research-related use involves (i) de-identified information (not PHI); (ii) limited data sets; (iii) reviews preparatory to research; or (iv) decedent information.

The Privacy Rule also permits a Covered Entity to obtain Patient Authorization to use or disclose PHI for future research purposes, provided the Patient Authorization meets certain criteria described in **Section 10.3** below.[9]

---

[6] Covered Entities may combine the informed consent form and the HIPAA authorization if certain requirements are met.

[7] 45 C.F.R. § 164.508(c).

[8] 45 C.F.R. § 164.512(i).

[9] *See* U.S. Department of Health and Human Services, Office for Civil Rights (OCR), *Guidance on HIPAA and Individual Authorization of Uses and Disclosures of Protected Health Information for Research* issued June 1, 2018 (the "Guidance"), *available at* https://www.hhs.gov/sites/default/files/hipaa-future-research-authorization-guidance-06122018%20v2.pdf. The 21st Century Cures Act of 2016, Pub. L. 114-255, Sec. 2063(b), required OCR to issue the guidance to clarify the circumstances under which an authorization would be deemed to sufficiently describe the future research purposes, whether an annual notice or reminder of the right to revoke was needed, and mechanisms by which an individual may revoke authorization.

10.2 Patient Authorization for Research

To use or disclose PHI for research using a Patient Authorization, the Covered Entity must obtain a written authorization that satisfies the requirements of 45 C.F.R. § 164.508. The core elements required for a valid authorization include the following:

- a description of the information to be used or disclosed that identifies the information in a specific and meaningful fashion;
- the name or other specific identification of the person(s), or class of persons, authorized to make the requested use or disclosure;
- the name or other specific identification of the person(s), or class of persons, to whom the Covered Entity may make the requested use or disclosure;
- a description of each purpose of the requested use or disclosure; the statement "at the request of the individual" is a sufficient description of the purpose when an individual initiates the authorization and does not, or elects not to, provide a statement of the purpose;
- an expiration date or an expiration event that relates to the individual or the purpose of the use or disclosure; the statement "end of the research study," "none," or similar language is sufficient if the authorization is for a use or disclosure of PHI for research, including the creation and maintenance of a research database or research repository;[10]
- the individual's right to revoke the authorization in writing and either (i) the exceptions to the right to revoke and a description of how the individual may revoke the authorization, or (ii) to the extent that the information is included in the entity's Notice of Privacy Practices, a reference to the Notice;
- the consequences to the individual of a refusal to sign the authorization (for instance, the individual may not be able to participate in the research if he or she refuses to sign the authorization, subject to the requirements of a Covered Entity's ability to condition treatment, enrollment, or eligibility for benefits on failure to obtain an authorization);
- the potential for information to be disclosed pursuant to the authorization or subject to redisclosure by the recipient and therefore no longer protected;
- signature of the individual and date; signature can be by personal representative if a description of that person's authority to act is included.

The Patient Authorization must be written in plain language and the individual must be provided with a copy of the signed authorization. A sample HIPAA Authorization is attached as **Exhibit 10.2**.

When the Patient Authorization is for a future research, the description of "each purpose" does not need to specify each specific future study if the particular studies to be conducted are

[10] 45 C.F.R. § 164.508(c)(1)(iv).

not yet determined, so long as the authorization "adequately describe[s] such purposes such that it would be reasonable for the individual to expect that his or her [PHI] could be used or disclosed for future research."[11] The Patient Authorization may allow the Covered Entity to use or disclose an individual's PHI for its own research purposes or disclose PHI to another entity for that entity's research activities.

In describing the right to revoke, an authorization for future research should explain that revocation will limit a Covered Entity's own continued use of the PHI, but that the PHI may continue to be used by other parties to whom the PHI was disclosed prior to the date of revocation. The Covered Entity may require individuals to use a standard revocation form, but the U.S. Department of Health and Human Services, Office for Civil Rights (OCR) "encourages" Covered Entities to consider offering alternative revocation options to make it easier for an individual to revoke, such as an electronic form on an electronic health record patient portal.[12] In addition, OCR permits a Covered Entity to cease using and disclosing PHI pursuant to an authorization based on an individual's oral request if the Covered Entity chooses to do so.[13]

Even if an individual revokes his or her authorization, the Covered Entity may continue to use or disclose PHI obtained prior to an individual's revocation to the extent the entity has taken action in reliance on the authorization.[14] Where the research is conducted by the Covered Entity, the entity could continue using or disclosing an individual's PHI post-revocation as necessary to maintain the integrity of the research (*e.g.*, to account for the withdrawal, to report adverse events, etc.).

A Patient Authorization for the use and disclosure of PHI for a particular research study may be combined with a consent to participate in the research, and may condition the provision of research-related treatment on the individual signing the Patient Authorization (Conditioned Authorization). A Covered Entity also may combine a Conditioned Authorization with a Patient Authorization to use PHI for future research (Compound Authorization), provided that the Compound Authorization clearly differentiates between the conditioned research component and the "unconditioned" future research component and the document affords the individual the opportunity to separately "opt in" to participation in the future research.[15]

10.3 Use/Disclosure without Patient Authorization

10.3.1 Waiver or Alteration of Authorization Requirements

A Covered Entity may use or disclose PHI for research purposes pursuant to a waiver or alteration of the Patient Authorization by an IRB or privacy board.[16] A waiver of the authoriza-

---

[11] See the Guidance and 78 Fed. Reg. 5566, 5612 (Jan. 25, 2013).

[12] See the Guidance, p. 5.

[13] *Id.*

[14] 45 C.F.R. § 164.508(b)(5)(i).

[15] 45 C.F.R. § 164.508(b)(3)(i).

[16] 45 C.F.R. § 164.512(i)(1)(i).

tion requirements would allow the researcher to use or disclose the PHI without the patient's authorization. An alteration would allow the researcher to use or disclose the PHI with an authorization that lacks or modifies some of the elements discussed above in **Section 10.2**.

The Privacy Rule recognizes that some institutions may not have IRBs, or that some IRBs may not have the expertise needed to review research that requires consideration of risks to privacy. Thus, the Privacy Rule permits Covered Entities to accept documentation of a waiver or alteration of a Patient Authorization from an alternative body (i.e., a privacy board) that could have fewer members or members with different expertise than IRBs. The Privacy Rule further clarifies that the Covered Entity does not need to create an IRB or privacy board. The IRB or privacy board could be created by the Covered Entity or the recipient researcher, or it could be an independent board. To meet the regulatory requirements, a privacy board must:

- have members with varying backgrounds and the professional competence necessary and appropriate to review the effect of the research protocol on the individual's privacy rights and related interests;
- include at least one member who has no affiliation with the Covered Entity, is not affiliated with the research sponsor, and is not related either to the Covered Entity or the Sponsor; and
- have no member participating in review of a research project in which the member has a conflict of interest.[17]

For approval of a waiver or alteration by a privacy board at a convened meeting, at least one member who satisfies the criteria for being unaffiliated with the Covered Entity or the research sponsor must be present, which differs from the IRB requirement of a non-scientific member having to be present at the convened meeting.[18]

The IRB/privacy board may approve a waiver or alteration of the Patient Authorization, provided it has obtained documentation of *all* of the following:[19]

- identification of the IRB or privacy board and the date on which the waiver or alteration was approved;
- a statement that the IRB or privacy board has determined that the waiver or alteration, in whole or in part, satisfies the three criteria in the Privacy Rule (discussed below);
- a brief description of the PHI for which use or access has been determined to be necessary by the IRB or privacy board;
- a statement that the waiver or alteration has been reviewed and approved under either full review or expedited review procedures; and

[17] 45 C.F.R. § 164.512(i)(1)(i)(B).

[18] 45 C.F.R. § 164.512(i)(2)(iv)(B); 45 C.F.R. § 46.108(b); and 21 C.F.R. § 56.108(c).

[19] 45 C.F.R. § 164.512(i)(2).

- the signature of the chair or other member, as designated by the chair, of the IRB or privacy board, as applicable.

The three criteria discussed above regarding the makeup of a privacy board must be satisfied for an IRB or privacy board to approve a waiver or alteration under the Privacy Rule:

- the use or disclosure of PHI must involve no more than minimal risk to the privacy of individuals, based on at least the presence of the following elements:
  - an adequate plan to protect identifiers from improper use and disclosure;
  - an adequate plan to destroy the identifiers at the earliest opportunity consistent with the conduct of the research, unless there is a health or research justification for retaining the identifiers or such retention is otherwise required by law; and
  - adequate written assurances that the PHI will not be reused or disclosed to any other person or entity, except:
    - as required by law;
    - for authorized oversight, or
    - for other research for which the use and disclosure of the PHI would be permitted under the Privacy Rules.
- the research could not practicably be conducted without the waiver or alteration; and
- the research could not be practicably conducted without access to and use of the PHI.[20]

The IRB or privacy board must use its judgment as to whether the waiver criteria have been satisfied. Several of the waiver criteria are closely modeled on the Pre-2018 Common Rule's criteria for the waiver of informed consent and for the approval of a research study, although there is a different primary focus on privacy. Thus, it is anticipated that IRBs have experience in making the necessary subjective assessments of risks. A sample waiver of Patient Authorization is found in **Exhibit 10.3.1**.

10.3.2 Review Preparatory to Research

The Privacy Rule permits a Covered Entity to allow a researcher to access and use PHI without an authorization or waiver of authorization for reviews preparatory to research if the Covered Entity obtains from the researcher assurance that:

- the use or disclosure is sought solely to review the PHI as necessary to prepare a research protocol or for similar purposes preparatory to research;
- no PHI is removed from the Covered Entity; and
- the use of or access to the PHI is necessary for research purposes.[21]

[20] 45 C.F.R. § 164.512(i)(2)(ii).

[21] 45 C.F.R. § 164.512(i)(1)(ii).

This provision might be used, for example, to design a research study or to assess the feasibility of conducting a study. It should not be used for the recruitment of research subjects.

10.3.3 Decedent Information

The Privacy Rule also permits a Covered Entity—without an authorization or waiver of authorization—to allow a researcher to access and use PHI that contains only decedent information if the Covered Entity obtains from the researcher:

- a representation that the use or disclosure is only for research on the PHI of the decedents;
- documentation of death of such individuals, if required by the Covered Entity; and
- a representation that the PHI involved is necessary for research purposes.[22]

10.3.4 Limited Data Sets with a Data Use Agreement

A data use agreement is an agreement entered into by the Covered Entity and the researcher in which the Covered Entity may disclose a limited data set to the researcher for purposes relating to research, public health, or health care operations.[23] A limited data set excludes specific direct identifiers of the individual, the individual's relatives or household members, and his or her employers. A limited data set may include zip codes; elements of dates (including dates of service, dates of birth and death); and geographic subdivisions (except street address). A limited data set ***may not*** include names, medical record numbers, health plan beneficiary numbers, device or serial numbers, or biometric identifiers. This is a partial list of prohibited items. The Privacy Rule sets forth 18 identifiers that may not be included.[24] Accordingly, this provision may have limited utility for device manufacturers who wish to compare outcomes for two different models of a device.[25]

A data use agreement is similar to a business associate agreement, except that the former commits the recipient to use the information received for activities concerning research, health care operations of the Covered Entity, or public health.[26] Data use agreements also prohibit the recipient from identifying or contacting the study subjects.[27] Such agreements must:

- establish the permitted uses and disclosures of the limited data set by the recipient, consistent with the purposes of the research, and which may not include any use or disclosure that would violate the Privacy Rule if done by the Covered Entity;
- establish who is permitted to use or receive the limited data set; and

[22] 45 C.F.R. § 164.512(i)(1)(iii).

[23] 45 C.F.R. § 164.514(e)(4).

[24] 45 C.F.R. § 164.514(e)(2).

[25] 45 C.F.R. § 164.514(e)(2).

[26] 45 C.F.R. § 164.514(e)(3).

[27] 45 C.F.R. § 164.514(e)(4)(ii)(C)(5).

- require the recipient to agree to the following:
  - not to use or disclose the information other than permitted by the data use agreement or as otherwise required by law;
  - use appropriate safeguards to prevent the use or disclosure of the information, other than as provided for in the data use agreement;
  - report to the Covered Entity any use or disclosure of the information not provided for in the data use agreement (of which the recipient becomes aware);
  - ensure that any agents, including a subcontractor, to whom the recipient provides the limited data set agree to the same restrictions and conditions that apply to the recipient with respect to the limited data set; and
  - not to identify the information or contact the individual.[28]

Covered Entities cannot simply rely on a data use agreement. They must also act to ensure compliance with the agreement, breaches are reported, and reasonable steps are taken if the Covered Entity becomes aware of an activity or practice that violates the data use agreement. Reasonable steps may include discontinuing the disclosure to the recipient and reporting the problem.[29] A sample data use agreement is at **Exhibit 10.3.4**.

10.3.5 De-Identification of PHI

If the information is de-identified, no Patient Authorization is required, as the information is no longer PHI so long as it remains de-identified. De-identified information must meet one of two criteria: (i) information has been stripped of all 18 personal identifiers listed in the Privacy Rule, and the Covered Entity does not have actual knowledge that the information could be used, alone or in conjunction with other available information, to identify the individual; or (ii) a person with appropriate knowledge of and experience with generally accepted statistical and scientific principles and methods for rendering information not individually identifiable determines and documents that there is only minimal risk that the information could not reasonably be used, alone or in conjunction with other available information, to identify an individual.[30]

PHI is considered de-identified when, under criterion (i) above, a Covered Entity removes the following 18 personal identifiers from the information:

1. names;
2. all geographic subdivisions smaller than a state;
3. all elements of dates except for years (unless years becomes an identifier);
4. telephone numbers;

---

[28] 45 C.F.R. § 164.514(e)(4)(ii).

[29] 45 C.F.R. § 164.514(e)(4)(iii).

[30] 45 C.F.R. §§ 164.502(d) and 164.514(a) and (b).

5. fax numbers;
6. e-mail addresses;
7. Social Security numbers;
8. medical records numbers;
9. health plan beneficiary numbers;
10. account numbers;
11. certificate/license numbers;
12. vehicle identifiers and serial numbers;
13. device identifiers and serial numbers;
14. Web Universal Resource Locators (URLs);
15. Internet Protocol address numbers;
16. biometric identifiers;
17. full face photographic images; and
18. any other unique identifying number, characteristic, or code.

The Covered Entity also must have no actual knowledge that the information could be used to identify an individual.[31]

Codes may be used to re-identify PHI that has been de-identified if the code cannot be used to identify individuals, is kept secure and is not used for any other purpose, and if the Covered Entity does not disclose the mechanism for re-identification.[32]

10.4 Recruitment

HHS has clarified that recruitment of subjects for research is "research"—not marketing or health care operations activity—and is subject to the general Patient Authorization requirements.[33] Where a Covered Entity wants to disclose information to a third party for purposes of recruitment, the Covered Entity will need to obtain (i) a Patient Authorization or (ii) a partial waiver of the Patient Authorization from an IRB or privacy board.

While HHS has indicated that Covered Entities may continue to discuss with patients the option of enrolling in a clinical trial, the HIPAA regulations do not address whether Covered Entities can review on-site medical records to identify potential enrollees for particular clinical trials, as this would involve "use" of PHI. Commentary suggests that identification and recruitment of potential enrollees by workforce members may be allowed under the "reviews preparatory to research" exception in 45 C.F.R. § 164.512(i)(l)(ii), but it does not permit the researcher to remove PHI from the Covered Entity's site. Remote access to a Covered Entity's

[31] 45 C.F.R. § 164.514(b)(2).

[32] 45 C.F.R. § 164.514(c).

[33] 67 Fed. Reg. 53230–31 (Aug. 14, 2002).

PHI for preparatory research activities is not considered removal so long as the researcher does not copy or retain the PHI.[34] A researcher who is not an employee of a Covered Entity or a member of its workforce may not use the "preparatory to research" provision to contact prospective research subjects. To contact prospective subjects, there must be a partial waiver of individual authorization under 45 C.F.R. § 164.512 (i)(1)(i).

10.5 Minimum Necessary Standard

A Covered Entity must make reasonable efforts to limit the use and disclosure of, or requests for, PHI to the minimum necessary to accomplish the intended purpose of the use, disclosure, or request.[35] For research purposes, the minimum necessary standard applies to:

- limited data sets;
- use/disclosure of PHI preparatory to research;
- use/disclosure of decedent PHI; and
- use/disclosure with IRB or privacy board waiver of Authorization.

The minimum necessary standard does NOT apply to de-identified health information (not PHI) or to use/disclosure pursuant to a Patient Authorization.

10.6 Accounting of Disclosures

In general, the Privacy Rule gives individuals the right to receive an accounting of certain disclosures of PHI made by a Covered Entity, including disclosure under waiver or alteration of authorization, use/disclosure of PHI preparatory to research, use/disclosure of decedent PHI, or for use/disclosure for public health purposes.[36] Generally speaking, this accounting must include disclosures of PHI that occurred during the six years prior to the individual's request for an accounting, and the accounting also must include specified information regarding each disclosure. A more general accounting is permitted for subsequent multiple disclosures to the same person or entity for a single purpose.[37] Among the types of disclosures that are exempt from this accounting requirement are research disclosures made pursuant to an individual's authorization and disclosures of the limited data set to researchers with a data use agreement.

The following elements must be recorded for each disclosure:

- date of disclosure;
- name of person/entity that received the PHI and, if known, the address of such entity/person;
- brief description of the PHI disclosed; and

[34] Pub. L. No. 114-255, Sec. 2063.

[35] 45 C.F.R. § 164.502(b)(2) and 164.514(d).

[36] 45 C.F.R. § 164.528.

[37] 45 C.F.R. § 164.528(b)(3).

- brief statement of the purpose of the disclosure that reasonably informs the individual of the basis for the disclosure.

In addition, for disclosures of PHI for research purposes in which the individual's authorization is not required and that involve at least 50 records, the Privacy Rule allows a simplified accounting of such disclosures by Covered Entities. Under this simplified accounting provision, Covered Entities may provide individuals with a list of all protocols for which the subject's PHI may have been disclosed under 45 C.F.R. § 164.512(i), as well as the researcher's name and contact information. Other requirements related to this simplified accounting provision are found at 45 C.F.R. § 164.528(b)(4).

10.7 Business Associate Considerations

HHS does not consider research activities to be covered functions; therefore, the business associate provisions of the Privacy Rule do not apply in the research context. This means that disclosures by a Covered Entity to a researcher for research purposes, as permitted by the Privacy Rule, do not require a business associate agreement; this remains true even in instances where the Covered Entity has hired the researcher to perform research on the Covered Entity's own behalf because, according to HHS, research is not a covered function or activity.[38]

Conversely, when a Covered Entity hires a researcher who is not an employee or workforce member to perform a HIPAA function, the Covered Entity must ensure the services are provided in a manner that complies with the Privacy Rule requirements for business associates, as well as the federal regulations for the protection of human subjects and the Covered Entity's research policies and procedures. For example, a researcher who is not an employee or workforce member may assist the Covered Entity in de-identifying PHI so it can be used in a research study or for another research purpose. Alternatively, a Covered Entity may contract with a research entity to contact patients to obtain a Patient Authorization to participate in research. In addition to the Privacy Rule considerations, when a researcher assists a Covered Entity in performing a HIPAA function, the Covered Entity must consider the ethical implications of this dual role.

10.8 Public Health Activities

In the research context, the exception for public health disclosures means that a Covered Entity may disclose PHI to a research sponsor if such information relates to the quality, safety, and effectiveness of the sponsor's products, so long as the disclosures are for legitimate public health purposes and not for commercial purposes.[39]

---

[38] 67 Fed. Reg. 53252 (Aug. 14, 2002).

[39] 67 Fed. Reg. 53228 (Aug. 14, 2002); *see also* 45 C.F.R. § 164.512(b)(i).

Chapter 11

Payment to Research Subjects

Valerie H. Bonham

Amy K. Dow

Introduction

Payment is frequently offered as an incentive to participate in research for the purposes of eliminating barriers involving financial sacrifice by subjects, expressing appreciation for subjects' participation, offering compensation for the time and inconvenience associated with participation, and motivating individuals who would otherwise lack interest in such activities.[1] The amount and schedule of payments should be provided to the Institutional Review Board (IRB) at the time of the initial review.[2] IRBs should be concerned about whether certain types and amounts of payment are fair and whether payment will have an impact on a subject's ability to evaluate the risks and voluntarily consent.[3]

Federal regulations governing research do not provide specific guidance on payment to research subjects. The regulations do, however, require that informed consent be obtained "only under such circumstances that provide the prospective subject or representative sufficient opportunity to consider whether or not to participate and that minimize the possibility of coercion or undue influence."[4] Undue influence may exist when an offer of payment is so attractive that it impairs a subject's ability to evaluate the risks or his or her ability to exercise proper judgment.[5] On occasion, findings in compliance audits of research institutions, which were conducted by the Office for Human Research Protections (OHRP), have included allegations that the amount or structure of payments to research subjects constituted improper

---

[1] *See, e.g.*, Elizabeth Ripley *et al.*, *Why Do We Pay? A National Survey of Investigators and IRB Chairpersons*, 5 J. Empirical Res. on Hum. Res. Ethics 43, 54 (2010); Leah E. Hutt, *Paying Research Subjects: Historical Considerations*, 12 Health L. Rev. 16, 16 (2003).

[2] FDA Information Sheet: Payment to Research Subjects, FDA (last updated Jan. 25, 2018), (hereafter *FDA Information Sheet: Payment to Subjects*), *available at* https://www.fda.gov/RegulatoryInformation/Guidances/ucm126429.htm.

[3] OHRP Informed Consent Frequently Asked Questions #6–10, OHRP (hereafter *OHRP Informed Consent Frequently Asked Questions*), *available at* https://www.hhs.gov/ohrp/regulations-and-policy/guidance/faq/informed-consent/index.html.

[4] 21 C.F.R. § 50.20; 45 C.F.R. § 46.116(a).

[5] OHRP IRB Guidebook, Chapter 3: Basic IRB Review, OHRP, *available at* http://wayback.archive-it.org/org-745/20150930182812/http://www.hhs.gov/ohrp/archive/irb/irb_chapter3.htm.

inducement in violation of the Pre-2018 Common Rule.[6] IRBs should be sensitive to the fact that undue inducements can result in inequitable subject recruitment, especially in economically depressed individuals.

11.1 Appropriate Payment

Regulations contain little guidance with respect to the amount of payment that may be provided to research subjects, leaving IRBs with little choice but to make often subjective decisions regarding the acceptability of proposed subject payments. These determinations are sometimes guided by little more than IRB members' personal opinions of whether a given payment amount will exert undue influence on the intended subject population under the circumstances.[7] As a result, several researchers have conducted surveys of IRBs and investigators to assess the amounts of payments for common research procedures.[8] Empirical research suggests that few IRBs have established systems for tracking payments across studies, resulting in payment amounts that may vary widely from study to study.[9] The lack of available guidance around appropriate payment levels is exacerbated by individual differences in the perceptions regarding the influence of a given financial incentive. Social science research suggests that even among individuals of similar socioeconomic status, the amount of a payment sufficient to influence decision-making varies widely from individual to individual.[10]

To address the lack of regulatory guidance regarding appropriate payments and to ensure consistency within their institutions, some IRBs have established payment schedules setting forth acceptable ranges for subject payments. These institutions have determined the amounts that may be paid to research subjects for study participation, including appropriate payment amounts for specific procedures. The amounts of payments under these schedules tend to increase as the procedures become more invasive, risky, and inconvenient for subjects.

11.2 Factors to Consider

A number of factors may be considered by IRBs tasked with approving subject payments. These factors will frequently be influenced by the intended purpose of the payment

[6] Scott Burris & Jen Welsh, *Regulatory Paradox: A Review of Enforcement Letters Issued by the Office for Human Research Protection*, 101 NW. U. L. REV. 643, 664 (2007).

[7] *See* Grady, Christine, *Payment of Clinical Research Subjects*, 115 J. CLIN. INVEST., 1681, 1681 (2005); Weise, Kathryn L., Smith, Martin L., et al, *National Practices Regarding Payment to Research Subjects for Participating in Pediatric Research*, 110 PEDIATRICS 577, 579 (2002); White, Tracie, *Just Another Lab Rat*, STANFORD MED. MAGAZINE (Summer 2008), *available at*: http://stanmed.stanford.edu/2008summer/just_another_lab_rat.html.

[8] *See, e.g.*, Dinora Dominguez *et al.*, *Commonly Performed Procedures in Clinical Research: A Benchmark for Payment*, 33 CONTEMP. CLINICAL TRIALS 860 (2012); Elizabeth Ripley *et al.*, *Why Do We Pay? A National Survey of Investigators and IRB Chairpersons*, 5 J. EMPIRICAL RES. ON HUM. RES. ETHICS 43, 54 (2010); Gail E. Henderson, *The Ethics of HIV "Cure" Research: What Can We Learn from Consent Forms?*, 31 AIDS RES. & HUM. RETROVIRUSES 56, 60 (2015).

[9] Weise, Kathryn L., Smith, Martin L., et al, *National Practices Regarding Payment to Research Subjects for Participating in Pediatric Research*, 110 PEDIATRICS 577, 580 (2002).

[10] Grady, *supra* note 7, at 1683-84.

as reimbursement for costs, an incentive to encourage participation, a token of appreciation, compensation for the subject's time and inconvenience, or a combination of these factors. For example, some IRBs have determined that only payments intended to offset the costs of clinical trial participation are acceptable.[11] These IRBs take the position that the purpose of subject compensation is simply to make the subject's participation in research revenue-neutral, eliminating a barrier that may prevent many, especially lower-income individuals, from participating in research.[12] Under these circumstances, payments should approximate the costs of a subject's participation. This may include only direct, out-of-pocket costs, such as parking, transportation and meals, or may include other costs such as lost income from time away from work and child care costs arising from research participation. Payments intended to reimburse subjects for direct costs incurred in connection with their participation in a clinical trial are widely accepted by IRBs as appropriate.[13]

Other IRBs take the position that subjects should be compensated for their contribution to the clinical trial and treat subjects as independent contractors who should be compensated for their services.[14] These IRBs may determine the appropriateness of the compensation as a factor of the prevailing wage in the area or as a multiple of the minimum wage. Still other IRBs utilize a market model, basing compensation levels on the amounts necessary to incentivize participation in the research.[15]

Depending upon the views of the IRB, the factors that may be considered in determining whether a given payment is appropriate may include the following:

- **Costs of participation.** The out-of-pocket expenses attributable to participation in the research, are frequently a primary consideration when determining the appropriateness of a payment. These may include parking and transportation costs, costs of meals if study visits are lengthy, and even overnight stays, if necessary. IRBs may also consider lost income, childcare expenses, and other costs directly related to the subject's participation in the study. Where the intent of the payment is solely reimbursement, this may be the only factor considered by the IRB.
- **Time commitment.** The amount of time required for study participation is often a factor in the amount subjects should be paid for their participation. The time required is relevant both in terms of the subject's lost income and, if the intent of the IRB is to compensate subjects for their services, as a means of quantifying the value of the services provided.

---

[11] *Id.* at 1685.

[12] *Id.*

[13] Emily Largent and Holly Fernandez Lynch, *Paying Research Participants: Regulatory Uncertainty, Conceptual Confusion, and a Path Forward*, 17 YALE J. HEALTH POL'Y L. & ETHICS 61, 75 (2017); *see also* Ezekiel J. Emanuel *et al.*, *What Makes Clinical Research Ethical?* 283 JAMA 2701, 2706 (2000).

[14] Grady, *supra* note 7, at 1685.

[15] *Id.*

- **Inconvenience.** Related to the amount of time required for participation is the amount of inconvenience suffered by subjects as a result of study participation. This may include overnight stays, frequent study visits, fasting requirements, preparations for procedures, diary completion and other information gathering tasks, and specimen collection requirements such as 24-hour urine collection. While difficult to quantify, inconvenience is often a factor to be considered, particularly when the intent of the payment is as an incentive for subjects to participate.[16]
- **Discomfort.** Where study procedures may cause subjects to experience discomfort, this fact frequently bears on the amount of the payment provided. More invasive and uncomfortable procedures are likely to result in increased payments, especially when the payment is intended to encourage participation.[17]
- **Degree of risk.** Particularly where the payment is a recruitment incentive, the degree of risk may be considered by the IRB in determining whether the payment is appropriate. ***A note of caution:*** Regulations and ethical imperatives demand that payments must not exert undue influence on research subjects.[18] Thus, payments should not be large enough to cause a subject to accept risks of study participation if he or she would not have accepted those risks absent the payment. Empirical research suggests that some IRBs require a decrease in payment amounts for studies involving greater risk.[19] This may result from concern that the potential harm to subjects requires greater caution to assure that the amount of payment does not cause a subject to participate where he or she might not have without the payment.
- **Potential benefit.** Some IRBs report decreasing subject payment amounts for studies in which subjects are more likely to experience clinical benefit from participation.[20] If the intent of the payment is to encourage enrollment, it stands to reason that lower payments may be sufficient where subjects' decisions to participate arise from self-interested desire to benefit from the research. In addition, FDA Information Sheets expressly state that, "Financial incentives are often used when health benefits to subjects are remote or non-existent."[21] Commentators have argued, however, that the ethical considerations are greatly reduced where subjects stand to benefit from participation in research.[22] In these instances, there is little

[16] Elizabeth Ripley *et al.*, *Why Do We Pay? A National Survey of Investigators and IRB Chairpersons*, 5 J. Empirical Res. on Hum. Res. Ethics 43, 54 (2010).

[17] Laura B. Dunn & Nora E. Gordon, *Improving Informed Consent and Enhancing Recruitment for Research by Understanding Economic Behavior*, 293 JAMA 609 (2005).

[18] *See, e.g.*, 21 C.F.R. § 50.20; 45 C.F.R. § 116(a). *See also* OHRP IRB Guidebook, Chapter 3: OHRP Informed Consent Frequently Asked Questions #6–10, OHRP, *available at* http://wayback.archive-it.org/org-745/20150930182812/http://www.hhs.gov/ohrp/archive/irb/irb_chapter3.htm.

[19] Weise, *supra* note 9, at 579.

[20] *Id.*

[21] *FDA Information Sheet: Payment to Research Subjects.*

[22] Grady, *supra* note 7, at 1681.

risk that a payment will encourage participation of a subject who is likely to benefit from the study.

11.3 Types and Method of Payment

In addition to considering whether the amount of a payment is appropriate, IRBs must consider whether the type and method of payment may unduly influence subjects' decisions to participate in the research. Most frequently, payments to research subjects consist of monetary compensation. In other instances, cash equivalents such as gift cards may be provided. Particularly in the context of pediatric research, savings bonds may also be provided as compensation to research subjects. Regardless of the form of payment, IRBs should be aware that payments to research subjects may represent reportable income.

Regulations of the Internal Revenue Service (IRS) require that any compensation to an individual by an institution in excess of $600 in any calendar year must be reported to the IRS as miscellaneous income.[23] Payments must be recorded at the time they are made and if the $600 threshold is reached, must be reported on IRS Form 1099.[24] As a result, many institutions require the collection of necessary demographic information, including social security numbers, for any subject who will receive a payment in connection with a research study. It is advisable that the consent form contain appropriate disclosures regarding the potential for reporting of study payments to the IRS, and permits subjects to waive payments at their option.

To avoid tax consequences and for other reasons, some institutions permit only small gifts and other items of minimal value to be given to research subjects. The intent of these items, such as t-shirts, coffee mugs, toys or videos for subjects who are children, and other items may be as a token of appreciation for the subject's participation. IRBs that generally approve only payments to reimburse subjects for out-of-pocket expenses may, however, make exceptions for these items. ***A note of caution:*** Where the research is regulated by FDA, subjects may not be compensated with coupons or vouchers for the investigational product once it is approved.[25]

11.4 Timing of Payment

FDA regulations require that the IRB consider at the time of initial review "both the amount of payment and the proposed method and timing of disbursement to assure that neither are coercive nor present undue influence."[26] *FDA Information Sheets: Payments to Research Subjects* provides specific guidance regarding the timing of payments to research subjects. This guidance states:

---

[23] I.R.C. § 6041, *codified at* 26 U.S.C. § 6041.

[24] 2018 Instructions for Form1099-MISC (Oct. 12, 2017), U.S. Dept. of the Treasury, IRS, *available at:* https://www.irs.gov/pub/irs-pdf/i1099msc.pdf.

[25] FDA Institutional Review Boards Frequently Asked Questions—Information Sheet, Question #50, FDA (Jan. 25, 2016), *available at* https://www.fda.gov/RegulatoryInformation/Guidances/ucm126420.htm#IRBOrg.

[26] *FDA Information Sheets: Payment to Research Subjects*; 21 C.F.R. § 50.20.

> Any credit for payment should accrue as the study progresses and not be contingent upon the subject completing the entire study. Unless it creates undue inconvenience or a coercive practice, payment to subjects who withdraw from the study may be made at the time they would have completed the study (or completed a phase of the study) had they not withdrawn. For example, in a study lasting only a few days, an IRB may find it permissible to allow a single payment date at the end of the study, even to subjects who had withdrawn before that date.[27]

In order to avoid undue influence over subjects' decisions to continue participation in a study once they are enrolled, prorated payments, such as payments for all completed study visits or all study procedures for which a subject would have been compensated if he or she completed the trial, should be made, regardless of the reasons for the subject's withdrawal.

The FDA guidance also addresses the propriety of bonus payments for study completion, providing:

> While the entire payment should not be contingent upon completion of the entire study, payment of a small proportion as an incentive for completion of the study is acceptable to FDA, providing that such incentive is not coercive. The IRB should determine that the amount paid as a bonus for completion is reasonable and not so large as to unduly induce subjects to stay in the study when they would otherwise have withdrawn. All information concerning payment, including the amount and schedule of payment(s), should be set forth in the informed consent document.[28]

Similarly, OHRP guidance provides that, "in studies of considerable duration or that involve multiple interactions or interventions . . . payment [should] be prorated for the time of participation in the study rather than delayed until study completion, because the latter could unduly influence a subject's decision to exercise his or her right to withdraw at any time."[29] This guidance goes on to state, as an example, that for a study lasting for six months, there might be monthly or bi-monthly payments.[30]

11.5 Children and Minors

The same considerations regarding payment to adults apply to children; however, the analysis when children are involved is somewhat more complicated. Children may be more susceptible to influence by offers of payment or other forms of remuneration depending on age, maturity, and life experiences. Children are less likely to be able to perform a meaningful evaluation of the risks and benefits when offered payment or some other form of remuneration. Payment may be made to the parents instead, as reimbursement for expenses associated with

---

[27] *FDA Information Sheets: Payment to Research Subjects.*

[28] *Id.*

[29] *OHRP Informed Consent Frequently Asked Questions*, #7.

[30] *Id.*

participation in the trial; however, some even caution against this. The American Academy of Pediatrics takes the position that "serious ethical questions arise when payment is offered to adults acting on behalf of minors in return for allowing minors to participate as research subjects."[31] A possible compromise might consist of offering the parents some compensation to offset expenses associated with the trial and by providing the child with some small token gesture of appreciation.[32] Regardless, consent must always be obtained in accordance with the regulations concerning parental consent and assent of the child.[33]

11.6 Incapacitated Subjects

Others also may be vulnerable and unable to make informed decisions about enrollment in research, much less have the ability to accept payment for participation. As with children, the same concerns exist when the individual consenting is not the study subject. Consent should be obtained only under circumstances in which the legal representative has been provided with sufficient opportunity to consider whether the subject should participate, and only under circumstances in which the possibility of coercion or undue influence has been minimized.[34]

11.7 Non-Resident Aliens

Providing payments to non-resident alien subjects as compensation for research participation may present additional challenges. Federal tax laws impose tax withholding requirements for persons who are not U.S. citizens, which will result in reduced payment amounts for these subjects.[35] Some institutions exclude non-residents aliens from study participation for this reason. If it is anticipated that non-resident aliens may participate in the study, the consent form should disclose the information that will be collected, the fact that information may be reported to the IRS, and the requirement to withhold taxes from payments. Institutions may wish to permit potential subjects to forgo payments at their option to avoid applicable tax implications.

[31] *Guidelines for the Ethical Conduct of Studies to Evaluate Drugs in Pediatric Populations*, American Academy of Pediatrics Committee on Drugs, 95 Pediatrics 286 (Feb. 1995), *available at* http://pediatrics.aappublications.org/content/pediatrics/95/2/286.full.pdf.

[32] Amdur, Robert and Bankert, Elizabeth, Institutional Review Board Member Handbook, 2d. ed., Jones and Bartlett, 111 (2007).

[33] 45 C.F.R. § 46.408(a); 21 C.F.R. § 50.55.

[34] 45 C.F.R. § 46.116; 21 C.F.R. § 50.20.

[35] *See* General Revisions of Regulations Relating to Withholding of Tax on Certain U.S. Source Income Paid to Foreign Persons and Related Collection, Refunds and Credits; Revision of Information Reporting and Backup Withholding Regulations; and Removal of Regulations Under Part 35a and of Certain Regulations Under Income Tax Treaties, T.D. 8734, I.R.B. 1997-44, 5, IRS (Nov. 3, 1997), *available at* https://www.irs.gov/pub/irs-irbs/irb97-44.pdf.

Chapter 12

Conflict of Interest Issues

Dale H. Cowan

Introduction

Conflicts of Interest (COIs) may arise in three different settings: 1) the activities and judgments of members of Institutional Review Boards (IRBs); 2) the activities of investigators submitting proposals for research involving human subjects; or 3) the relationships of institutions that establish, control, and monitor IRBs and the research conducted by members of their staff.

12.1 Conflicts of Interest Defined

A conflict of interest (COI) has been defined as "a set of conditions in which professional judgment concerning a primary interest (such as a patient's welfare or the validity of research) tends to be unduly influenced by a secondary interest (such as financial gain).[1] COIs represent the potential for biased judgment, but they are not an indicator of the likelihood or certainty that such judgments or compromises will occur.[2] The Committee on Conflict of Interest in Medical Research, Education, and Practice—appointed in 2007 by the Institute of Medicine (IOM) (now the National Academy of Medicine)—defines conflicts of interest as "a set of circumstances that creates a risk that professional judgment or actions regarding a primary interest will be unduly influenced by a secondary interest."[3] Primary interests include promoting and protecting the integrity of research, the quality of medical education, and the welfare of patients.[4] Secondary interests include financial interests as well as other interests such as publication pressure, prestige, scientific reputation, and career advancement.[5] It is relevant to note that COIs are ubiquitous, denote a state of affairs, and do not indicate the occurrence of any improper behavior or scientific misconduct.[6]

---

[1] Dennis F. Thompson, *Understanding Financial Conflicts of Interest*, 329 NEW ENG. J. MED. 573 (1993).

[2] CD DeAngelis et al., *Reporting Financial Conflicts of Interest and Relationships Between Investigators and Research Sponsors,* 286(1) J. AM. MED. ASSOC. 89 (2001).

[3] COMM. ON CONFLICT OF INTEREST IN MED., RESEARCH, EDUC., & PRACTICE, INST. OF MED., CONFLICT OF INTEREST IN MEDICAL RESEARCH, EDUCATION, AND PRACTICE, CH.2 (Bernard Lo & Marilyn J. Field eds., 2009) [hereafter *Inst. of Med. COI*], *available at* https://www.ncbi.nlm.nih.gov/books/NBK22937/.

[4] *Id.*

[5] R. Horton, *Conflicts of Interest in Clinical Research: Opprobrium or Obsession?*, 349 LANCET 1112 (1997).

[6] J.J. Cohen, *Trust Us to Make A Difference: Ensuring Public Confidence in the Integrity of Clinical Research,* 76(2) ACAD. MED. 209 (2009).

12.2 Regulations and Policies Affecting Activities and Judgments of Members of IRBs

Regulations issued by the Department of Health and Human Services (HHS) that delineate the organization, management, and operation of IRBs include a section that addresses the requirements for IRB membership at 45 C.F.R. § 46.107. Sub-paragraph (e) of those requirements states "No IRB may have a member participate in the IRB's initial or continuing review of any project in which the member has a conflicting interest, except to provide information requested by the IRB."[7] This requirement, which was included in the 2018 Common Rule issued on January 17, 2017,[8] applies to all research involving human subjects conducted or sponsored by more than 15 federal agencies that have signed on to the 2018 Common Rule. Identical language is included in regulations issued by the Federal Food and Drug Administration (FDA) at 21 C.F.R. 56.107(e).[9]

Published studies have shown that IRBs vary greatly in their policies and practices with regard to COIs of their members who review and approve research protocols.[10] This is due to the fact that HHS policy ". . . provides no standards on what constitutes a meaningful COI, nor does it suggest policies and procedures to protect IRB-related activities from conflicts."[11] For example, there is no specification, with respect to financial conflicts, that denotes the dollar amount that creates a potential conflict, or to whom a conflict should be reported. The options for reporting include reporting to the IRB Chair or reporting to an independent committee established by the institution for the express purpose of monitoring COIs.

Individual institutions can adopt policies that provide guidance for identifying and reporting COIs. The simplest and least helpful policies are those that merely restate the regulations issued by HHS. An example of a more detailed policy is that of The Cleveland Clinic Foundation (CCF) in Cleveland, OH, which states in relevant part:

> IRB members are responsible to inform the IRB Chair of any conflicts and cannot participate in the review of projects involving their conflicting interest. Any member who has a conflict of interest is not allowed to vote and is required to leave the room during discussion unless requested by the IRB Chair to provide information during the discussion phase only. An abstaining member with a conflict of interest does not count toward quorum and will be recorded in the meeting minutes.
>
> IRB members annually disclose and update as necessary conflict of interest relationships with the COI Administrator in compliance with the CCF Conflict of

[7] 45 C.F.R. § 46.107(e) (2017).

[8] At the time of publication, the effective date of the Revised Common Rule is January 21, 2019. Research commenced before that date will be regulated under the pre-2018 Common Rule unless the institutional review board overseeing the research decides to apply the Revised Common Rule. Research starting after January 21, 2019 will be regulated under the 2018 Common Rule. 83 Fed. Reg. 28497 (Jun. 19, 2018).

[9] 21 C.F.R. § 56.107(e) (2017).

[10] C. Vogeli et al., *Policies and Management of Conflicts of Interest within Medical Research Institutional Review Boards: Result of a National Study*, 84(4) ACAD. MED. 488 (2009).

[11] *Id.*

Interest Policy. IRB members must reveal any real or potential financial or non-financial conflict of interest to the IRB Chair prior to the review of research including studies, unanticipated problems or non-compliance at convened meetings and abstain from review if conflicted. Members conducting expedited review are also required to abstain from review of any project in which they are conflicted.

IRB members must declare if they or any immediate family member (spouse and dependent children) have any personal financial conflicts of interest with the study, investigator, or sponsor including involvement in the design, conduct, products, or services being tested or reporting of the research prior to any discussion...The threshold of a conflict of interest is at least as stringent as the level of a researcher conflict of interest.[12]

When adopting policies regarding COIs, it is important, particularly with respect to financial COIs, for institutions to identify specific thresholds (*e.g.*, dollar amounts) that trigger disclosure of the COI.

12.3 Regulations and Policies Affecting Investigators Submitting Proposals for Research Involving Human Subjects

On May 12, 2004, HHS released its *Final Guidance Document on Conflict of Interest*,[13] which applies to human subjects research conducted or supported by HHS or regulated by FDA. *The Final Guidance* states:

> "The Department recommends that in particular, IRBs, institutions, and investigators consider whether specific financial relationships create financial interests in research studies that may adversely affect the rights and welfare of subjects. These entities may find it useful to include the following questions in their deliberations:
>
> - What financial relationships and resulting financial interests could cause potential or actual conflicts of interest?
> - At what levels should those potential or actual financial conflicts of interest be managed or eliminated?
> - What procedures would be helpful, including those to
>   - collect and evaluate information regarding financial relationships related to research,
>   - determine whether those relationships potentially cause a conflict of interest, and

[12] Permission for use granted by The Cleveland Clinic Foundation per communication from Bridget C. Howard, JD, Executive Director, IRB, The Cleveland Clinic Foundation.

[13] 69 Fed. Reg. 26393, 26395 (2004); *see also* U.S. DEP'T OF HEALTH AND HUMAN SERVS., FINANCIAL CONFLICT OF INTEREST: HHS GUIDANCE (2004) (May 5, 2004) [hereafter *HHS COI Guidance*], *available at* https://www.hhs.gov/ohrp/regulations-and-policy/guidance/financial-conflict-of-interest/index.html.

  - determine what actions are necessary to protect human subjects and ensure that those actions are taken?
- Who should be educated regarding financial conflict of interest issues and policies?
- What entity or entities would examine individual and/or institutional financial relationships and interests?[14]

A variety of methods or combinations thereof may be effective in managing or eliminating COIs.

> In establishing and implementing methods to protect the rights and welfare of human subjects from conflicts of interest created by financial relationships of parties involved in research, the Department recommends that IRBs, institutions engaged in research, and investigators consider the [following] questions:
>
> - Does the research involve financial relationships that could create potential or actual conflicts of interest?
>   - How is the research supported and financed?
>   - Where and by whom was the study designed?
>   - Where and by whom will the resulting data be analyzed?
> - What interests are created by the financial relationships involved in the situation?
> - Do individuals or institutions receive any compensation that may be affected by the study outcome?
> - Do individuals or institutions involved in the research:
>   - have any proprietary interests in the product, including patents, trademarks, copyrights, or licensing agreements?
>   - have an equity interest in the research sponsor and, if so, is the sponsor a publicly held company or non-publicly held company?
>   - receive significant payments of other sorts? (*e.g.*, grants, compensation in the form of equipment, retainers for ongoing consultation, or honoraria)
>   - receive payment per participant or incentive payments, and are those payments reasonable?
> - Given the financial relationships involved, is the institution an appropriate site for the research?
> - How should financial relationships that potentially create a conflict of interest be managed?
> - Would the rights and welfare of any human subjects be better protected by any or a combination of the following:
>   - reduction of the financial interest?
>   - disclosure of the financial interest to prospective subjects?

[14] *HHS COI Guidance.*

- separation of responsibilities for financial decisions and research decisions?
- additional oversight or monitoring of the research?
- an independent data and safety monitoring committee or similar monitoring body?
- modification of role(s) of particular research staff or changes in location for certain research activities, *e.g.*, a change of the person who seeks consent, or a change of investigator?
- elimination of the financial interest?[15]

12.4 Regulations and Policies Affecting Institutions that Establish, Control, and Monitor IRBs and the Research Conducted by Members of Their Staff

In addition to members of IRBs and investigators, institutions may have relationships that can be the source of conflicts of interest. In recognition of this, HHS, in its *Financial Conflict of Interest: HHS Guidance* (2004)[16] stated that:

> institutions engaged in HHS conducted or supported human subjects research consider whether the following actions or other actions would help ensure that financial interests do not compromise the rights and welfare of human research subjects.
>
> Actions to consider:
>
> - Establishing the independence of institutional responsibility for research activities from the management of the institution's financial interests.
> - Establishing conflict of interest committees (COICs) or identifying other bodies or persons and procedures to
>   - deal with individuals' or institutional financial interests in research or verify the absence of such interests and
>   - address institutional financial interests in research.
> - Establishing criteria to determine what constitutes an institutional conflict of interest, including identifying leadership positions for which the individual's financial interests are such that they may need to be treated as institutional financial interests.
> - Establishing clear channels of communication between COICs and IRBs.
> - Establishing policies on providing information, recommendations, or findings from COIC deliberations to IRBs.
> - Establishing measures to foster independence of IRBs and COICs.
> - Determining whether particular individuals should report financial interests to the COIC. These individuals could include IRB members and staff and appropriate officials of the institution, along with investigators, among those who report financial interests to COICs.

---

[15] *Id.*

[16] *Id.*

- Establishing procedures for disclosure of institutional financial relationships to COICs.
- Providing training to appropriate individuals regarding financial interest requirements.
- Using independent organizations to hold or administer the institution's financial interest.
- Including individuals from outside the institution in the review and oversight of financial interests in research.
- Establishing policies regarding the types of financial relationships that may be held by parties involved in the research and circumstances under which those financial relationships and interests may or may not be held."[17]

Additional actions to consider include:

- Regarding IRB review, "determining the kind, amount, and level of detail of information to be provided to research subjects regarding funding and financial interests"[18]
- Regarding the investigator, "using special measures to modify the informed consent process when a potential or actual financial conflict exists."[19]

A report from the COIC about whether a conflict exists can be made to the IRB without the IRB receiving details that might prejudice its review of any proposed research.

In its report on *Conflict of Interest in Medical Research, Education, and Practice*, the IOM made several specific recommendations in line with the 2004 Guidance issued by the HHS.[20] Recommendations relevant to this discussion are:

- To manage identified conflicts of interest and monitor implementation of management recommendations, institutions should create a conflict of interest committee.
- As part of their conflict of interest policies, institutions should require individuals covered by their policies, including senior institutional officials, to disclose financial relationships with pharmaceutical, medical device, and biotechnology companies to the institution on an annual basis and when an individual's situation changes significantly.

Other recommendations pertain to educating faculty, students, residents, and fellows regarding conflict of interest issues, and convening a broad-based consensus development process to establish a standard content, format, and procedures for the disclosure of financial relationships with industry.

---

[17] *Id.*

[18] *Id.*

[19] *Id.*

[20] *Inst. of Med. COI*; *HHS COI Guidance*.

Chapter 13

Billing for Clinical Trial Services: General Overview

Eve Brunts

Introduction

Health care providers who participate in human subjects research typically need to assess payment for clinical trial services by research sponsors and third party payers in order to ensure that: (i) from a human subjects protection perspective, a subject participating in clinical trials is aware of the clinical trial costs that he or she will incur; (ii) from a financial perspective, there is adequate compensation for any clinical trial services provided; and (iii) from a billing compliance perspective, clinical trial services are billed to third party payers, sponsors, and subjects only if appropriate. Responsibility for the costs of all clinical trial services should ideally be determined prior to the start of the clinical trial, and allocation of that responsibility should be documented consistently in the clinical trial agreement and informed consent documents as well as communicated internally to personnel involved in both research and billing of clinical trial services.

Informed consent documents must address what additional costs the subjects may incur if they participate in the clinical trial. The informed consent process and documents should also address with regularity the clinical trial services that will be paid for by the sponsor, covered by insurance, and services that must be paid for by the subject (if any), including responsibility for payment for services necessary to diagnosis or treat a research-related injury. Institutional Review Boards (IRBs), as part of the review of informed consent documents, may be expected to ensure those portions of the consent form are accurate and do not raise potential compliance concerns.

13.1 Basic Coverage Principles

Research sponsors do not always offer to pay for all clinical services. Sponsors may, for example, decline to pay for services that might be covered by third party payers as medically necessary services if provided outside the clinical trial. Once an individual enrolls in a clinical trial, however, coverage for services provided as part of the clinical trial, even if those services are generally considered medically necessary, may be limited. Understanding applicable coverage principles allows health care providers to evaluate whether all clinical trial services are likely covered by either the sponsor or a third party payer.

Some basic principles generally apply to coverage clinical trial services across third party payers:

- A health care provider should not bill a third party payer for any items or services for which the sponsor has agreed to pay;
- A health care provider should not bill a third party payer for any items provided free of charge by the sponsor, such as drugs and devices;
- A health care provider should bill a third party payer only for services that are medically necessary to diagnose or treat a patient's condition; and
- A health care provider may not bill a third party payer for any items which the informed consent documents indicate are being provided at no cost to the subject.

Specific coverage standards for clinical trial services by third party payers such as Medicare, Medicaid, and private health plans vary.

13.2 Medicare

Different Medicare coverage principles apply to different types of clinical trials: (i) clinical trials covered under Medicare Clinical Trial Policy; (ii) clinical trials covered under the investigational device exemption (IDE) regulations; and (iii) all other clinical trials. Special coding requirements also apply to clinical trial services covered under the Medicare Clinical Trial Policy or IDE regulations.

13.2.1 Medicare Clinical Trial Policy

Medicare Clinical Trial Policy[1] mandates coverage of the "routine costs" of "qualifying clinical trials." These defined terms establish the scope of coverage under the Medicare Clinical Trial Policy.

A "qualifying clinical trial" must meet four criteria.

- The purpose of the trial must be the evaluation of an item or service that falls within a Medicare benefit category (*e.g.*, physician services, durable medical equipment, diagnostic tests) and is not statutorily excluded from coverage (*e.g.*, cosmetic surgery, hearing aids).

[1] For the current Medicare Clinical Trial Policy (Medicare National Coverage Determinations (NCD) Manual, § 310.1) and related information, *see* CMS, Medicare Clinical Trial Policies, *available at*, https://www.cms.gov/Medicare/Coverage/ClinicalTrialPolicies/index.html?redirect=/ClinicalTrialPolicies/ (last visited June 28, 2018).

- The trial must have a therapeutic intent (*i.e.*, the trial must assess the effect of the intervention on patient outcome) and not be designed exclusively to test toxicity or disease pathophysiology.
- Trials of therapeutic interventions must enroll patients with a diagnosed disease rather than healthy volunteers. Trials of diagnostic interventions, however, may enroll healthy patients in order to have a proper control group.
- The trial must either have certain desirable characteristics or be "deemed" to have those desirable characteristics. Qualifying clinical trials "deemed" to have desirable characteristics include trials that: (i) are funded by federal agencies such as the National Institutes of Health (NIH) or are supported by centers or cooperative groups that are funded by those federal agencies;[2] or (ii) are conducted under an investigational new drug application (IND) or are exempt from having an IND.[3] Currently, only clinical trials "deemed" to have desirable characteristics may be qualifying clinical trials as the Centers for Medicare and Medicaid Services (CMS) has yet to implement a mechanism for determining whether other clinical trials have desirable characteristics.

If a clinical trial is a qualifying clinical trial, Medicare will cover the "routine costs" of that clinical trial. Routine costs expressly include:

- items and services typically provided absent a clinical trial (*e.g.*, standard of care);
- items and services required solely for the provision of the investigational item or service (*e.g.*, administration of a non-covered chemotherapeutic agent);
- items and services required for the clinically appropriate monitoring of the effects of the item or service, or the prevention of complications; and
- items and services needed for reasonable and necessary care arising from the provision of the investigational item or service, particularly the diagnosis and treatment of complications.

Routine costs expressly exclude:

- the investigational item or service itself, unless the item or service is otherwise covered outside a clinical trial;
- items and services provided solely to satisfy data collection and analysis needs and that are not used in the direct clinical management of the patient (*e.g.*, monthly computed tomography scans for a condition usually requiring only a single scan); and

---

[2] Those federal agencies are: NIH, Centers for Disease Control and Prevention (CDC), Agency for Healthcare Research and Quality (AHRQ), Centers for Medicare & Medicaid Services (CMS), Department of Defense (DOD), and Department of Veterans Affairs (VA).

[3] *See* 21 C.F.R. § 312.2.

- items and services customarily provided by the research sponsors free of charge for any enrollee in the trial.

Under the Medicare Clinical Trial Policy (Policy), Medicare will also pay for items and services that are medically necessary for the diagnosis or treatment of complications arising from the provision of an investigational item or service, regardless of whether the clinical trial giving rise to the complication is a qualifying clinical trial. The Policy addresses coverage with evidence development; more specifically, the Policy acknowledges that CMS may, through the National Coverage Determination (NCD) process, provide coverage for items and services in a clinical trial for which there is some evidence of significant medical benefit, but the evidence is insufficient to support a medical necessity determination.

13.2.2 Investigational Device Exemption (IDE) Studies

Medicare limits coverage of medical devices investigated in clinical trials and/or services associated with the use of such devices if those devices have not yet been approved by the Food and Drug Administration (FDA) for marketing on the ground that the safety and efficacy of the devices have not been proven.[4] Medicare may, however, cover certain investigational devices and/or associated services if the devices are used in a clinical trial under an IDE and the clinical trial has been approved by the CMS. Medicare coverage depends in part on the category of the device as determined by the FDA. The FDA will categorize the device as Category A or Category B when issuing an IDE to the research sponsor.[5]

Category A (experimental) devices are those devices "for which 'absolute risk' . . . has not been established (that is, initial questions of safety and effectiveness have not been resolved) and the FDA is unsure whether the device type can be safe and effective."[6] Category A devices are not eligible for Medicare coverage. Medicare, however, covers routine care services furnished in an FDA-approved Category A IDE clinical trial as long as CMS determines that the Medicare coverage criteria are met.[7]

Category B (non-experimental/investigational) devices are those devices for which "initial questions of safety and effectiveness of that device type have been resolved" or "it is known that the device type can be safe and effective because, for example, other manufacturers have

---

[4] *See* 42 U.S.C. § 1395y(m); 42 C.F.R. §§ 405.201–405.215; 42 C.F.R. § 411.15(o); and Medicare Benefit Policy Manual, ch. 14 (Medical Devices), *available at* https://www.cms.gov/Regulations-and-Guidance/Guidance/Manuals/Internet-Only-Manuals-IOMs-Items/CMS012673.html.

[5] An IDE from the FDA is required to undertake a clinical investigation of a medical device that has not yet been approved or cleared for marketing. An IDE may or may not be required to investigate a medical device that is already on the market. If an IDE is issued, the coverage principles for Category A and Category B devices apply, depending on the categorization. If an IDE from the FDA is not required (*i.e.*, because the medical device under investigation is a non-significant risk device), Medicare Administrative contractors apply the same coverage principles, where appropriate, as are applied to Category A and Category B devices. Medicare Benefit Policy Manual, ch. 14 § 30.

[6] 42 C.F.R. § 405.201(b).

[7] *Id.* § 405.211.

obtained FDA approval with clearance for that device type."[8] Category B devices are eligible for Medicare coverage.[9] Medicare covers a Category B IDE device and routine care items and services furnished in an FDA-approved Category B IDE clinical trial as long as CMS determines that the relevant Medicare coverage criteria are met.[10]

Providers or sponsors seeking Medicare coverage for either Category A or Category B IDE clinical trials must submit a request packet to CMS that includes a request letter that describes the scope and nature of the IDE clinical trial including how the clinical trial meets the Medicare coverage IDE clinical trial criteria as well as supporting documentation such as the protocol.[11] A listing of all CMS-approved Category A and B IDE clinical trials are posted on the CMS website and published in the Federal Register.[12] Approval covers the IDE clinical trial, so each health care provider participating in the clinical trial and submitting claims does not need to obtain separate approval.

13.2.3 Other Clinical Trials

Coverage for services provided in clinical trials that do not fall within the scope of the Clinical Trials NCD or the IDE regulations will depend on local Medicare contractors' discretion (subject to Medicare general coverage principles).

13.3 Medicaid

Medicaid coverage of clinical trial services is not established by CMS, but is instead determined by each state. Coverage may therefore vary across state Medicaid programs. States may limit coverage of "experimental" or "investigational" or "research" services on the grounds that the services are not medically necessary.[13] Those limits affect coverage of clinical trial services. Some state mandated benefit laws applicable to clinical trial services (and discussed below under **Section 13.4** Private Health Plans) may apply to Medicaid and provide for coverage of certain clinical trial services.[14] Limits may be contained in law, regulations, the state Medicaid plan approved by CMS, or administrative guidance and will be state specific.

---

[8] *Id.* § 405.201(b).

[9] *Id.* § 405.205.

[10] *Id.* § 405.207.

[11] *Id.* § 405.211; CMS, MLN Matters MM8921 (Jan. 1, 2015). Medicare coverage criteria address, for example, the purposes of the clinical trial, the design of the clinical trial, compliance with federal human subjects protection requirements, the dissemination of clinical trial results, and generalizability of results to the Medicare beneficiary population. *See* CMS, Approved IDE Studies [hereafter *Approved IDE Studies*], *available at* https://www.cms.gov/Medicare/Coverage/IDE/Approved-IDE-Studies.html (last visited June 28, 2018).

[12] *See* Approved IDE Studies.

[13] For example, the California Medicaid program does not cover "experimental" services. "Investigational services" may be covered under certain circumstances but only if the services are "not performed as part of a research study protocol" and there is a "reasonable expectation" of a medical benefit to the patient. Cal. Code Regs. tit. 22, § 51303.

[14] *See, e.g.*, Cal. Welf. & Inst. Code § 14132.98.

13.4 Private Health Plans

Coverage of clinical trial services by private health plans is determined by: (i) federal law mandating coverage of certain services; (ii) state laws mandating coverage of certain services (to the extent not preempted by Employee Retirement Income Security Act of 1974 (ERISA)[15] for self-funded employer health plans); and/or (iii) the decision of the health plan to offer additional benefits not mandated by law.

13.4.1 Federal Law

Federal law requires certain health plans to provide coverage of certain clinical trial services.[16] Specifically, health plans may not: (i) deny a "qualified individual" the right to participate in an "approved clinical trial;" (ii) deny, limit or impose conditions on the coverage of "routine patient costs" of items and services provided in connection with such a clinical trial; or (iii) discriminate against a "qualified individual" due to the individual's participation in such a clinical trial.

"Routine patient costs" is defined broadly to include all items and services that are typically covered for a qualified individual not in a clinical trial (consistent with the plan coverage), except the following:

- the investigational item, device, or service;
- items and services provided solely for data collection and analysis and not used in the patient's direct clinical management; and
- services that are clearly inconsistent with "widely accepted and established standards of care" for the diagnosis.[17]

The mandated coverage extends only to "qualified individuals," which covers individuals who are participants under the health plan and are eligible to participate in an "approved clinical trial" for the treatment of cancer or another life-threatening disease or condition as set forth in the trial protocol. In addition, a health care professional who is a participating provider in the health plan has determined that the individual's participation in the clinical trial is appropriate based on the clinical trial protocol and the individual's condition *or* the individual provides medical and scientific information that establishes that participation in the trial is appropriate based on the trial protocol and the individual's condition.

The mandated coverage also extends only to an "approved clinical trial," which is a Phase I-IV clinical trial aimed at preventing, detecting or treating cancer or another life-threatening

[15] 29 U.S.C. §§ 1001–1003.

[16] 42 U.S.C. § 300gg-8; *See* Dep't of Labor, FAQs About Affordable Care Act Implementation (Part XV), Q3 (Apr. 29, 2013), *available at* https://www.dol.gov/sites/default/files/ebsa/about-ebsa/our-activities/resource-center/faqs/aca-part-xv.pdf; CMS, The Ctr. for Consumer Info. & Ins. Oversight, Affordable Care Act Implementation FAQs-Set 15, *available at* https://www.cms.gov/CCIIO/Resources/Fact-Sheets-and-FAQs/aca_implementation_faqs15.html (last visited June 28, 2018).

[17] 42 U.S.C. § 300gg-8(a)(2)(B).

disease or condition (*i.e.*, a disease or condition from which death is probable if the course of the disease or condition is not interrupted). Such trial must be:

- funded or approved by certain federal agencies or departments specified in the law or conducted by cooperative groups/centers of those agencies and departments (*e.g.*, the Centers for Disease Control and Prevention, Agency for Healthcare Research and Quality, NIH, and CMS); or
- conducted under an IND that is reviewed by the FDA or a drug trial that is exempt from IND application requirements.

13.4.2 State Laws

Many states have mandated benefit laws that require health plans to cover services provided in certain clinical trials.[18] The scope of these laws varies, but the laws often address coverage of services in clinical trials involving treatments for cancer or other life-threatening diseases. The laws may also limit coverage to clinical trials that meet specific standards (*e.g.*, source of funding), including some laws that incorporate standards from the Medicare Clinical Trial Policy.

13.4.3 Health Plan

Coverage of clinical trial services will otherwise vary by health plan. General standards addressing coverage of medically necessary services or exclusion of experimental and investigational services may determine the scope of coverage. Some health plans, however, have adopted specific criteria for coverage of clinical trial services.[19]

13.5 Research-Related Injuries

General coverage principles may apply to the diagnosis and treatment of research-related injuries as those services are not part of a clinical trial. Such services may be treated instead as standard of care services subject to general medical necessity and other coverage principles. As noted above, the Medicare Clinical Trial Policy mandates coverage of services that are medically necessary for the diagnosis or treatment of complications arising from the provision of an investigational item or service.

A research sponsor's agreement to pay for research-related injury services may implicate Medicare coordination of benefit rules, known as Medicare secondary payer (MSP) rules. MSP

[18] For example, Maryland requires health plans to cover patient care costs (essentially the costs of treatments that would otherwise be covered if not provided in connection with a clinical trial) for clinical trials that involve treatment for cancer or any other life-threatening condition. The clinical trials must approved by NIH, an NIH cooperative group, FDA, the VA or the IRB of an institution in Maryland which has a multiple project assurance contract approved by the Office of Protection from Research Risks of the NIH. There must be no other clearly superior non-investigational treatment alternative and there is a reasonable expectation that the treatment will be at least as effective as the non-investigational alternative. Md. Code Ann., Ins. § 15-827.

[19] *See, e.g.*, Aetna, *Clinical Trials, Coverage of Routine Patient Care Costs*, Policy No. 0466 (eff. Aug. 3, 2001) (last visited June 28, 2018), *available at* http://www.aetna.com/cpb/medical/data/400_499/0466.html.

rules limit coverage for services to diagnose and treat research-related injuries that would otherwise be covered by Medicare. These MSP rules apply when both Medicare and another insurer are responsible for payment. The MSP rules apply to promises by a research sponsor to pay for subject injuries because CMS takes the position that a research sponsor making such a promise is a liability insurer subject to the MSP rules. Under the MSP rules, if a liability insurer has responsibility for the payment of a health care service, then the liability insurer must generally be billed before Medicare.[20] Medicare will only pay as a secondary payer even if the liability insurer has agreed to pay for services only if the services are not covered by Medicare.

Sponsors that assume responsibility for payment for research-related injuries may also have reporting obligations under MSP requirements. Liability insurers (which CMS has interpreted to include sponsors) that are responsible for paying for health care services on behalf of Medicare beneficiaries must report such payments to CMS or pay a penalty.[21]

IRBs should consider whether informed consent documents addressing research-related injuries include promises by the sponsor to pay for services if Medicare and other third party payers do not pay. Any such proposed language should be carefully reviewed by legal counsel.

13.6 Cost-Shares

When clinical trial services are covered by third party payers, subjects may still have cost-share obligations (*e.g.*, copayments, deductibles, and coinsurance). If so, IRBs should ensure that informed consent documents are clear that subjects retain this payment responsibility.

Payment by sponsors of cost-sharing obligations or the waiver of cost-sharing obligations by clinical sites can raise potential compliance concerns under fraud and abuse laws. When such actions involve federal health care program beneficiaries, such actions could be perceived as inducements to subjects to obtain the services. Any such proposed payments or waivers should be carefully reviewed by legal counsel.

---

[20] 42 U.S.C. § 1395y(b)(2)(A); 42 C.F.R. §§ 411.20–411.39.

[21] 42.U.S.C. § 1395y(b)(8); Dep't Health & Human Services & Centers for Medicare & Medicaid Services, MMSEA Section 111 Medicare Secondary Payer Mandatory Reporting, Liability Insurance (Including Self-Insurance), No-Fault Insurance, and Workers' Compensation User Guide, Ch. III: Policy Guidance, § 6.5 (ver. 5.3 Dec. 15, 2017) (last visited June 28, 2018), *available at* https://www.cms.gov/Medicare/Coordination-of-Benefits-and-Recovery/Mandatory-Insurer-Reporting-For-Non-Group-Health-Plans/Downloads/New-Downloads/NGHPUserGuideVer53Ch3Policy.pdf.

Chapter 14

Use of Biospecimens an
Research and Research

Gabrielle Goldstein

Michele R. Goodman

Alice K. Marcee

Introduction

Human biospecimens and private information are of increasing importance to the research community. Researchers, health care institutions, and institutional review boards (IRBs) are encountering research studies involving these materials with mounting frequency. This reflects shifts in the broader research environment. New and innovative technologies and leaps in computational power have changed the magnitude of how information and biospecimens are collected and used for research purposes. "Big data" initiatives and sophisticated analytics are the keys to personalized medicine, and these require access to large sets of health data and biospecimens.

Studies using these materials often do not involve direct interaction with research participants; instead, researchers access and analyze information from medical records, claims data, and biospecimens collected and stored for diagnostic or research purposes. The risks to participants posed by these sorts of research projects are different than in more traditional, interventional research. This is because risks in data and biospecimen studies are largely informational, rather than physical. In other words, the principal harms that could arise in the context of these studies are often in relation to the inappropriate release or use of information, rather than risks posed by direct intervention. At the same time, public expectations are shifting towards a more participatory paradigm, in which research participants are actively involved in research design and conduct, and want to be informed about and asked for their permission when their materials are used in research.

These developments in research design, capacity, and public expectations create challenges and opportunities for IRBs. IRBs and research institutions must balance the expectations and desires of participants with those of researchers. Regulators have taken these changes into account, resulting in updates referred to as the 2018 Common Rule that address the use of biospecimens and data in research. In accordance with these regulations, the analysis that IRBs [redacted] and biospecimen studies often hinges on the *identifiability* [redacted] stored, and used in research.

[redacted] Sections below, IRBs will continue to play a key role in ensuring that [redacted] confidentiality safeguards are in place for research involving biospeci- [redacted] information. However, regulators have recognized that IRBs may not have [redacted] to fulfill this obligation, particularly in an age of rapid technological [redacted] innovation. To assist IRBs, the Department of Health and Human Services [redacted] issue guidance on appropriately protecting subjects' privacy and confidentiality, [redacted] should incorporate such guidance in IRB procedures and guidelines as appropriate.

[redacted] **Section 14.1** of this chapter sets out key definitions that drive the analysis regarding whether research involving biospecimens and data constitutes "human subjects research" necessitating IRB oversight. These definitions generally hinge upon the *identifiability* of the materials. **Section 14.2** discusses the types of studies that often involve biospecimens and data – namely, prospective collection of materials for research, and secondary use of materials for research. Taking a deeper dive into secondary use, **Section 14.3** then discusses three exemptions to the research regulations in the context of secondary use of identifiable biospecimens and data. **Section 14.4** discusses the research repositories of biospecimens and data, and the chapter concludes with some practical considerations for IRBs.

IRBs should note that the terms "tissue," "specimen," and "biospecimen" are often used interchangeably, as are "bank" and "repository." Similarly, the terms "data" and "private information" are often used interchangeably. A biospecimen is defined broadly, referring to any biological specimen obtained from patients or human research subjects. This includes, for example, fixed, frozen, or fresh pathology or autopsy specimens, blood, urine, saliva, bone marrow, semen, breast milk, or any purified DNA, RNA, proteins, cell lines, or clones.

14.1 Key Definitions

14.1.1 Nonidentified Biospecimens and Nonidentified Private Information

Under the 2018 Common Rule, researchers and their institutions continue to have flexibility with regard to the use of data and biospecimens that are not "identifiable." Under the Pre-2018 Common Rule, "identifiable" means that the identity of the subject is or may readily be ascertained by the investigator or associated with the private information or biospecimen.[1] The Food and Drug Administration (FDA) has described "identifiable" biospecimens similarly, but expanded the scope to include consideration of whether the investigator *or any others associated with the investigation*, including the sponsor, are able to link the biospecimen to the subject from whom it was collected.[2]

[1] 45 C.F.R. § 46.102(f); 82 Fed. Reg. 7149 at 7260 (Jan. 19, 2017) (to be codified at 45 C.F.R. § __.102(e)(5), (e)(6)).

[2] FDA, Guidance on Informed Consent for In Vitro Diagnostic Device Studies Using Leftover Human Specimens that are Not Individually Identifiable (Issued Apr. 25, 2006), *available at* https://www.

Materials that are not identifiable include data that is *de-identified* and biospecimens and data that are unidentifiable or are coded such that the researcher cannot access information that would allow him or her to identify the person from whom the biospecimen or data derives.[3] Such data and biospecimens generally do not meet the definition of "human subjects" under Pre-2018 Common Rule requirements and FDA regulations,[4] and also do not constitute "protected health information" under the HIPAA Privacy Rule.[5]

Specific research uses of such data and biospecimens do not generally require specific informed consent or HIPAA authorization. However, institutions housing such materials and IRBs overseeing their use in research often establish institutional requirements for the maintenance and use of these materials, which may include IRB determination of exemption or categorization as not human subjects research activity, discussed in more detail in **Section 14.3**.

14.1.2 Identifiable Biospecimens and Identifiable Private Information

The use of identifiable biospecimens and identifiable private information (*e.g.*, medical records) in research presents somewhat more significant ethical, legal, and policy issues, and few topics have garnered more attention in the research community.

To help IRBs and others assure the rights of individuals when their identifiable biospecimens or identifiable data are used in research, federal departments and agencies have been working to modernize and enhance available guidance and applicable requirements. One primary focus of these efforts is clarifying when biospecimens and data become "identifiable," as described above in **Section 14.1.1**.

The concept of identifiability became more complex with the discovery that genetic data could in some circumstances be traced back to the individuals from whom it was obtained.[6] To address this issue, the Pre-2018 Common Rule requirements require federal agencies, in consultation with appropriate experts, to (i) review collaboratively[7] the meaning of "identifiable," initially and at least once every four years, and to (ii) assess whether certain analytic technologies or techniques should be considered to generate identifiable private information or

fda.gov/downloads/medicaldevices/deviceregulationandguidance/guidancedocuments/ucm071265.pdf.

[3] HHS Office of Human Research Protection, Guidance on Research Involving Coded Private Information or Biological Specimens (Oct. 16, 2008), *available at* https://www.hhs.gov/ohrp/regulations-and-policy/guidance/research-involving-coded-private-information/index.html.

[4] 45 C.F.R. § 46.102(f); 21 C.F.R. §§ 50.1-.56; 21 C.F.R. §§ 56.101-.124; *see also* FDA, Nonbinding Recommendations for Informed Consent for In Vitro Diagnostic Device Studies Using Leftover Human Specimens that are Not Individually Identifiable (Issued Apr. 25, 2006), *available at* https://www.fda.gov/downloads/medicaldevices/deviceregulationandguidance/guidancedocuments/ucm071265.pdf.

[5] 45 C.F.R. § 164.502(d).

[6] *See* Amy L. McGuire & Laura M. Beskow, *Informed Consent in Genomics and Genetic Research*, 11 Ann. Rev. Genomics Hum. Genetics 361 (2010).

[7] In furtherance of efforts to harmonize guidance among federal departments and agencies. *See* 82 Fed. Reg. 7149, 7160 (Jan. 19, 2017).

biospecimens.[8] Federal agencies will make a list of these technologies and techniques available and will update it periodically. IRBs should be sure to reference this list and the most recent guidance available to keep pace with the evolving concept of identifiability.

Researchers' interaction with identifiable biospecimens or data typically occurs in one of two different ways, each of which is discussed below. The nature and scope of IRB review required may vary depending on the research use.

14.2 Types of Research Studies Involving Identifiable Biospecimens and Data

14.2.1 Primary or Prospective Research Use

Primary or prospective research uses are those for which the identifiable biospecimens or data were initially collected. Such research uses include collection for a specific research study or for storage in a repository for future research use (as discussed in **Section 14.4** below). IRB review is required for these research uses. IRBs should review the proposed informed consent to ensure it contains any basic or additional statements required to inform subjects as to how their biospecimens or private information might be used. Specifically, the Pre-2018 Common Rule requirements require that the informed consent for primary or prospective research involving identifiable biospecimens or identifiable private information include:

(i) a statement that identifiers might be removed from the identifiable biospecimens or identifiable private information, and that the non-identified biospecimens and information could be used for future research or distributed to other investigators without additional informed consent; or

(ii) a statement that the subject's biospecimens or information will not be used for future research, even if the identifiers are removed.[9]

When appropriate based on the research protocol, the informed consent must also include:

(iii) a statement that the subject's biospecimens (even if non-identified) may be used for commercial profit and whether the subject will or will not share in the commercial profit;

(iv) a statement regarding whether clinically relevant research results, including individual research results, will be disclosed to subjects, and if so, under what conditions; and

(v) whether the research will or might include whole genome sequencing.[10]

---

[8] 82 Fed. Reg. 7149 at 7260 (Jan. 19, 2017) (to be codified at 45 C.F.R. § __.102(e)(7)). For example, the preamble to the 2018 Common Rule requirements notes an expectation that whole genome sequencing will be assessed for its ability to re-identify information or biospecimens. *See* 82 Fed. Reg. 7149, 7169 (Jan. 19, 2017).

[9] 82 Fed. Reg. 7149 at 7266 (Jan. 19, 2017) (to be codified at 45 C.F.R. § __.116(b)(9)).

[10] 82 Fed. Reg. 7149 at 7266 (Jan. 19, 2017) (to be codified at 45 C.F.R. § __.116(c)).

14.2.2 Secondary Research Use

Investigators may wish to use identifiable biospecimens or data for a research purpose other than the research or clinical purpose for which they were initially collected. This would be considered a secondary research use of such biospecimens or data. For example, investigators may seek to use identifiable biospecimens or data, which they initially collected or that were collected by another investigator, to study a new research question. Investigators may also be interested in using identifiable biospecimens or data collected initially for a clinical or other non-research purpose, such as a lab test or biopsy. Therefore, informed consent for storage and use in research may not have been obtained when the biospecimens or data were collected, or was obtained for a different research purpose.

Investigators have several options to address the issue of informed consent when seeking IRB approval for a secondary research use of identifiable biospecimens or data. An investigator may request IRB approval for new research requiring study-specific consent, as described above in **Section 14.2.1**, or a determination that the research is within the scope of a previously-approved consent. Or, an investigator may request that the IRB waive the requirement to obtain informed consent, as discussed in **Chapter 9**, **Sections 9.8.2 and 9.8.3.**[11] The Pre-2018 Common Rule requirements also include an additional waiver criterion for research involving identifiable biospecimens or data—a finding that the research could not practicably be carried out without using such biospecimens or data in an identifiable format, also discussed in **Chapter 9**, **Section 9.8.2** (in the "Added by the 2018 Common Rule" section).[12] It is recommended that IRBs consider the following when applying the waiver criteria: (i) whether there are adequate protections in place to protect the privacy of subjects and maintain confidentiality (*e.g.*, coding procedures, control of and access to data, honest broker mechanisms); (ii) the level of risk; (iii) the risk of introducing bias into the research; (iv) the investigator's ability to locate or contact subjects; (v) potential anxiety or confusion for subjects; (vi) the number of subjects; (vii) the length of time since the biospecimens or data were first collected; and (viii) the likelihood that subjects would object to the proposed secondary use, based on the purpose of the original collection.[13]

[11] With regard to FDA-regulated research, current FDA regulations allow exception from the general requirements for informed consent only in life-threatening situations or for emergency research, when certain conditions are met. 21 C.F.R. §§ 50.23, .24. However, in furtherance of the FDA's obligation to harmonize FDA regulations with the 2018 Common Rule requirements, the FDA has stated that it will revise its informed consent regulations to provide for waiver or alteration of informed consent requirements under appropriate safeguards. Until such regulations are issued, the FDA does not intend to object to an IRB approving waived or altered informed consent requirements under the 2018 Common Rule requirements criteria. *See* FDA, IRB Waiver or Alteration of Informed Consent for Clinical Investigations Involving No More Than Minimal Risk to Human Subjects (July 2017), *available at* https://www.fda.gov/downloads/RegulatoryInformation/Guidances/UCM566948.pdf.

[12] 82 Fed. Reg. 7149 at 7267 (Jan. 19, 2017) (to be codified at 45 C.F.R. § __.116(f)(3)(iii)). The FDA has indicated that as it revises its regulations to harmonize with the 2018 Common Rule requirements, it will consider adding this new criterion in any waiver provision. *See* FDA, IRB Waiver or Alteration of Informed Consent for Clinical Investigations Involving No More Than Minimal Risk to Human Subjects (July 2017), n.6.

[13] OHRP, Attachment D: FAQ's Terms and Recommendations on Informed Consent and Research Use of Biospecimens (July 20, 2011), *available at* https://www.hhs.gov/ohrp/sachrp-committee/recommendations/2011-october-13-letter-attachment-d/index.html.

In addition, the Pre-2018 Common Rule requirements provide for certain exemptions related to secondary research use of identifiable biospecimens or data. These exemptions are discussed in **Section 14.3** below.

14.3 Secondary Research Use of Identifiable Biospecimens or Data–Exemptions

The Pre-2018 Common Rule requirements provide three exemptions from the overall requirements of the regulations in the context of the secondary research use of identifiable biospecimens and data. The first two exemptions are with regard to the storage, maintenance, and use of such materials, when broad consent is obtained and the IRB undertakes a limited review. The third exempts certain specific secondary uses of such materials, and does not require consent for such uses.

It should be noted that currently, these exemptions are not available for FDA-regulated research, such as research using leftover biospecimens for investigational device studies. As noted in **Section 14.2.2**, however, the FDA intends to harmonize its regulations with the 2018 Common Rule requirements to promote consistency in the regulation of human subjects research.

14.3.1 Exemptions for Storage, Maintenance, and Use: Broad Consent and Limited IRB Review

The 2018 Common Rule requirements introduced the option of obtaining a broad consent (as discussed in **Chapter 9**, **Section 9.3.4**) for the secondary research use of identifiable biospecimens or data. This option is reflected in a pair of exemptions that are subject to limited IRB review. IRBs will be responsible for reviewing the adequacy of both the consent and the privacy and confidentiality protections in place.

The first is an exemption for the storage or maintenance of identifiable biospecimens or data for secondary research use.[14] The exemption requires that an IRB conduct a limited review to make the following determinations: (i) broad consent for the storage, maintenance, and secondary research use of identifiable biospecimens or data is obtained in accordance with applicable requirements; (ii) broad consent is appropriately documented or waiver of documentation is obtained; and (iii) if there is a change made for research purposes in the way the identifiable biospecimens or data are stored or maintained, there are adequate provisions to protect the privacy of subjects and to maintain the confidentiality of data.

Regarding the change in storage or maintenance described in (iii) above, IRBs need only review the aspects of storage and maintenance that are changed for research purposes.[15] Examples of changed aspects include moving identifiable biospecimens or data from one electronic

[14] 82 Fed. Reg. 7149 at 7262 (Jan. 19, 2017) (to be codified at 45 C.F.R. § __.104(d)(7)).

[15] Additionally, the institution where the identifiable biospecimens or identifiable private information are stored or maintained will need to consider what other protections might be appropriate, including with regard to other legal or regulatory requirements and institutional policies. *See* 82 Fed. Reg. 7149, 7198 (Jan. 19, 2017).

or physical storage location to another, storing them longer than they otherwise would have been stored, placing them in a registry or repository to serve as a resource for investigators, or providing electronic or physical access to investigators.[16]

The second exemption is for research involving use of identifiable biospecimens or data for which broad consent is required.[17] This exemption will often work in conjunction with the first exemption referenced above. To qualify for the second exemption, the following criteria must be met: (i) broad consent for the storage, maintenance, and secondary research use of identifiable biospecimens or data is obtained in accordance with applicable requirements; (ii) broad consent is appropriately documented or waiver of documentation was obtained; (iii) the IRB conducts a limited review to make a determination that there are adequate provisions to protect the privacy of subjects and to maintain the confidentiality of data, and determines that the research to be conducted is within the scope of the broad consent; and (iv) the investigator does not include returning individual research results to subjects as part of the study plan.[18]

14.3.2 Exemption: No Consent Required

Under the 2018 Common Rule requirements, there also is an exemption for the secondary research use of identifiable biospecimens or data for which consent is not required,[19] unlike the exemptions requiring broad consent as discussed in **Section 14.3.1** above. This exemption is applicable when at least one of the following criteria are met: (i) the identifiable biospecimens or data are publicly available; (ii) the information is recorded by the investigator in such a way that the identity of the subjects cannot readily be ascertained, and the investigator does not contact subjects or try to re-identify subjects; (iii) the secondary research use is regulated under HIPAA;[20] or (iv) the secondary research use is conducted by or on behalf of a federal entity and involves the use of federally generated nonresearch information provided that the original collection was subject to specific federal privacy protections and continues to be protected.

This exemption may apply when an investigator wishes to use medical records or biospecimens stored in a clinical department, such as a pathology lab. The identifiable biospecimens or data that the investigator is seeking need not exist at the initiation of the research study. Rather,

---

[16] *Id.*

[17] 82 Fed. Reg. 7149 at 7263 (Jan. 19, 2017) (to be codified at 45 C.F.R. § __.104(d)(8)).

[18] This would not prevent the investigator from returning individual research results when required by law regardless of whether or not such return is described in the study plan. *Id.*; *see also* 82 Fed. Reg. 7149, 7199 (Jan. 19, 2017).

[19] 82 Fed. Reg. 7149 at 7262 (Jan. 19, 2017) (to be codified at 45 C.F.R. § __.104(d)(4)).

[20] Under HIPAA, where appropriate, it is required to obtain the individual's authorization for future research use of protected health information, or a waiver of that authorization by an IRB or a HIPAA Privacy Board. Accordingly, this criterion is based on the assumption that consent should be unnecessary. *See* 82 Fed. Reg. 7149, 7194 (Jan. 19, 2017). Note that, under HHS's current interpretation of the HIPAA Privacy Rule, authorization can be obtained from an individual for use and disclosure of protected health information for future, unknown research purposes, so long as the authorization describes the future research such that the individual would reasonably expect his or her protected health information to be used for future research purposes (HIPAA Omnibus Rule, 79 Fed. Reg. 5566, Jan. 25, 2013; 80 Fed. Reg. 53972, Sept. 8, 2015).

the exemption would still apply if the research involves biospecimens or data that are added during the course of the study.[21]

14.4 Biospecimen and Data Repositories for Research

As mentioned above, human biospecimens and data have become more important to biomedical research over time. These materials are collected, stored, and used in a few ways. Such data and biospecimens may be obtained through routine clinical care and treatment, collected for the purpose of conducting a specific research project, or collected prospectively for unspecified, future research purposes. These materials may be compiled into clinical repositories, or repositories specifically created for research. Some repositories serve more than one purpose. This section focuses on research repositories created for use by multiple investigators, for repeated use, and/or for future research.

IRBs are involved with biospecimen and data repositories at three separate stages. The first stage is the point at which biospecimens and data are collected. The second stage involves the storage and management of the biospecimens and data. The final stage comes when investigators would like to use biospecimens and/or data from the repository for a specific research protocol.

14.4.1 Research Repository Defined and Described

Research and other organizations have developed a variety of different types of repositories for maintaining and distributing human data and biospecimens. Non-research repositories at, for instance, health care organizations, include data and biospecimens collected for non-research purposes (such as for clinical treatment), and those collected in databases such as medical records and hospital pathology departments. Study-specific repositories include data and biospecimens that were collected for a specific research project. General use or central repositories include biospecimens and data collected for prospective, future research. This section focuses on creation and use of research repositories.

A research "repository" is a facility for storing biospecimens or data, in this case, for future research use. Biospecimen repositories may contain unidentifiable biospecimens, biospecimens linked to a code that could be used to identify individuals, or biospecimens accompanied by a compendium of associated identifiable information. Repository activities involve three components: (i) the collection of the biospecimens and/or data; (ii) the storage and management of the biospecimens and data; and (iii) the release of biospecimens and/or data to recipient investigators.[22]

---

[21] *See* 82 Fed. Reg. 7149, 7192 (Jan. 19, 2017).

[22] OPRR Issues to Consider in the Research Use of Stored Data or Tissue (Aug. 19, 1996) [hereafter *OPRR Stored Data or Tissue*], *available at* https://www.hhs.gov/ohrp/regulations-and-policy/guidance/issues-to-consider-in-use-of-stored-data-or-tissues/index.html.

Under current regulations, each research use of biospecimens and/or private information that meets the definition of human subjects research under FDA regulations and the Pre-2018 Common Rule requirements requires some degree of IRB oversight. As discussed above, this often hinges on the *identifiability* of the materials. The 2018 Common Rule requirements have provided streamlined options for some of these activities, as discussed in **Section 14.3**. Research organizations and other institutions are increasingly creating repositories of data and biospecimens that are available for secondary research use. According to federal guidance, the creation of such repositories is considered a "research" project when such repositories will include identifiable private information or biospecimens.[23] Thus the creation and operation of such research repositories is governed by HHS and HIPAA regulations and requires IRB oversight and approval. Repositories of unidentifiable biospecimens and data may not constitute human subjects research, but institutions often establish parameters for collection, storage, and use of such materials as a matter of institutional policy and best practice.

14.4.2 Collection of Biospecimens and Data for Storage in a Repository

The establishment of biospecimen and data repositories that involve the collection of identifiable biospecimens and/or data for research purposes must be reviewed and approved by an IRB. The IRB should determine if the biospecimen repository is research, exempt research, qualifies for expedited review, or requires review by the full committee.

See **Chapter 2**, **Section 2.3.2** for a discussion of research activities that are exempt. Note that, under the 2018 Common Rule, an IRB may use an expedited review process to review research for which limited IRB review is a condition of exemption.[24]

Expedited review may be appropriate in some circumstances, including when (i) blood samples are collected by finger stick, heel stick, ear stick, or venipuncture; (ii) biospecimens are collected prospectively for research purposes by noninvasive means; or (iii) data, documents, records, or biospecimens were collected or will be collected for nonresearch purposes, in each case unless the IRB reviewer determines that the study involves more than minimal risk.[25]

While some tissue repositories may be exempt, exempt subject to limited IRB review, or simply not considered human subjects research activities (in the case of certain repositories of

---

[23] HHS Office for Protection from Research Risks, Issues to Consider in the Research Use of Stored Data or Tissue (Nov. 7, 1997), *available at* https://www.hhs.gov/ohrp/regulations-and-policy/guidance/issues-to-consider-in-use-of-stored-data-or-tissues/index.html; OHRP, Coded Private Information or Specimens Use in Research, Guidance (2008) (Oct. 16, 2008), *available at* https://www.hhs.gov/ohrp/regulations-and-policy/guidance/research-involving-coded-private-information/index.html.

[24] 82 Fed. Reg. 7149 at 7264 (Jan. 19, 2017) (to be codified at 45 C.F.R. §__.110(b)(iii)).

[25] OHRP, OHRP Expedited Review Categories (1998), Categories of Research that May be Reviewed by an IRB Through an Expedited Procedure (Nov. 9, 1998), *available at* https://www.hhs.gov/ohrp/regulations-and-policy/guidance/categories-of-research-expedited-review-procedure-1998/index.html; 82 Fed. Reg. 7149 at 7264 (Jan. 19, 2017) (to be codified at 45 C.F.R. §__.110(b)(i)). Final Rule requires that the Secretary of HHS review the list of categories of research that may be reviewed by expedited procedure at least every 8 years (82 Fed. Reg. 7149 at 7264 (Jan. 19, 2017) (to be codified at 45 C.F.R. §___.110(a)).

unidentifiable materials), the organization housing the repository should still take an active role in setting parameters for the formation of all repositories. While reviewing the request to establish a tissue repository, the IRB and/or institutional administration should establish conditions under which data and biospecimens may be accepted into the repository and how they may be shared.[26] The type of biospecimens and the process for collecting the biospecimens should be reviewed. For instance, will the biospecimens be collected solely for research purposes or will the collection be part of a clinical procedure with excess tissue going to the repository?

Written informed consent and HIPAA authorization should be obtained, unless a waiver of informed consent and waiver of or an exception to HIPAA authorization is approved by the IRB. See **Chapter 9**, **Section 9.3** for a discussion of more specific informed consent requirements for primary and prospective collection of identifiable materials for future research, including new elements that must be included in the informed consent forms under the 2018 Common Rule. See also **Chapter 9**, **Section 9.3.4** for a discussion of broad consent, which may be utilized in the context of prospective and primary collections of such materials. In addition to the standard required elements for informed consent and HIPAA authorization, it is a best practice for research repository consents to contain a clear description of (i) the operation of the repository; (ii) the specific types of research to be conducted if known or anticipated; (iii) the conditions under which data and biospecimens will be released to recipient investigators; and (iv) procedures for protecting the privacy of participants and maintaining the confidentiality of data.[27] If genetic research is anticipated, information should be included about the potential consequences and legal protections under the Genetic Information and Nondiscrimination Act of 2008 (Public Law 110-233) and state law.

Finally, IRBs should consider whether a Certificate of Confidentiality should be obtained for the repository as an additional method to protect privacy. Certificates of Confidentiality protect identifiable research information from forced or compelled disclosure. Investigators and others who have access to research records are able to refuse to disclose identifying information on research participants in civil, criminal, administrative, legislative, or other proceedings, whether federal, state, or local, with certain exceptions. Certificates of Confidentiality help to minimize risks to subjects by adding an additional level of protection for maintaining confidentiality of private information.[28]

14.4.3 Storage of Biospecimens and Management of Data in a Research Repository

The IRB has a continuing obligation to oversee the storage and management of the research repository. Unless exempt from IRB review, or approved via expedited review,[29] continuing review should be conducted by the IRB no less than annually with reports of the number of

---

[26] *OPRR Stored Data or Tissue.*

[27] *Id.*

[28] *Id.*

[29] 82 Fed. Reg. 7149 at 7264 (Jan. 19, 2017) (to be codified at 45 C.F.R. § __.109(f)).

participants from whom data and/or biospecimens were collected along with all other materials generally required for continuing review of studies. Recall that, as described in **Chapter 9, Section 9.3.4** the 2018 Common Rule requirements provide an exemption for the storage and maintenance of identifiable biospecimens or identifiable private information for secondary research uses, following a limited IRB review and in accordance with broad consent requirements.[30] Note also that this limited review can be accomplished through expedited review.[31] This pathway can be utilized in operating a research repository with identifiable biospecimens and data when the applicable regulatory requirements are met.

In all cases, IRBs should ensure that the research repository's privacy protections and security measures continue to meet legal and ethical standards. For instance, using a locked file cabinet with limited personnel having access to keys may have been appropriate to protect data in the early 1990s; however, today, it is appropriate and best practice to use an encrypted computer system with a firewall and sophisticated password requirements.

14.4.4 Disclosure and Release of Biospecimens and/or Data from Research Repository to Recipient Investigators

How and under what circumstances biospecimens and/or data may be provided to recipient investigators should be addressed in IRB-approved standard operating procedures and/or the repository's operating protocol. Note that, as described in **Chapter 9, Section 9.3.4**, the 2018 Common Rule requirements provide two exemptions for the use of identifiable biospecimens or identifiable private information for secondary research uses.[32]

In terms of distributing research repository materials, housing institutions should enter into usage agreements with external recipients (*e.g.*, researchers outside the institution) and should have policies in place governing internal recipients (*e.g.*, researchers from another department within the institution). For transfer of data externally, this may involve a data use agreement or other form of data sharing agreement. For transfer of biospecimens externally, this may involve a Material Transfer Agreement between the housing institution and the recipient institution, with the particular researchers from each institution named in the agreement. These usage agreements should specify the conditions under which the biospecimens and/or data may be used and the responsibilities of the recipient investigator and, if appropriate, his or her employing institution. Regardless of the form of agreement, the contract with the recipient should contain specific provisions regarding ownership of materials; limits on usage; confidentiality protections; publication rights; rights to inventions and research results; and legal liability as a result of the use or misuse of the material. Additionally, as a matter of policy, some housing institutions may approve the transfer of data and/or biospecimens only when the request is accompanied by proof of an IRB-approved protocol.

---

[30] 82 Fed. Reg. 7149 at 7261 (Jan. 19, 2017) (to be codified at 45 C.F.R. § ___.104(d)(7)).

[31] 82 Fed. Reg. 7149 at 7264 (Jan. 19, 2017) (to be codified at 45 C.F.R. § ___.110(b)(1)(iii)).

[32] 82 Fed. Reg. 7149 at 7263 (Jan. 19, 2017) (to be codified at 45 C.F.R. § ___.104(d)(8)); 82 Fed. Reg. 7149 at 7262 (Jan. 19, 2017) (to be codified at 45 C.F.R. § ___.104(d)(4)).

14.5 Practical Considerations and Best Practices

14.5.1 Research Repository Operations and Governance

As described earlier, research with non-identifiable biospecimens and data does not require IRB oversight and approval, subject to institutional requirements; however, it would still be beneficial and best practice for repositories of non-identifiable biospecimens and data to undergo some institutional oversight.

Typically, each research repository will have a director or principal investigator who will develop a set of standard operating procedures (SOPs) specifying the conditions under which data and biospecimens may be added to, maintained by, and transferred from, the repository. These SOPs are typically approved by the overseeing governing body and the IRB, and they set out the requirements for informed consent and authorization for inclusion of materials in the repository. Once the repository is approved by the overseeing IRB, individual research uses of repository materials may not require individual IRB oversight and approval, as long as such requests comply with the repository's SOPs.

As a matter of best practice, the repository's housing institution will often establish a repository review committee or similar committee, which will oversee access to the repository, make decisions about the allocation of resources, and sometimes serve as an initial forum to resolve disputes. This committee may be comprised of representative stakeholders who use, contribute to or are otherwise affected by the repository's activities.

14.5.2 Information Technology

Institutional review boards will continue to play a key role in ensuring that adequate privacy and confidentiality safeguards are in place for research involving biospecimens and private information, and HHS will issue guidance on appropriately protecting subjects' privacy and confidentiality. In the meantime, IRBs should ensure that such safeguards include modern security measures such as data encryption, control over access (physical and electronic), and firewalls, as appropriate.

IRBs and institutions should also review the research repositories' systems for tracking biospecimens and associated information, as well as the form of consent provided and any limitations on such consent. As research repositories grow in volume and complexity, such systems will be critical for successful operation and management of the repository and compliance with applicable regulatory requirements and institutional policies. For example, if broad consent for the use of identifiable biospecimens and data is obtained or refused, such consent or refusal must be tracked over the subject's lifetime. It may also be useful for research repository systems to include or link to IRB approvals and subjects' medical records.

Creation, Storage, Use of Biospecimens and Data

	Identifiable* materials	Unidentifiable+ materials
Collection of materials / "creation" of research repository	IRB review and approval required. New informed consent form language required (__.116(b)(9) and __.116)(c))**	Not "human subjects research" but subject to institutional requirements and community best practices
Storage/Maintenance of materials	Exemption from human subjects research (HSR) after limited IRB review & broad consent standards met (__.104(d)(7))**	Not "human subjects research" but subject to institutional requirements and community best practices
Use of materials	Exemption from HSR with limited IRB review & broad consent standards met (___.104(d)(8))**	Not "human subjects research" but subject to institutional requirements and community best practices
	Exemption from HSR, no consent required in certain circumstances (___.104(d)(4))**	

* 2018 Common Rule requirements definition: the identity of the subject is or may readily be ascertained by the investigator or associated with the private information or biospecimen.

FDA definition: the identity of the subject is or may readily be ascertained by the investigator *or any others associated with the investigation*, including the sponsor, or associated with the private information or biospecimen.

\+ 2018 Common Rule requirements definition: data that is *de-identified* and biospecimens and data that are unidentifiable or are coded such that the researcher cannot access information that would allow him or her to identify the person from whom the biospecimen or data derives.

FDA definition: data that is *de-identified* and biospecimens and data that are unidentifiable or are coded such that the researcher *or any others associated with the investigation*, including the sponsor, cannot access information that would allow him or her to identify the person from whom the biospecimen or data derives.

** Currently applicable only to 2018 Common Rule requirements-regulated research (not FDA-regulated research).

Chapter 15

Secondary Findings in Genomic Research: Ethics, Law, and Practicality

Ann T. Hollenbeck

Katherine B. Steuer

Introduction

Secondary findings arise when a test is performed for one purpose and returns additional results which are unrelated to that purpose. This problem is well-known in imaging studies: obtain a diagnostic image for one purpose but see a concerning lesion nearby, for instance.[1] With the advent of genomics[2] research, however, a higher frequency of secondary findings in this context is anticipated.[3] Genomic testing using next generation sequencing (NGS) technologies is being adopted rapidly in both the research and clinical contexts, revealing many previously unknown genetic variants. Knowledge of variants that are linked with diseases or other clinical differences can sometimes help in tailoring appropriate medical care. Genomic sequencing, however, generates data about the entire collection of a person's genes, not just the specific gene or panel of genes of interest when the test is ordered. The scope of the data sometimes gives rise to these secondary findings.

Under what circumstances should secondary findings, also known as incidental findings in research results be returned to a research participant? Both the Presidential Commission for the Study of Bioethical Issues and the American Society for Human Genetics (ASHG) advise

---

[1] Jeffrey R. Botkin, John W. Belmont, Jonathan S. Berg, Benjamin E. Berkman, Yvonne Bombard, Ingrid A. Holm, Howard P. Levy, Kelley E. Ormond, Howard M. Saal, Nancy B. Spinner, Benjamin S. Wilfond and Joseph D. McInerney, American Society of Human Genetics Position Statement, *Points to Consider: Ethical, Legal and Psychosocial Implications of Genetic Testing in Children and Adolescents*, THE AM. J. OF HUMAN GENETICS 97, 6 (2015) (ASHG Position Statement).

[2] Genomic testing in both the research and clinical contexts can determine the person's complete DNA sequence using laboratory testing and extensive analysis. "Genome-scale sequencing" includes either whole-genome or whole-exome sequencing. *Id.* at 8.

[3] Presidential Commission for the Study of Bioethical Issues, *Anticipate and Communicate: Ethical Management of Incidental and Secondary Findings in the Clinical, Research, and Direct-to-Consumer Contexts*, at 2, *available at* https://bioethicsarchive.georgetown.edu/pcsbi/sites/default/files/FINALAnticipateCommunicate_PCSBI_0.pdf (Anticipate and Communicate). *But see* Sebastian Schuol, Christoph Schickhardt, Stefan Wiemann, Claus R. Bartram, Klaus Tanner, Roland Eils, Benjamin Meder, Daniela Richter, Hanno Glimm, Christof von Kalle and Eva C. Winkler, *Opinion: So rare we need to hunt for them: reframing the ethical debate on incidental findings*, GENOME MEDICINE 2105 7:83 (Reframing), at 3-4 (arguing that incidental findings are relatively rare).

investigators to have a plan for disclosing and managing secondary and incidental findings (collectively, secondary findings)[4] and to include that plan as part of the protocol submitted to the Institutional Review Board (IRB) for review.[5] In turn, IRBs are expected to evaluate investigators' plans to assess their adequacy.[6] This raises the question of what an IRB should require by way of policy and in its reviews of research protocols. This chapter discusses matters an IRB should consider addressing in its policies on secondary findings and challenges that may arise in the review of research protocols that are likely to result in secondary findings.

The Pre-2018 Common Rule[7] requires investigators to disclose the risks and benefits of participating in research, including, when appropriate, the possibility of currently unforeseeable risks.[8] "It could be argued that, at a minimum, this requirement obligates investigators to disclose the fact that significant findings might be discovered during the course of the research and whether or not those will be offered to subjects and/or their physicians."[9] Under the 2018 Requirements (2018 Requirements)[10] an additional element of informed consent must be included when appropriate—namely a statement as to whether clinically relevant research results, including individual results, will be disclosed to subjects, and if so, under what conditions.[11]

The return of secondary findings has prompted much analysis and debate in part because it is at the intersection of research and clinical care. The IRB's role is essential in formulating policy and reviewing investigator plans regarding secondary findings. An IRB should be prepared to: (i) ensure the investigator addresses secondary findings in the protocol when relevant; (ii) set a general institutional standard for disclosure criteria; (iii) develop informed consent templates and approve the consent language regarding secondary findings; (iv) approve and oversee the process for secondary findings review and disclosure; (v) review and approve disclosure of secondary findings when appropriate; and (vi) monitor the safety of secondary findings disclosures. Investigators and IRBs, working collaboratively, will better effectively manage these complex issues and their evolution.

---

[4] Anticipate and Communicate, *supra* note 3, at 5; *See* ASHG Position Statement, *supra* note 1, at 9 ("When secondary findings are likely to be generated in the conduct of pediatric research, ASHG recommends that investigators develop an IRB-approved plan to manage such findings.")

[5] Anticipate and Communicate, *supra* note 3, at 13, 14.

[6] Anticipate and Communicate, *supra* note 3, at 15.

[7] 45 C.F.R. Part 46. The Pre-2018 Common Rule was updated on January 19, 2017, effective in part January 19, 2019. Federal Policy for the Protection of Human Subjects, 82 Fed. Reg. 7149 (Jan. 19, 2017).

[8] 45 C.F.R. § 46.116(a)(2), (a)(3) and (b)(1).

[9] Amy L. McGuire, Bartha Maria Knoppers, Ma'n H. Zawati, and Ellen Wright Clayton, *Can I be sued for that? Liability risk and the disclosure of clinically significant genetic research findings,* 24 GENOME RESEARCH 719, 720 (2014) (*Can I be sued for that?), available at* http://www.ncbi.nlm.nih.gov/pmc/articles/PMC4009601/.

[10] 82 Fed. Reg. 7149 (January 19, 2017).

[11] 82 Fed. Reg. at 7256 and 7266 (to be codified in 45 C.F.R. § 46.116(c)(8)). Additionally, the consent form for research involving biospecimens must, under the 2018 Requirements, state whether the research will or might include whole genome sequencing, defined to mean sequencing of a human germline or somatic specimen with the intent to generate the genome or exome sequence of that specimen. 45 C.F.R. § 46.116(c)(9).

15.1 Non-Return of Secondary Findings

If some kinds of secondary findings can be anticipated but will not be shared, these should be identified in the investigator's plan and the informed consent. For example, the IRB's policy should require telling participants if a discovery of adoption, non-paternity, or consanguinity will or will not be revealed.[12] If the investigator does not wish to return any findings, or any secondary findings, to participants, the reasons for this decision should be stated in the investigator's plan after anticipating the kinds of secondary findings that may result. IRB policy should then facilitate IRB discussion and review, including its rationale for approval or non-approval, and should require the informed consent to explain the "no returns" plan to participants. The IRB should seek to ensure that investigators are not shirking any ethical duty by not returning secondary findings to participants.

15.2 Returning Secondary Findings

The IRB's policy should require the investigator's plan to address returning secondary findings. The plan should include details about which kinds of secondary findings will be returned, under what circumstances, and to whom. Further issues that the IRB should require the plan to consider are discussed below. Many of the highlighted legal and ethical issues arise in research with adults and children, but the challenges are particularly vexing in the pediatric context.[13]

15.2.1 Clinical Actionability

Consensus appears to be emerging that only clinically "actionable" results should be returned—meaning only those secondary findings that an individual or practitioner can make use of or act upon for health, personal, reproductive, or clinical decision making.[14] More nar-

[12] ASHG Position Statement, *supra* note 1, at 13–15. Revealing misattributed parentage can have substantial ethical implications. *Id.*

[13] ASHG Position Statement, *supra* note 1, at 1.

[14] Michael P. Mackley, Benjamin Fletcher, Michael Parker, Hugh Watkins, and Elizabeth Ormondroyd, *Stakeholder Views on Secondary Findings in Whole-Genome and Whole-Exome Sequencing: A Systematic Review of Quantitative and Qualitative Studies*, GENET. MED. 19:3, at 283–293 (Mar. 2017), *available at* https://www.ncbi.nlm.nih.gov/pmc/articles/PMC5447864/; S. Wolf, W. Burke and B. Koenig, *Mapping the Ethics of Translational Genomics: Situating Return of Results and Navigating the Research-Clinical Divide.* J. OF LAW, MEDICINE & ETHICS, 43: 486–501 (2015), at 488, doi: 10.1111/jlme.12291 (Mapping the Ethics of Translational Genomics); Gail P. Jarvik, Laura M. Amendola, Jonathan S. Berg, Kyle Brothers, Ellen W. Clayton, Wendy Chung, Barbara J. Evans, James P. Evans, Stephanie M. Fullerton, Carlos J. Gallego, Nanibaa' A. Garrison, Stacy W. Gray, Ingrid A. Holm, Iftikhar J. Kullo, Lisa Soleymani Lehmann, Cathy McCarty, Cynthia A. Prows, Heidi L. Rehm, Richard R. Sharp, Joseph Salama, Saskia Sanderson, Sara L. Van Driest, Marc S. Williams, Susan M. Wolf, Wendy A. Wolf, eMERGE Act-ROR Committee and CERC Committee, CSER Act-ROR Working Group, and Wylie Burke, *Return of Genomic Results to Research Participants: The Floor, the Ceiling, and the Choices In Between*, 94 AM J. HUMAN GENETICS 818, 821 (2014) (The Floor, the Ceiling); *also see* Ellen Wright Clayton, *Incidental Findings in Genetics Research Using Archived DNA*, J. LAW MED ETHICS 2008, 286-292, *available at* https://www.ncbi.nlm.nih.gov/pmc/articles/PMC2576744/pdf/nihms73001.pdf (Incidental Findings in Genetics Research Using Archived DNA); Chimene Kesserwan, Lainie Friedman Ross, Angela R. Bradbury, "The Advantage and Challenges of Testing Children for Heritable Predisposition to Cancer," *2016 ASCO Educational Book, available at* https://meetinglibrary.asco.org/content/160621-176.

rowly, "actionability" can also mean "there are established therapeutic or preventative or other available actions that have the potential to change the clinical course of the disease."[15] If secondary findings are clinically actionable, investigators are much more likely to feel that they have an ethical duty, founded on the principle of beneficence, to disclose the findings.[16] Thus, the plan should require investigators to assess whether the action can be taken to reduce the risk to the participant (or others), and whether serious consequences could arise from not learning and acting on the information.[17]

Even in the clinical (non-research) setting, this subject is evolving. In 2013, the American College of Medical Genetics and Genomics (ACMG) urged analysis and reporting on potentially damaging but not diagnostically related variations in a set of 56 genes that have been associated with the risk of various medical conditions.[18] This approach sparked criticism and debate, including about what genes should be on the list of genes that should be disclosed to patients and whether patients should be able to refuse results.[19] In 2014, based on feedback from its members, ACMG revised its guidelines to allow clinical sequencing patients to opt-out of receiving information on alterations not related to the diagnosis at hand.[20] More recently, the American Society of Human Genetics (ASHG) recommended in the clinical context that pediatric genomic secondary findings be offered "only when the information has clear clinical utility for the child and/or his family members" after a robust informed consent process.[21] But in the clinical context, ASHG advised that parents must be told if a secondary finding would have "urgent and serious implications for a child's health or welfare, and effective action can be taken to mitigate that threat."[22] In October 2016, ACMG revised its list of 56 genes to remove one gene and add four genes,[23] and articulated a process for curating and updating this list over time.

---

[15] Fabsitz, *et al.*, *Ethical and Practical Guidelines for Reporting Genetic Research Results To Study Participants: Updated Guidelines from an NHLBI Working Group*, CIRC. CARDIOVASC. GENET. 2010 Dec 1; 3(6): 574–580.

[16] Anticipate and Communicate, *supra* note 3, at 30.

[17] Washington University Institutional Review Board, "Guidelines for reviewing studies involving genetic research," *available at* https://hrpo.wustl.edu/wp-content/uploads/2015/04/2015-04-03-Guidelines-for-reviewing-studies-involving-genetic-research-revised-12_06_2011-2.pdf.

[18] *See* ACMG recommendations for reporting of incidental findings in clinical exome and genome sequencing, 15 GENETICS IN MEDICINE 565-574 (2013) (ACMG's Incidental Findings Recommendation) *available at* https://www.nature.com/gim/journal/v15/n7/full/gim201373a.html.

[19] *E.g.*, Lanie Friedman Ross, Mark A. Rothstein, Ellen Wright Clayton, *Mandatory Extended Searches in All Genome Sequencing: Incidental Findings, Patient Autonomy, and Shared Decision Making*, 310 J. AM. MEDICAL ASS'N, 367-68 (2013).

[20] *See* ACMG's statement concerning its revised Policy Statement at https://www.acmg.net/docs/Release_ACMGUpdatesRecommendations_final.pdf; *ACMG Policy Statement: Updated Recommendations Regarding Analysis and Reporting of Secondary Findings in Clinical Genome-Scale Sequencing*, 17 GENETICS IN MEDICINE 68-69 (2014), *available at* https://www.nature.com/gim/journal/v17/nl/full/gim2014151a.html.

[21] ASHG Position Statement, *supra* note 1, at 9.

[22] ASHG Position Statement, *supra* note 1, at 9. ASHG concluded that genome-scale sequencing is not indicated for "screening in healthy children."

[23] Sarah S. Kalia *et al.*, *Recommendations for reporting of secondary findings in clinical exome and genome sequencing, 2016 update (ACMG SF v2.0): a policy statement of the American College of Medical Genetics*

Even had ACMG not softened its position requiring receipt (without opt-out) of certain secondary findings in the clinical context, many posit that these requirements should not be applied in the research context given the different goals and duties of research.[24] Challenging this view, however, are those who press for the return of all secondary findings because, even if not actionable now, secondary findings could be actionable in the future or may have health or reproductive implications for the participant or patient and his or her family.[25] Others propose a standard of "personal utility" to replace clinical utility as the measure,[26] potentially adding a more subjective element. Significantly, assessing whether results will be returned requires consideration of how likely a given gene mutation is to result in a phenotypic change such as development of disease (or penetrance).[27]

15.2.2 Reproductive Implications for the Participant or Family Members

When a child research participant tests positive for some mutations, this may reveal that one or both parents are carriers of the condition. This information may significantly impact each parent's desire to have additional children, as well as the patient's decisions later in life. Thus, the investigator's plan for returning secondary findings should address whether carrier status and other reproductive implications will be returned.

---

and Genomics, GENET. MED., Nov. 17, 2016, at 1, https://www.nature.com/gim/journal/v19/n2/full/gim2016190a.html.

[24] The Floor, the Ceiling, at 820; Distinctions Between Research and Clinical Care at 106-07, 109. *See also* ASHG Position Statement, *supra* note 1, at 9 ("Clinicians have a primary obligation to act in the best interests of their patient; researchers must protect the welfare of subjects but are primarily charged with the production of generalizable knowledge."); Reframing, at 5; Susan M. Wolf, Rebecca Branum, Barbara A. Koenig, Gloria M. Peterson, Susan A. Berry, Laura M. Beskow, Mary B. Daly, Conrad V. Fernandez, Robert C. Green, Bonnie S. LeRoy, Noralane M. Lindor, P. Pearl O'Rourke, Carmen Radecki Breitkopf, Mark A. Rothstein, Brian Van Ness, Benjamin S. Wilfond, *Returning a Research Participant's Genomic Results to Relatives: Analysis and Recommendations*, J. LAW. MED. ETHICS, 440-463, at 441, 446 (Fall 2015) (Returning Results to Relatives) (discussing return of research results, generally); Chimene Kesserwan, Lainie Friedman Ross, Angela R. Bradbury, "The Advantage and Challenges of Testing Children for Heritable Predisposition to Cancer," *2016 ASCO Educational Book, available at* http://meetinglibrary.asco.org/content/160621-176 ("There currently is no consensus list of actionable genes for obligatory disclosure in the research setting."). *See also* Anticipate and Communicate, *supra* note 3, at 23-24; *see also* Wylie Burke, Barbara J. Evans, and Gail P. Jarvik, *Return of Results: Ethical and Legal Distinctions Between Research and Clinical Care*, 166 AM. J. MEDICAL GENETICS PART C SEMINARS IN MEDICAL GENETICS 105 (2014) (Distinctions Between Research and Clinical Care).

[25] *See* American College of Medical Genetics and Genomics' Board of Directors' Policy Statement: *Clinical utility of genetic and genomic services: a position statement of the American College of Medical Genetics and Genomics* (2015) and *available at* https://www.acmg.net/docs/ACMG_Position_Statement_Clincial_Utility_of_Genetic_and_Genomic_Services_AOP.pdf; *see also* Returning Results to Relatives, *supra* note 24, at 444.

[26] *See* Jeffrey R. Botkin, *Ethical Issues in Pediatric Genetic Testing and Screening for Current Opinion in Pediatrics*, CURR. OPIN. PEDIATR. 28(6):700–704 (Dec. 2016), *available at* https://www.ncbi.nlm.nih.gov/pmc/articles/PMC5300789/.

[27] *See* Kimberly J. Johnson and Sara Gehlert, Return of results from genomic sequencing: A policy discussion of secondary findings for cancer predisposition, Vol. 2, Issue 3, J. CANCER POLICY, pp. 75-80 (2014) (Policy Discussion) *available at* http://ac.els-cdn.com/S2213538314000150/1-s2.0-S2213538314000150-main.pdf?_tid=a3b70e46-e66d-11e6-8dcd-00000aab0f02&acdnat=1485727105_615234fbc286aeaf41c9992a5cd19639; Washington University Institutional Review Board, "Guidelines for reviewing studies involving genetic research," (requiring investigators' plans to consider whether there is evidence linking the mutation (or other genetic finding) to a disease phenotype and the "penetrance of the phenotype").

If there is any plan to provide these results to the family, such as in the pediatric context, implications of this plan should be addressed directly, including the likelihood of the condition developing. Learning that one is a carrier of a serious disease can be concerning to a participant and his/her family members. Thus, potential emotional distress is a possible risk of participation in the genomic research that should be included in the plan and disclosed in the informed consent.[28] But for some families at high risk for genetic diseases, "the baseline uncertainty about risk status can cause psychosocial distress in the absence of genetic testing."[29]

15.2.3 Disclosure to Relatives

Parents and more distant relatives may ask the investigator for a research participant's genomic test results, including secondary findings, because of their reproductive or other health implications. A majority of authors of an extensive ethical analysis on this issue concluded that it might be ethical for researchers to offer genomic information to a research participant's relatives "in the exceptional circumstances of discovering highly pathogenic and actionable variants that the relative is likely to carry, and whose disclosure is highly likely to avert imminent harm."[30] In any event, researchers should anticipate that relatives may make these requests, determine participant preferences for sharing this information, and address the issue of sharing in compliance with federal and state health information confidentiality laws (*e.g.*, HIPAA). Researchers should also ask participants to identify a representative to make decisions about these issues if the participant is unable to do so or is deceased.[31]

15.2.4 Deceased Research Participants

The investigator's plan should grapple with the possible return of secondary findings to family members of a deceased research participant because of the potential reproductive or other impacts to them or to their offspring. Some ethical bases for returning these results to family members are beneficence and the duty to warn. These values also suggest that the investigator's plan address, before disclosure, the appropriate resources to explain and provide proper follow-up, for example, via genetic counseling.[32] Some posit that this duty depends on the closeness of the relationship between the researcher and the deceased participant, *i.e.* whether the researcher also acted in the role of physician to the participant/patient.[33] Others propose disclosing these findings only if the surviving relative explicitly asks.[34] Ideally, the

[28] Anticipate and Communicate, *supra* note 3, at 39, 40.

[29] ASHG Position Statement, *supra* note 1, at 7.

[30] Returning Results to Relatives, *supra* note 24, at 448.

[31] Returning Results to Relatives, *supra* note 24, at 448; Boers et al, *Postmortem disclosure of genetic information to family members: Active or passive?*, TRENDS IN MOLECULAR MEDICINE 21(3):148-153 (MARCH 2015), *available at* https://www.researchgate.net/publication/273154989_Postmortem_disclosure_of_genetic_information_to_family_members_Active_or_passive.

[32] *Id.* at 67.

[33] Lauren C. Milner, Emily Y. Liu, & Nanibaa' A. Garrison, *Relationships Matter: Ethical Considerations for Returning Results to Family Members of Deceased Subjects*, 13 AM. J. OF BIOETHICS, 66, 66-67 (2013).

[34] Boers et al., Postmortem disclosure of genetic information to family members: Active or passive?

informed consent or HIPAA authorization signed by participants will give permission for disclosures of secondary findings to family members in these circumstances. Refer to **Chapter 10** for a discussion of HIPAA authorizations.

When this is not possible, the plan must address whether HIPAA and the Common Rule permit release of the secondary findings. HIPAA applies even to the medical information of decedents—generally, HIPAA protects the individually identifiable health information about decedents for 50 years following the date of death.[35] HIPAA, however, allows sharing of decedents' health information for research purposes in certain situations.[36] Under the Common Rule, a deceased research participant is no longer a "human subject"[37] and thus not under the IRB's oversight; however, the plan should address the potential death of research participants. In discussing the return of intended results (not specifically secondary findings) in pediatric genomic research, a "preventative ethics approach should … address the risks of non-disclosure, be sensitive to timing [following the death of a child], take study design and the types of results being disclosed into account, and be responsive to ethical concerns."[38] Thus, it is "essential to anticipate possible research results and have a clear protocol for return of results after the death of pediatric research participants."[39] The same considerations hold for return of results and secondary findings in the adult population.

15.2.5 Secondary Findings from Analyzing Previously Stored Tissue Samples

Under the Pre-2018 Common Rule, IRBs have enjoyed the freedom to waive consent requirements for some research that uses samples that are stored from previous clinical or research uses.[40] Additionally, if the stored samples are de-identified and thus considered not to involve "human subjects" consistent with 45 C.F.R. § 46.101(b)(4), this research will not fall under the IRB's purview. As a result of these exceptions, participants may not know that their samples, including DNA, are being used in research. Giving participants the choice of whether or how their stored and de-identified samples are used in research was not the norm in the recent past,[41] and it is probably not the norm now under these regulatory standards. But

---

[35] 45 C.F.R. §160.103, definition of "protected health information," paragraph (2)(iv).

[36] 45 C.F.R. § 164.512(i)(1)(iii). In clinical situations, HIPAA allows sharing of protected health information after death with personal representatives of the decedent, and with the decedent's family members who were involved in their care, if not inconsistent with the decedent's wishes. 45 C.F.R. § 164.510(b)(5).

[37] 45 C.F.R. § 46.102(f) ("Human subject means a living individual …") (to be renumbered 45 C.F.R. § 46.102(e)(1) in the 2018 Requirements).

[38] Sarah Scollon, Katie Bergstrom, Laurence B. McCullough, Amy L. McGuire, Stephanie Gutierrez, Robin Kerstein, D. Williams Parsons, Sharon E. Plon, *Pediatric Cancer Genetics Research and an Evolving Preventative Ethics Approach for Return of Results after Death of the Subject*, J. LAW MED. & ETHICS Fall 2015, 529-537, at 536 (Preventative Ethics, at 534).

[39] *Id.* at 536.

[40] *See* 45 C.F.R. § 46.116(d) (alteration or waiver of some or all informed consent requirements) and §46.408(c) (waiver of requirement for parental permission for research participation).

[41] Incidental Findings in Genetic Research Using Archived DNA, *supra* note 14, at 292.

analysis of the consent form under which the sample was gathered is necessary.[42] Publicly available IRB policies revealed one academic medical center that requires IRB review of all proposals for genomic research in part due to the possibility of re-identification of individuals and family members.[43]

An investigator's plan for returning secondary findings should take into account whether or not the use of the samples was known to the participants, as returning results will be more complex, and will raise more ethical issues, if the participants will be surprised that their samples were used. The plan also should address any restrictions in the informed consent, which may contain various promises (such as not to contact the participants, not to share information, etc.). If the informed consent under which the samples were obtained does not address these issues up front, the IRB might consider mandating in its policy that such instances be presented to the IRB or a subcommittee of the IRB for case-by-case review of the legal, ethical, and practical issues occasioned by a desire to return secondary findings.

The 2018 Requirements will impose additional requirements for the use of biospecimens, at least if not previously stored. Briefly, the new rule will require informed consents for the use of identifiable biospecimens to state that either the biospecimen might be de-identified and used for future research, or that it will not be used in research at all.[44] Broad consent for secondary (but not primary) research on identifiable biospecimens will be allowed, but the IRB should review any studies that would propose to return results (presumably including secondary findings).[45] Notably, the 2018 Requirements do not address whether all biospecimens are inherently "identifiable" in the context of current genomic analytic technology when interfaced with publicly available databases. Instead, the 2018 Requirements require the fifteen agencies and departments covered by the 2018 Requirements to assess every four years whether new scientific and technology developments should change the classification of biospecimens as "identifiable."[46]

15.2.6 Results from Non-CLIA Laboratories

The Clinical Laboratory Improvement Amendments of 1988 (CLIA) apply to laboratories that examine "materials derived from the human body for the purpose of providing information for the diagnosis, prevention, or treatment of any disease or impairment of, or the assessment of the health of, human beings."[47] The CLIA regulations are generally understood to restrict

---

[42] Washington University Institutional Review Board, "Guidelines for reviewing studies involving genetic research," *available at* https://hrpo.wustl.edu/wp-content/uploads/2015/04/2015-04-03-Guidelines-for-reviewing-studies-involving-genetic-research-revised-12_06_2011-2.pdf.

[43] *Id.*

[44] 82 Fed. Reg. at 7266 (to be codified at 45 C.F.R. § 46.116(b)(9)).

[45] 82 Fed. Reg. at 7266 (to be codified at 45 C.F.R. § 46.116(d)); 82 Fed. Reg. at 7199.

[46] 82 Fed. Reg. at 7260 (to be codified at 45 C.F.R. § 46.102(e)(7). *See also* note 11.

[47] 42 U.S.C. § 263a(a).

return of patient-specific, individual results obtained in a non-CLIA research laboratory.[48] This restriction arises from concerns about the validity and accuracy of results obtained in a laboratory that does not meet all of CLIA's stringent requirements, including for analytic test validation[49] and staff qualifications and training, which could result in both false positives and false negatives.[50] Thus, IRBs should require investigators analyzing samples in non-CLIA labs to determine how these results will be handled.

15.2.7 FDA Regulation of Laboratory Developed Tests and Next Generation Sequencing

The FDA announced in 2014 draft guidance that it will expand oversight of laboratory developed tests (LDTs), requiring investigational device exemptions for a broader group of "home brew" tests that are used in human subject research before results can be returned.[51] It offered a risk-based approach.[52] FDA later stated that it would delay issuing a final guidance to allow for further discussion with stakeholders.[53] FDA reiterated its commitment to a risk-based approach, but is considering certain exceptions and "grandfathering" of tests that are already in use.[54]

FDA has also issued a discussion paper and two guidance documents addressing its fairly flexible approach to next generation sequencing technologies.[55] The discussion paper recog-

---

[48] The CLIA regulations do not apply to "[r]esearch laboratories that test human specimens but do not report patient specific results for the diagnosis, prevention or treatment of any disease or impairment of, or the assessment of the health of individual patients." 42 C.F.R. § 493.3(b)(2). This is widely, but not universally, taken to mean that results from non-CLIA research laboratories may not be returned to patients or research participants. *See* Anticipate and Communicate, *supra* note 3, and sources cited therein, at 81-82. *See also* SACHRP, Attachment C: Return of Individual Results and Special Consideration of Issues Arising from Amendments of HIPAA and CLIA, *available at* https://www.hhs.gov/ohrp/sachrp-committee/recommendations/2015-september-28-attachment-c/index.html. *But see* The Floor, the Ceiling, *supra* note 14, at 823; Distinctions Between Research and Clinical Care, *supra* note 24, at 107-08; Fabsitz, *et al.*, *Ethical and Practical Guidelines for Reporting Genetic Research Results To Study Participants: Updated Guidelines from an NHLBI Working Group*, CIRC. CARDIOVASC. GENET. 2010 Dec 1; 3(6): 574–80.

[49] 42 C.F.R. § 493.1253.

[50] *E.g.*, 42 C.F.R. §§ 493.1443, 493.1449, 493.1461, 493.1469, 493.1489.

[51] FDA, *Draft Guidance for Industry, Food and Drug Administration Staff, and Clinical Laboratories, Framework for Regulatory Oversight of Laboratory Developed Tests* (Oct. 3, 2014), *available at* https://www.fda.gov/downloads/MedicalDevices/DeviceRegulationandGuidance/GuidanceDocuments/UCM416685.pdf.

[52] *Id.* at 9-10.

[53] FDA, "Discussion Paper on Laboratory Developed Tests (LDTs)," January 13, 2017, at 1, *available at* https://www.fda.gov/downloads/MedicalDevices/ProductsandMedicalProcedures/InVitroDiagnostics/LaboratoryDevelopedTests/UCM536965.pdf.

[54] *Id.* at 3, 4.

[55] FDA, Optimizing FDA's Regulatory Oversight of Next Generation Sequencing Diagnostic Tests—Preliminary Discussion Paper (Dec. 29, 2014), *available at* https://www.fda.gov/downloads/medicaldevices/newsevents/workshopsconferences/ucm427869.pdf (NGS Discussion Paper); Guidance, Considerations for Design, Development, and Analytical Validation of Next Generation Sequencing (NGS)—Based In Vitro Diagnostics (IVDs) Intended to Aid in the Diagnosis of Suspected Germline Diseases (Apr.13, 2018), *available at* https://www.fda.gov/downloads/medicaldevices/deviceregulationandguidance/guidancedocuments/ucm509838.pdf; Guidance, Use of Public Human Genetic Variant Databases to Support Clinical Validity for Next Genetic and Genomic-Based In

nized that, unlike typical in vitro diagnostic tests (IVDs) that "detect only a single or a defined number of substances to diagnose one or several specified conditions, NGS tests can identify an essentially unlimited number of variants based on the over 3 billion base pairs that compose the human genome. Evaluating whether each data point is accurately measured would take years and thus delay the public's access to the benefits of this technology."[56] FDA stated that it desired to explore whether and how to communicate about less characterized genetic variants to patients.[57]

When analytic validity is not clearly established, IRBs should consider the extent to which test results derived from NGS genomic or genetic tests or LDTs should be shared with participants.[58]

15.3 Ethical Considerations in Returning Results

The ethical underpinnings of whether to disclose secondary findings are complex and must be balanced. The duty to disclose secondary findings is founded on ethical concepts of respect for persons (autonomy), beneficence (duty to help/assist), and non-maleficence (the duty to avoid harm and/or the duty to rescue). For adult and emancipated minor participants, this ethical stance should be balanced with participants' right not to know, based on respect for persons (autonomy). A participant may not wish to learn of any genetic risks of developing a future disease. Should this participant's autonomous desire not to know trump what the investigator may feel is an ethical duty under the principle of beneficence to advise the participant of, for example, a genetic mutation that could influence reproductive planning? These ethical considerations make clarity in the informed consent document of critical importance.

For children, the ethical analysis can be even more challenging.[59] Whether or not predictive testing for adult onset conditions should be conducted during childhood continues to be debated.[60] Genome-scale sequencing in children is now being considered for "diagnostic testing, predictive testing for childhood-onset conditions, pharmacogenetic testing, and test-

---

Vitro Diagnostics (Apr. 13, 2018), *available at* https://www.fda.gov/downloads/MedicalDevices/DeviceRegulationandGuidance/GuidanceDocuments/UCM509837.pdf.

[56] NGS Discussion Paper, *supra* note 55, at 2.

[57] *Id.* at 2, 7.

[58] *See* The Children's Hospital of Philadelphia, "Policy on Reporting Incidental Findings from Research Procedures," *available at* https://irb.research.chop.edu/sites/default/files/documents/IRBSOP903.pdf. (Mar. 11, 2013).

[59] In July 2015, the American Society of Human Genetics (ASHG) set forth its current opinion on the ethical, legal and social issues concerning genetic testing in children. *See also* ASHG Position Statement, *supra* note 1.

[60] American Academy of Pediatrics and American College of Medical Genetics and Genomics, *Ethical and Policy Issues in Genetic Testing and Screening of Children*, PEDIATRICS 2103; 131:620-622; Chimene Kesserwan, Lainie Friedman Ross, Angela R. Bradbury, "The Advantage and Challenges of Testing Children for Heritable Predisposition to Cancer," *2016 ASCO Educational Book, available at* https://meetinglibrary.asco.org/content/160621-176; Jeffrey R. Botkin, *Ethical Issues in Pediatric Genetic Testing and Screening for Current Opinion in Pediatrics*, CURR. OPIN. PEDIATR. 28(6):700–704 (Dec. 2016), *available at* https://www.ncbi.nlm.nih.gov/pmc/articles/PMC5300789/.

ing in children with cancer to inform diagnosis or therapy" in both the research and clinical contexts.[61] Should beneficence, non-maleficence, and the "best interests" of the child outweigh the autonomy of parents who desire not to know of secondary findings that are actionable and could impact the child's health or well-being? Many would say that parents should not be allowed to refuse (in the research or clinical contexts) secondary findings that could impact their child's health during childhood.[62] The IRB should require that the investigator consider this issue in the secondary-findings plan and informed consent. It may be that an investigator's plan for some studies would preclude participation of children whose parents refuse receipt of actionable secondary findings. Opting-in to receipt of genomic results, however, should not be a requirement for participating in studies with therapeutic benefit, such as tumor sequencing in order to select the appropriate chemotherapy.[63]

If genomic secondary findings reveal in a child a condition that is not actionable now but that could affect the child's future lifestyle choices or reproductive decisions, which principles should control? In this instance, beneficence and non-maleficence may counsel that the results not be returned in order to preserve the child's right to an "open future"—a future not clouded by knowledge of the secondary findings and a future in which the child as an adult may decide if he or she wants to learn of the secondary findings.[64] If the investigator plans not to return such secondary findings, parents should not be offered these results because their decision to receive them will not be respected. Yet they need to be advised of this plan at the outset in order to assess the risks and benefits of taking part in the research.[65] Although hotly debated, some hold that these secondary findings should be available to parents because they could affect current family planning or life choices of the parents and even other family members.[66]

A further issue in the pediatric context is the role of older children and adolescents in this decision-making. Unless waived, their assent must be obtained for research.[67] Issues that the investigator's plan may need to address include assent from adolescents before testing as to what kinds of secondary findings will and will not be provided, subsequent adolescent refusal to receive actionable secondary findings, and demands to know those that the parents refuse.[68] The IRB may, for example, require that the parents and adolescent agree in order to have both parental permission and adolescent assent to the research and to the plan for return or non-return of secondary

---

[61] ASHG Position Statement, *supra* note 1, at 8.

[62] The Floor, the Ceiling, *supra* note 14, at 822.

[63] *Id.* at 822.

[64] *Id.* at 821.

[65] Preventative Ethics, *supra* note 38, at 535.

[66] ACMG recommendations for reporting of secondary findings in clinical exome and genome sequencing, *available at* https://www.nature.com/gim/journal/v15/n7/full/gim201373a.html; Mapping the Ethics of Translational Genomics, *supra* note 14, at 496.

[67] 45 C.F.R. § 46.408(a); *see also* 45 C.F.R. §§ 46.404, 46.405(c), 46.406(d), 407(b)(iii).

[68] *See generally* Ellen Wright Clayton *How Much Control Do Children and Adolescents Have over Genomic Testing, Parental Access to Their Results, and Parental Communication of those Results to Others?*, J. LAW, MED. & ETHICS (2015), 538-544.

findings, perhaps with an exception for findings that are highly actionable during adolescence and with serious risk of harm if not addressed. For pediatric participants, "[t]he informed consent process and procedures for returning genomic research results to pediatric patients and their families must be a particularly flexible process, involving the parents and adjusting to the increasing capacity of the patient's ability to assent, and eventually consent upon the age of majority."[69]

15.4 Method and Timing of Disclosure

The investigator's plan must address how and when disclosure is likely to be made. The problems—including surprise and embarrassment—of the "cold call" to participants to give results or secondary findings from studies that a participant is unaware of can be dramatic.[70] Plans for explanations, counseling, and other advising should be determined in advance. "Given the lack of consensus on how to best return actionable genetic results, and given the concerns about the complexity of genetic information, many research programs have elected to use genetic providers, such as trained genetic counselors to communicate individual research results."[71] If there is no budget for providing such follow-up plans, the plan should specify that secondary findings will not be returned or should require a clear statement to participants that no assistance in understanding and dealing with the secondary findings will be provided. This likely increases the risk of participation in the research.

15.5 Informed Consent

As discussed, IRBs are charged with ensuring an appropriate, understandable informed consent document.[72] Thus, the IRB policy addressing return of secondary findings should require that the consent form and communications be clear about the possibility of secondary findings, what kind of findings will be analyzed (or omitted from the analysis), any plan to return or not to return those findings, and whether the participants will be given a choice of receipt.[73] In addition to emotional risks such as knowing of a mutation causing fear of the condition developing, discussed above, risks that must be considered include the risk to privacy and the risk of genetic discrimination. The structure and contents of the consent form in this context deserves careful scrutiny, and are detailed further in **Chapter 9**.

A plan not to return secondary findings should be justified to the IRB separately, and should be explained to participants in the informed consent document. Informed consent, of

---

[69] Preventative Ethics, *supra* note 38, at 536.

[70] Incidental Findings in Genetics Research Using Archived DNA, *supra* note 14, at 1.

[71] Chimene Kesserwan, Lainie Friedman Ross, Angela R. Bradbury, "The Advantage and Challenges of Testing Children for Heritable Predisposition to Cancer," *2016 ASCO Educational Book, available at* https://meetinglibrary.asco.org/content/160621-176; *see also* Yale University Institutional Review Boards, IRB Policy 720, "Incidental Findings with Possible Health and Safety Significance for Research Participants," *available at* https://your.yale.edu/policies-procedures/policies/720-irb-policy-720-incidental-findings-possible-health-and-safety.

[72] 45 C.F.R. § 46.116.

[73] *See* Incidental Findings in Genetics Research Using Archived DNA, *supra* note 14, at p. 2.

course, is not just a document; it is also discussion and communication of these complex issues between the investigator and the participants or their legal decision-makers.

Finally, if there was no plan for the return of secondary findings or if the plan failed to account for certain results, IRBs generally require investigators to seek IRB approval for any desired return of the secondary finding.[74]

Disclosure is among the chief ways to secure and maintain the trust of participants and members of the public who might in the future participate in the research enterprise; preservation of this trust should guide IRBs in setting policies that direct the contents of the informed consent documents in the genomics context.[75]

[74] *E.g.,* Yale University Institutional Review Boards, IRB Policy 720, "Incidental Findings with Possible Health and Safety Significance for Research Participants," *available at* https://your.yale.edu/policies-procedures/policies/720-irb-policy-720-incidental-findings-possible-health-and-safety; Stony Brook Research Human Subjects Standard Operating Procedure 17.9, "SBU Guidance on the Management of Incidental Findings in Human Research," *available at* https://research.stonybrook.edu/human-subjects-standard-operating-procedures/sbu-guidance-management-incidental-findings-human.

[75] Mapping the Ethics of Translational Genomics, *supra* note 14, at 496.

Chapter 16

Typical Areas of IRB Noncompliance

Jacqueline A. Holz

Introduction

Institutional Review Boards (IRBs) often can be noncompliant when performing the duties assigned to them by the federal regulations. This noncompliance or alleged noncompliance has not only been evidenced in litigation, but also documented in guidance issued by regulatory agencies as set forth below. Legal counsel can use this information to assist the IRB in structuring its review and meeting process to be compliant with federal and state requirements.

In addition to the more standard regulatory agency guidance, the Office for Human Resarch Protections (OHRP) provides access to webinars that may assist legal counsel in enabling the IRB to better understand and be compliant with relevant state and federal regulations.[1]

16.1 Inadequate IRB Review at Convened Meetings

OHRP has expressed concern that when IRBs are reviewing protocol applications and amendments, little substantive review takes place.[2] According to the OHRP, IRBs appear to review only minimal information regarding (i) risks to subjects and how they are minimized; (ii) human subject recruitment and enrollment procedures; (iii) the equitable selection of human subjects; (iv) provisions to protect the privacy of human subjects and maintain the confidentiality of data; and (v) additional safeguards to protect the rights and welfare of human subjects who are likely to be vulnerable.[3]

According to the OHRP Inspector General, "IRBs across the country are inundated with protocols" and the workload of the average IRB has increased to the point that they are unable to provide meaningful review.[4] As a result, some IRBs provide "only one to two minutes of

---

[1] *Mini-Tutorials*, OHRP (last visited June 29, 2018), https://www.hhs.gov/ohrp/education-and-outreach/online-education/mini-tutorials/index.html.

[2] *Types of Determinations*, OHRP (Feb. 4, 2009), https://www.hhs.gov/ohrp/compliance-and-reporting/types-of-determinations/index.html (last visited June 29, 2018) [hereafter *2009 OHRP Compliance Report*]. Note that although the report is dated 2009, examples of determination letters are also provided, dated through 2016.

[3] *Id.*

[4] *Institutional Review Boards: A Time for Reform*, Dep't of Health & Human Servs. Office of Inspector General, (June 1998), https://www.oig.hhs.gov/oei/reports/oei-01-97-00193.pdf [hereafter *OIG: Time for Reform*].

review per study."[5] Overwork has also resulted in IRBs being preoccupied with form over substantive review of the initial protocols, adverse events, and continuing reviews.[6] As one critic stated, "IRBs are spending too much time editing informed consent forms and too little time analyzing the risks and potential benefits posed by research."[7] Expedited review can present its own set of compliance challenges. OHRP has cited IRBs for using expediting initial and continuing review and protocol amendments when full IRB review, as opposed to expedited review, is appropriate. In addition, IRBs have been cited for failing to inform the full IRB of approvals made using expedited review and for allowing a non-IRB member to perform expedited review.[8]

16.1.1 Engaging in Appropriate Review of Research Protocols and Amendments

Legal counsel can assist the IRB by educating members about the appropriate process for review of research protocols and amendments. The IRB members should engage in substantive discussions at IRB meetings. As stated above, OHRP has noted that some IRBs provide only one to two minutes of review per study, and in at least one of its determination letters, OHRP has noted that an IRB appeared not to have considered systematically and rigorously such issues as risks to subjects and how they are minimized, equitable selection of subjects and subject recruitment, privacy and confidentiality protections, and additional safeguards for subjects likely to be vulnerable to coercion or undue influence.[9]

A notable case involves a federal lawsuit filed by the participants in an investigational research study alleging the IRB members (among others) at the University of Oklahoma Health Science Center used excessive time-saving mechanisms and took only one hour for its meeting, including dinner.[10] The complaint alleged that given the number of active protocols, safety reports, and other matters to process, no deliberative review could have occurred during that time period. In another matter, an otherwise healthy 24-year old volunteer named Ellen Roche died during an asthma study at Johns Hopkins University, which later acknowledged the absence of serious discussion in IRB meetings about protocols.[11]

These findings should provide a warning sign to IRBs to assess the amount of time spent at the meeting (and prior to the meeting) by the IRB members and consultants for reviewing new protocols, amendments, adverse actions, and continuing review items. The initial IRB review can filter out clinical trials that are unsound or pose excessive risks, but only if a sufficient

[5] Beh, Hazel Glenn, *The Role of Institutional Review Boards in Protecting Human Subjects: Are We Really Ready to Fix a Broken System?* 26 LAW & PSYCHOLOGY REVIEW 1, 35 (Spring 2002).

[6] *See OIG: Time for Reform.*

[7] Weijer, Charles, *The Ethical Analysis of Risk,* 28 J.L. MED. & ETHICS 344 (2000); *see also* Beh, *supra* note 5.

[8] *2009 OHRP Compliance Report.*

[9] *See OIG: Time for Reform.*

[10] Robertson v. McGee, No. 01-CV-00G0H(M) (N.D. Okla.) (Jan. 29, 2001).

[11] Gina Kolata, *Johns Hopkins Admits Fault in Fatal Experiment*, NEW YORK TIMES (July 17, 2001), *available at* https://www.nytimes.com/2001/07/17/us/johns-hopkins-admits-fault-in-fatal-experiment.html.

amount of time is spent reviewing the protocol information, sufficient IRB expertise is available in the field where the study will be conducted, and the IRB members solicit information from the investigator in response to questions or concerns they have about the study. OHRP suggested in its review of the Johns Hopkins asthma study (Roche) that the IRB should have evaluated the safety of the study medication used to induce bronchospasm. The IRB should not be hesitant to table a clinical study pending the receipt of information necessary to support the safety of the study.

Too often, IRBs are on a tight time schedule and move quickly through their agenda. Legal counsel should take note of the time spent on each agenda item at the next IRB meeting. A comparison of the time devoted towards each item in the OHRP findings of noncompliance and the allegations that have been made in recent litigation could provide information that legal counsel can use in training the IRB members on this topic. This assessment will assist the IRB in determining whether the time spent would be considered reasonable by the regulatory authorities or a plaintiffs' attorney. It may be necessary to make adjustments to the IRB process to ensure that those individuals responsible for overseeing each aspect of the review process are spending an appropriate amount of time for the review. It may also be necessary to include others in the IRB membership, including representatives from administration, legal, research, and finance.

16.2 Inadequate IRB Records

Common OHRP findings of noncompliance indicate that IRB protocol records often fail to include all the information specified in the regulations.[12] Minutes lacked sufficient detail to show attendance at meetings and actions taken. The votes were not recorded in a manner that identified the number of members voting for, against, and abstaining (*e.g.*, Total = 15; Vote For = 14, Opposed = 0; Abstained = 1). Further, the records did not reflect the basis for requiring changes in or disapproving research and a written summary of controverted issues and their resolution. In numerous instances, it was difficult for OHRP to reconstruct a complete history of all IRB actions related to the review and approval of the protocol due to poorly maintained IRB files. In some instances, OHRP could not determine what the IRB actually approved.[13] In addition, OHRP found that institutions failed to retain IRB records and records relating to research for at least three years after completion of research. The records were not accessible for inspection and copying by authorized representatives of the U.S. Department of Health and Human Services (HHS) in a reasonable manner.[14]

16.2.1 Maintaining Appropriate IRB Records

Legal counsel should be familiar with regulations set forth by HHS and the Food and Drug Administration (FDA) relating to IRB records and retention of research and research-

[12] 45 C.F.R. § 46.115(a)(1), (3), (4) and (7); *see also* 21 C.F.R. § 56.115(a)(1), (3), (4), and (7).

[13] *2009 OHRP Compliance Report.*

[14] *Id.*

related records. It is not uncommon for IRB staff to look to legal counsel to determine whether minutes are appropriately drafted and contain sufficient detail to reflect the discussions at the meeting, especially for meetings where conflicts or hotly contested issues were discussed. It is not necessary to quote in the minutes the exact conversations of members. Summations of discussion should be sufficient, as long as they are accurate. To the extent that legal counsel works with the IRB or study coordinators to modify informed consent forms, all drafts should be forwarded to the IRB for inclusion in the IRB records. It is also important for legal counsel to work with the IRB to ensure that the records maintained are consistent with the requirements of the institution's IRB policies and procedures. Irregularities between policies and practices may catch the attention of a government inspector during an audit or inspection. Another area where the expertise of legal counsel is generally called upon is the retention of research and research-related records. To the extent state law requirements are more comprehensive or stringent than federal requirements, legal counsel will want to educate the IRB on the appropriate retention period.

Draft guidance has been prepared by the OHRP (November 2015) as recommendations or suggestions regarding regulatory requirements for IRB minutes preparation and maintenance.[15] The draft guidance, when finalized, will that require IRB minutes show the attendance, actions taken, votes taken as to these actions, basis for requiring changes or not approving research, and a "written summary" of what issues were in dispute and the related resolution as to those discussions.

16.3 Inadequate Expertise on IRB

HHS regulations require the adequacy of the IRB to be evaluated in light of the anticipated scope of the institution's research activities, the types of populations likely to be involved, and the size and complexity of the institution. The regulations further require that IRBs be sufficiently qualified through the diversity of the members, including consideration of race, gender, and cultural backgrounds and sensitivity to such issues as community attitudes.[16] OHRP has found that IRBs often did not have the background and expertise to review research based on failure to include members with sufficient understanding of cultural conditions, including social, economic, and political status, of the subject population.[17]

This finding was consistent with the 1998 OHRP Report which found that IRBs often lack the necessary expertise to adequate review specific protocols. This was further evidenced in another Johns Hopkins event. In October 2001, OHRP cited ongoing problems at Johns Hopkins and noted that at a June 23 meeting, one of the IRBs had reviewed and approved oncology

[15] *Draft Guidance on Minutes of Institutional Review Board Meetings*, OHRP (Nov. 5, 2015) https://www.hhs.gov/ohrp/regulations-and-policy/requests-for-comments/draft-guidance-minutes-2015/index.html (last visited June 29, 2018).

[16] 45 C.F.R. § 46.107(a); *see also* 21 C.F.R. § 56.107(a).

[17] *See 2009 OHRP Compliance Report*, *supra* note 2, at 37 and more recent sample determination letters provided on report website.

clinical trials without a member with oncology experience and background being present.[18] A related and common problem is that the IRB may lack a quorum because no nonscientific member is present at the full IRB meeting.[19]

16.3.1 Maintaining Adequate Expertise on the IRB

Compliance with this requirement is sometimes challenging depending on the size of the institution and its community. To the extent the IRB begins to review more protocols in a specified area, such as mental health, cardiology, oncology, etc., the IRB should consider adding a member that has expertise in that area. While the IRB chairperson is typically the individual who monitors expertise, this area can additionally be monitored by legal counsel to ensure compliance with the expertise requirements of the regulations. The IRB may, at its discretion, invite individuals with competence in special areas to assist in the review of issues that require expertise beyond or in addition to that routinely available on the IRB. These *ad hoc* individuals may not, however, vote with the IRB.

Another critical area for ensuring expertise is the education of IRB members. Institutions, as well as their IRB and physician investigators, should understand the requirements applicable to them to avoid noncompliance and possible adverse FDA or OHRP action. To assist with understanding these requirements, there must be an active educational component of the IRB. This may be accomplished by offering on-line educational program, attending local or national seminars addressing research issues, using an IRB handbook with an annual competency test, or including several educational sessions in the IRB meeting itself. Of particular concern, institutions should establish educational programs on financial conflict of interest as part of their educational requirements for clinical investigators and IRB members. Institutions should make their policies and procedures, including those for financial conflict of interest and related documents and forms, available online.

16.4 Deficient Informed Consent

Informed consent represents one of the most important requirements of ethical research and one of the most difficult areas for IRBs.[20] OHRP has noted instances where (i) required elements of informed consent were omitted; and (ii) the language was too complex to be understandable by the human subject or the human subject's legally authorized representative.[21] Further, there were instances where the informed consent form contained exculpatory lan-

[18] Steinbrook, Robert, M.D., *Controlling Conflict of Interest — Proposals from the Institute of Medicine*, (10.1056/NEJMp0810200) and published at NEJM.org (April 29, 2009); *see 2009 OHRP Compliance Report.*

[19] *2009 OHRP Compliance Report.*

[20] Cohen, Glen, *Administrative Developments: New Human Subject Research Guidelines for IRBs*, 28 JOURNAL OF LAW, MEDICINE AND ETHICS 305 (Fall 2000).

[21] *2009 OHRP Compliance Report supra* note 2, at 27, 29.

guage through which the subject or the subject's legally authorized representative was made to waive or appear to waive certain legal rights.[22]

16.4.1 Ensuring Appropriate Informed Consent

The authorities cited above indicate that the informed consent process is often flawed. The IRB should not hesitate to make inquiry of the investigator of the informed consent process that will be utilized. Researchers should be questioned to determine whether they spend a sufficient amount of time explaining the clinical trial and the risks, benefits and alternatives, if any, to the potential human subjects.

The IRB should consider having designated IRB members meet with the human subjects on a random basis to ask questions about the clinical trial to verify whether they actually understood the information provided to them. Based on the interviews, IRB professionals could counsel investigators about how to improve the informed consent process and enhance human subject protection.[23]

To the extent the institution has legal counsel, the IRB should request that counsel serve as a consultant to the IRB by attending meetings and reviewing the clinical study information, especially the informed consent document. Counsel will be familiar with the informed consent requirements for your state and can assist in identifying whether the risks and benefits are fully addressed. In many instances, especially in multi-state studies sponsored by the National Institutes of Health (NIH) and pharmaceutical companies, it may be difficult to obtain changes in the informed consent document. Legal counsel may need to negotiate with the company or the sponsor.

Some practical tips for improving the informed consent document include (i) making sure that the consent document is clear and organized; (ii) using understandable language (*e.g.*, replace technical words with more commonly understood lay terms where possible); (ii) using short, simple sentences; (iii) using pronouns (*e.g.*, "you" vs. "the human subject"); (iv) using an active voice; (v) using headings to separate different sections of the document; and (vi) using a readable font (*e.g.*, Times New Roman 12 to 14-point type). The use of lay members on the IRB to review the informed consent document for understandability cannot be overstated. For a more detailed discussion about understanding research informed consent, see **Chapter 9**.

16.5 Deficient Continuing Review

IRBs have faced much criticism with respect to their handling of the continuing review process. A 1998 statement issued by the HHS Office of Inspector General (OIG) was extremely critical of research oversight.[24] The 1998 OIG Report found that continuing reviews had become a low priority at many IRBs. It criticized IRBs for failing to conduct conscientious

[22] *Id.* at 30.

[23] Hoffman, Sharona, *Continued Concern: Human Subject Protection, The Institutional Review Board and Continuing Review*, 68 TENN. L. REV. 725, 760 (Summer 2001).

[24] *See OIG: Time for Reform.*

continuing reviews of research studies. Specifically, the 1998 OIG Report revealed that IRBs routinely reviewed only written reports that were submitted by investigators conducting the clinical trials. The IRBs did not visit research sites, oversee the informed consent process, or seek feedback from research participants. As a result, the continuing review process had basically become a self-reporting process by investigators and did not provide adequate oversight of approved research projects.[25]

In 1999, the OHRP criticized IRBs for failing to conduct substantive and meaningful continuing reviews.[26] A follow-up report issued by the OIG in April 2000 concluded that, in the intervening two years, only minimal progress had been made in strengthening continuing protections for human subjects.[27] The 2009 Compliance Oversight Activity report of the OHRP echoed these findings. It found that continuing review of research was not substantive and meaningful. It found that IRBs granted extensions beyond the expiration date of the study or failed to conduct the continuing review at least once per year.[28]

16.5.1 Improving Continuing Review

The IRB and investigators must plan ahead to meet required continuing review dates. If an investigator has failed to provide continuing review information to the IRB or the IRB has not reviewed or approved a research study by the continuing review date, the research must stop, unless the IRB finds that it is in the best interest of currently enrolled subjects to continue participating in the research.

Continuing IRB review of research must be substantive and meaningful. In conducting continuing review of research not eligible for expedited review, it is recommended that all IRB members receive and review a protocol summary and a status report on the progress of the research, including (i) the number of human subjects accrued; (ii) a summary of any adverse events or unanticipated problems involving risks to human subjects or others and any withdrawal of human subjects from the research or complaints about the research since the last IRB review; (iii) a summary of any relevant recent literature, findings obtained thus far, amendments or modifications to the research since the last review, any relevant multi-center trial reports, and any other relevant information, especially information about risks associated with the research; and (iv) a copy of the current informed consent form.

Primary reviewer systems may be employed so long as the full IRB receives the above information. Primary reviewers should also receive a copy of the complete protocol including

---

[25] Hoffman, *supra* at 23.

[26] Compliance Oversight Branch Division of Human Subject Protections Office for Protection from Research Risks, OHRP Compliance Activities: Common Findings and Guidance 1, 2 (1999) (this document is no longer available on the OHRP website).

[27] *Protecting Human Research Subjects: Status of Recommendations,* Dep't of Health & Human Servs. Office of Inspector General (Apr. 2000), https://oig.hhs.gov/oei/reports/oei-01-97-00197.pdf (last visited June 29, 2018).

[28] *2009 OHRP Compliance Report, supra* note 2, at 11-12.

any modifications previously approved by the IRB.[29] Furthermore, the IRB meetings should document the separate deliberations, actions, and votes for each protocol undergoing continuing review by the convened IRB.

Even where (i) the research is permanently closed to the enrollment of new subjects; and (ii) all subjects have completed all research-related interventions, continuing review is required as long as the research remains active for long term follow-up of subjects. Furthermore, continuing review is required where the remaining research activities are limited to data analysis.

16.6 Noncompliance with Policies and Procedures

OHRP has found that institutions do not have written IRB policies and procedures that adequately describe the activities required by HHS regulations. The policies and procedures do not sufficiently state the IRB process (i) for conducting its initial and continuing review of research and for reporting its findings and actions to the investigator and the institution; (ii) for determining which projects require review more often than annually and which projects need verification from sources other than the investigators that no material changes have occurred since previous IRB review; (iii) for ensuring prompt reporting to the IRB of proposed changes in a research activity—and for ensuring that such changes in approved research during the period for which IRB approval has already been given may not be initiated without IRB review and approval except when necessary to eliminate apparent immediate hazards to the subject; or (iv) for ensuring prompt reporting to the IRB, appropriate institutional officials, and department or agency head of (a) any unanticipated problems involving risks to subjects or others or any serious or continuing noncompliance with 45 C.F.R. Part 46 or the requirements or determinations of the IRB; and (b) any suspension or termination of IRB approval.

16.6.1 Maintaining Appropriate Policies and Procedures

Successful IRBs make use of written procedures that, in one way or another, cover a common core of topics. The FDA website has a Self Evaluation Checklist for IRBs that will assist legal counsel and the IRB in determining whether its policies (or standard operating procedures) sufficiently address all aspects of FDA regulations.[30] Since the written procedures should reflect the current processes, the written procedures should be reviewed on a regular basis and updated as necessary to remain current. FDA believes that when good procedures are developed, written, and followed, the rights and welfare of the subjects of research are more likely to be adequately protected. Legal counsel can be of great assistance to the IRB in reviewing, preparing and maintaining appropriate policies and procedures. Legal counsel is in a position to learn of changes to state and federal regulations, new guidance documents, and relevant case law. This information provides legal counsel with a unique perspective in

---

[29] *See 2009 OHRP Compliance Report.*

[30] *Institutional Review Board (IRB) Written Procedures: Guidance for Institutions and IRBs*, OHRP, FDA (May 2018), https://www.fda.gov/downloads/RegulatoryInformation/Guidances/UCM512761.pdf (last accessed June 29, 2018).

reviewing and drafting policies. HHS and FDA expect institutions to comply with their written policies. Institutions are often unaware that they are out of compliance until an inspector arrives. Periodic reviews of practices and policies by the IRB and legal counsel will assist in avoiding surprises when the inspector arrives.

In May 2018, FDA and OHRP issued *Institutional Review Board (IRB) Written Procedures: Guidance for Institutions and IRBs*, that is intended to help those tasked with administrative IRB written procedures duties. The 2018 guidance supersedes OHRP's July 1, 2011 *Guidance on Written IRB Procedures* and FDA's 1998 *Appendix H: A Self-Evaluation Checklist for IRBs*, (formerly part of FDA's *Information Sheet Guidance for IRBs, Clinical Investigators, and Sponsors*).[31]

16.7 Inadequate Oversight of Clinical Trials

One of the major problems with research is that IRBs cannot effectively monitor compliance with ethical requirements. Many IRBs have discretion at the beginning of the research process to approve, reject, and change research protocols. However, once a clinical trial has been approved, IRBs have very little power to ensure compliance with ethical standards they set out for researchers. There often is virtually little, if any, contact with the human subjects or the researcher once the study has been approved and is underway. In many ways, IRBs rely on the good faith of the researchers to police themselves, but in recent years, this policy has been fraught with violations.[32]

At the heart of this problem are deficiencies in funding and personnel available for oversight of clinical trials. A 1999 NIH report noted that, although IRB workloads have been increasing, resources have not been expanding at a proportional rate.[33]

16.7.1 Improving Clinical Trial Oversight

Clinical trial oversight is a challenging area for IRBs because the typical budget for an IRB may not allow for extra employees, space, or software to assist in IRB operations. Investing in these resources, however, will assist the IRB and institution avoid costly errors and cessations of clinical trials. One oversight mechanism that an IRB can adopt is the practice of audits. They can be as routine as an audit of random medical records to ensure informed consents are properly placed in the medical record of a research participant, or sending a representative of the IRB to observe the informed consent process with a potential participant. The IRB also has the option of conducting "for cause" or "not for cause" audits. The IRB may conduct, or have a third party conduct, periodic audits of clinical trials to ensure that the principal investigator is operating the research study in accordance with the protocol and IRB written policies and

[31] *Id.*

[32] Cohen, *supra* note 20, at 306.

[33] Mahoney, John D., *NIH Initiative to Reduce Regulatory Burdens: Identification of Issues and Potential Solutions*, 2 BIOLAW S:301, S:321 (1999), *available at* https://archives.nih.gov/asites/grants/06-17-2015/archive/grants/policy/regulatoryburden/index.html.

procedures; is in compliance with current FDA or other applicable regulations; and that written informed consent has been obtained. The audit may be study- or investigator-oriented.

Generally, little or no prior notice would be given to the investigator in a "for cause" audit since the IRB would need to act quickly. On the other hand, in a "not for cause" audit, it would appear reasonable to offer the Principal Investigator some advance notice (*e.g.*, 48 hours or a week) so that he/she can arrange for additional staff to accommodate the routine audit process.

The audit process will likely involve a review of the protocol and any modifications, Investigational Drug Brochure, the informed consent form, advertising materials, the files of the Principal Investigator, the files of the IRB, hospital medical records (for consent documentation purposes), case report forms, etc. Only as needed would there be interviews with the Principal Investigator, members of the study team, or research subjects.

OHRP has indicated that oversight might be necessary in connection with clinical trial websites. On September 20, 2005, OHRP issued guidance on IRB review of such websites.[34] This document provides guidance to IRBs about circumstances when review of clinical trial websites is necessary and some practical points to consider in the review process.

The FDA in its Recruiting Study Subjects—Information Sheet (last updated March 29, 2018), states that an IRB should review the "methods and material" that are being proposed to be used in the recruitment of study subjects.[35] This Information Sheet provides clarifying information as to when IRB review of the listing of clinical trial on the internet is advised.

16.8 Conflicts of Interests

As reflected in the "Fred Hutchinson" case[36]—where patients had died prematurely in two clinical trials at Seattle's Fred Hutchinson Cancer Research Center—and the University of Oklahoma case (mentioned earlier **Section 16.1.1**),[37] conflicts of interest must be avoided. Research must operate under the governing principle that it is performed without bias created by potential financial gain on the part of the researcher or institution. Financial relationships with sponsors or with innovative companies must be managed to ensure that scientific objectivity remains intact and subjects remain protected from unreasonable risk. At the same time, strong arguments can be made that too stringent management over financial inter-relationships will impede innovation and is unfair to the research community. Disclosure of these interests may help achieve the right balance. Currently, HHS and FDA regulations require recusal of

[34] *IRB Review of Clinical Trial Websites*, OHRP (Sep. 20, 2005), https://www.hhs.gov/ohrp/regulations-and-policy/guidance/clinical-trial-websites/index.html (last visited June 29, 2018).

[35] *Recruiting Study Subjects—Information Sheet*, FDA (last updated Mar. 29, 2018), https://www.fda.gov/RegulatoryInformation/Guidances/ucm126428.html (last visited June 29, 2018).

[36] Wilson, Duff & David Health, *Uninformed Consent, What Patients at 'The Hutch" Weren't Told About the Experiments in Which They Died,* SEATTLE TIMES, March 11-15, 2001, *available at* https://old.seattletimes.com/uninformed_consent/qa.html [hereafter *Seattle Times*].

[37] Robertson v. McGee, No. 01-CV-00G0H(M) (N.D. Okla.) (Jan. 29, 2001).

any IRB member with a financial interest in a project under review.[38] Both HHS and FDA require disclosure of financial interests meeting a certain threshold.[39] A complete discussion on conflicts of interest may be found at **Chapter 12**.

16.8.1 Avoiding Conflicts of Interest

The IRB should utilize an application for review form that requires all investigators to disclose any potential conflict of interest. Also, the IRB chair should inquire of the IRB members about whether they have any potential financial conflict of interest related to any of the protocols that the IRB is about to consider. The IRB should have clear procedures for recusal of IRB members, including the IRB Chair, from deliberating/voting on all protocols for which there is a potential or actual financial conflict of interest. Many IRBs remind their members of these policies at the outset of each meeting and incorporate this reminder in the minutes of the meeting. The IRB minutes should also specifically reflect such recusals as they occur during meetings.

16.9 Research Misconduct

Research misconduct includes fabrication, falsification, or plagiarism in proposing, performing or reviewing research, or in reporting research results. Research misconduct does not, however, include honest error or difference of opinion. Instances of research misconduct should be reviewed by the IRB and/or an institutional component set up for this purpose, perhaps within a compliance or internal audit function. Federal regulations govern how this is done for research supported by the Public Health Service of HHS.[40] A complete discussion of scientific misconduct in clinical research may be found in **Chapter 18**.

16.10 Reporting Noncompliance to OHRP

IRBs and research institutions often are concerned that reporting incidents of noncompliance to the OHRP will trigger an investigation. According to the OHRP, however, IRBs that do good-faith reporting are less likely to be targeted for a "not-for-cause evaluation."[41] Further, OHRP has stated that reporting incidents is important not only because the regulations require it, but also to foster a partnership with OHRP to assist in responding to and preventing incidents.

The Division of Compliance at OHRP conducted a review and analysis of 6,511 incident reports from institutions conducting research between January 1, 2008, and December 31,

---

[38] *See* 45 C.F.R. § 46.107(e); 21 C.F.R. § 56.107(e).

[39] 42 C.F.R. Part 50, Subpart F; 21 C.F.R. Part 54.

[40] 42 C.F.R. Part 93; *see also* HHS Office of Research Integrity at https://ori.hhs.gov/.

[41] Relias, '*Serious Noncompliance' the Leading Incident Reported to OHRP* (Feb. 1, 2017), *available at* https://www.ahcmedia.com/articles/139958-serious-noncompliance-the-leading-incident-reported-to-ohrp; *see also,* Ramnath K, Cheaves S, Buchanan L, *et al.*, *Incident Reports and Corrective Actions Received by OHRP* (Nov.-Dec. 2016) 38:6, *available at* https://www.thehastingscenter.org/irb_article/incident-reports-corrective-actions-received-ohrp/.

2014 and found that the incident type most frequently reported was "serious noncompliance," which often involved changes to the research protocol without IRB approval and breakdowns of the informed consent process. Overall, there were 2,943 instances of serious noncompliance and 583 instances of continuing noncompliance.[42]

This review provides a learning opportunity for other institutions and their legal counsel in mitigating risks in their IRB process. The issues of noncompliance can be used to analyze current processes and provide insight for education and training of IRB members, staff, and principal investigators.

---

[42] *Id.*

Chapter 17

IRB Compliance and Internal Audits

Mary Holloway Richard

Introduction

The maturation of the institutional review board (IRB) process necessarily includes a system of checks, balances, education and compliance. The layers of regulatory oversight of the product and device development process, the ever-important protections afforded to human subjects and the public, and the efforts to secure and maintain the integrity of data involved in clinical research rest upon a plethora of legal requirements. This is made more complex in a health care institution, such as a hospital, by the already layered administration that may encompass health care facilities with clinical research activities. The importance of an internal audit in achieving and maintaining regulatory compliance for research activities cannot be over-emphasized. The value of an internal audit plan is two-fold. First, having an audit plan in place requires the organization to maintain a list of requirements and risks tailored to the specific IRB and the perhaps unique research activities of the organization. Second, a viable audit plan demonstrates the organization's commitment to compliance in the area of clinical research. This chapter will provide the structure and essential elements for a process audit although a risk-based audit provides an alternative that may be attractive to the institution.[1]

17.1 Regulatory Requirements Create Benchmarks for IRB Audit

As discussed in more detail in **Chapter 2**, familiarity with the roles and responsibilities of the various participants or overseers of clinical research is imperative and begins with an awareness of the relevant laws. The Department of Health and Human Services (HHS) has authority for research conducted or supported by HHS, while the Food and Drug Administration (FDA) authority includes oversight of human subjects protection and of the IRB structure and process.[2] In the clinical research arena, the prior question is whether the research is exempt from federal regulatory review. For research governed by HHS, 45 C.F.R. § 101(b)(1)-(6) created six exemptions. Exemptions from FDA oversight exist for certain research that commenced before July 27, 1981, for emergency use of a test article with some restrictions, and for the evaluation of food quality and taste as covered in HHS regulations.[3]

[1] The authors recommend coordination of the IRB compliance plan with the institution's overall compliance plan.

[2] 21 C.F.R. Part 50; 21 C.F.R. Part 56.

[3] 21 C.F.R. § 56.104; 21 C.F.R. § 56.102(d).

It is also important to consult state law as some states may have adopted more stringent requirements than those of the federal regulatory schemes. Institutional and department policies and procedures reflect those legal requirements and, in turn, become the list of tasks comprising the internal audit of IRB operations. For example, the informed concept regulatory requirements[4] are translated into specific elements for dialogue with prospective subjects, forms that the subjects need to execute, and IRB deliberation. The elements of the compliance plan are discussed in greater detail in **Section 17.3** below.

17.2 Overview of Institutional Research as Initial Step in the Internal Audit of Clinical Research Activities: Authority for Project, Scope, and Scheduling

17.2.1 Identification of Individuals with Audit Responsibilities

The individual tasked with design and oversight responsibilities for the internal audit must be identified as early in the audit process as possible. This individual may be referred to as either the IRB Compliance Officer or Research Compliance Officer (CO).[5] The CO's responsibilities must be set out, and other key supporting individuals also must be identified. An Audit Committee may also be appointed. The scope and scheduling (annually or periodically, such as every three years) of the internal clinical research audit (Audit) shall be determined by the CO or as determined by institutional management. Scheduling may be prioritized according to identified risks, patient complaints, incidents such as never events, or regulatory complaints or citations.

17.2.2 The IRB's Internal and External Relationships System: Impact on the Compliance Review

Visualizing the process may be helpful, such as with flowcharts and diagrams representing the flow of information, billing and payment, documentation and preservation of data, and scheduling requirements. This is a good time for the CO to create timelines for certification, review, approval, IRB appointments and reappointments, periodic training of key personnel, and periodic and ongoing auditing activities. Another tool for eliciting needed information, the questionnaire, may provide a window into actual compliance[6] with existing procedures or requirements and help identify potential areas of duplication and miscommunication among participants.

For the internal IRB, it is important to place the clinical research compliance program within the corporate compliance program. The larger institutional compliance plan will provide a model for review of key personnel, activities within the annual report or other report, a

---

[4] 21 C.F.R. Part 50, Subparts B and D; 21 C.F.R. § 51.25; 45 C.F.R. § 46, Subpart A.

[5] This individual may be an internal or external auditor. Although reference is made to IRB Compliance Officer throughout this chapter, the intent is to include those persons to whom tasks related to IRB compliance activities are delegated.

[6] Compliance with existing internal procedures, federal statutes, regulations and guidelines, state law, ethical guidelines, and industry and clinical best practices.

listing of federal and state laws and regulations that apply to the larger institution and to clinical research activities, institutional standards and policies that may relate to clinical research, institution-wide record keeping, monitoring, enforcement, and discipline/correction alternatives.

Although this chapter focuses on compliance reviews of internal IRBs, external IRBs are increasingly relied upon. In fact, some sponsors require use of an external IRB for specific clinical trials. For this reason, it is important to acknowledge the need to review their operations and activities for compliance with federal and state laws and guidelines. Written agreements between the reviewing and relying entities should clarify their respective roles, rights, and responsibilities. The relying entity cannot delegate all of its responsibilities for clinical research under the various regulations. Rather, it is common for the relying entity to make certain reports (*e.g.*, deviations, unanticipated events, data safety monitoring, noncompliance with protocol deviations) to provide relevant local context issues, to enroll patients, and to obtain and document participant consent. The reviewing entity commonly provides minutes of meetings and communicates with the relying entity in support of applicable regulations and other guidelines. The reviewing entity can generally conduct all kinds of reviews (*e.g.*, initial, continuing, and modification reviews), and should provide for the IRB's assistance and support in engaging in such review activities, including proper make-up of the board and adherence to established procedures required by reporting. For systems or researchers relying upon independent IRBs to provide regulatory review and oversight of research activities, the compliance process cannot be entirely delegated.[7]

Finally, documentation related to delegation of duties is extremely important in the context of clinical research compliance. Delegation must be within the regulations and, where clinical research programs are accredited, within the guidelines set by those accrediting organizations. Documentation may be found in policies and procedures, clinical research review agreements (such as with external IRBs), and corporate board minutes, all of which lend themselves to transparency in the clinical research activities of the organization.

17.2.3 Beginning with Baseline Information: Policies, Procedures, and Key Participants

Following the initial step of identifying goals and objectives,[8] the CO shall identify and gather all relevant policies and procedures of both the clinical research being undertaken and of the internal audit (institutional, departmental, and regulatory).[9] Those include policies and procedures for a properly organized IRB, distinguishing between regulated research and exempt

[7] Ass'n for the Accreditation of Human Research Protection Programs, Inc., Evaluation Instrument for Accreditation, Standard I-2 (Oct. 3, 2016), *available at* https://admin.share.aahrpp.org/Website%20Documents/2016%20Evaluation_Instrument_for_Accreditation%202016-10-04.pdf. *See also* AAHRPP, Tip Sheet 24: Relying on an External IRB, *available at* https://admin.share.aahrpp.org/Website%20Documents/Tip_Sheet_24_Relying_on_An_External_IRB.PDF.

[8] These objectives may be departmental, institutional, or agency guidelines or requirements.

[9] OIG Work Plans that are issued annually by HHS and the Center for Medicare and Medicaid Services (CMS), and recent OIG audit findings provide up-to-date guidance for compliance activities.

activities, clinical trial review, informed consent, proper billing, reporting and record-keeping, and response to complaints or deficiencies. Some of these policies, such as billing and confidentiality policies, may have been created by those not directly involved with research. It is also important to be aware of noting policies and procedures required but not currently in place, as well as those in existence but not being followed. The CO must identify the key players in the clinical research process across the organization or system. Qualifications and training for the individuals fulfilling in those key roles (principal investigators, research coordinators, administrators, bioethicists, legal counsel, sponsors and regulators) must be established within the organization. Key players will likely include non-employed medical staff, employed medical staff, other employees and independent contractors, individuals with affiliation entities (such as with coordination by a national data base or registry), and sponsors. The CO will need to be familiar with the manner in which studies are catalogued and ensure that the record of IRB compliance is maintained within the institution or system.

The CO shall be responsible for identifying the pertinent policies. The time spent initially gathering relevant policies and procedures, albeit time-consuming depending on the history of clinical research in the institution, in all likelihood will speed the process along and facilitate creation of a workable system.

17.2.4 The Compliance Audit: Key Components

In establishing the compliance plan for an IRB, those tasked with the responsibility for designing such a plan will be well-served by having an organizational chart and the support of the organization's leadership, especially if an institution is just starting this process. The following preliminary activities will generate the initial information upon which to base the compliance plan and help design the audit. Audits come into play externally by regulatory bodies and internally as part of planned compliance efforts or as a response to weaknesses that need to be corrected.

1. Interviewing key personnel, such as the Corporate Compliance Officer, management over clinical research, key staff, IRB members, and the bioethics person is the first step in the process of developing a compliance plan;
2. Using questionnaires to determine if crucial policies are being followed. Those policies might relate to the process for applying for IRB review, the manner in which studies are analyzed prior to review, the makeup of the IRB, training/certification status of all key personnel, proper and consistent record keeping by the IRB, and a record of incidents/complaints/regulatory complaints and their resolution; and
3. Cataloguing research activities and the number of studies according to researcher, sponsor, disease category, those impacting vulnerable populations, and behavioral research. Identify research conducted or supported by HHS grant applications and consortia agreements.

4. Once data is gathered:
   a. Distinguish between research and other activities (quality) and identify exempt activities;[10] (See also checklists in **Exhibits 2.3.2(a)** and **2.3.2(b)** for sample exempt research checklists.)

   b. Determine whether necessary policies and procedures exist and whether they are sufficient;

   c. Identify whether the IRB is reviewing studies according to its policies and procedures;

   d. Confirm appropriate and current registration;

   e. Confirm issuance of reports as required to regulatory bodies;

   f. Determine whether there is a process in place to provide heightened review of clinical research involving vulnerable populations review (availability of experts for each group and selection of participants is compliant); and

   g. Identify whether coding and billing is being properly performed.

17.3 Elements of Institutional Compliance Plan

The institutional compliance plan may be organized any number of ways, but must contain the following basic components: (i) catalogue of the elements of applicable regulations; (ii) existing policies and procedures; (iii) identification of key players in clinical research; (iv) an understanding of system or organizational components involved in or impacting clinical research; (v) a compliance team in which each member's responsibilities are based on audit findings and other compliance activities; and (vi) the audit schedule. As each section of the compliance plan is written, it is important to include any forms that have been developed to memorialize activities. Some compliance plans organize policies and guidelines or procedures according to training and evaluation, subject protection, principal investigators, other clinical researchers, other employees, reimbursement (including coding and billing), response to identified deficiencies or risks, and the organization and operation of the internal IRB.[11] An effective compliance plan considers the following factors:

1. **Personnel:** Provide training and periodic re-training (training logs, evaluation of materials); impart knowledge of and cultivate familiarity with laws, regulations and policies that apply to clinical research; identify the best approach to communicate with employees and staff to keep them updated. Address certification of clinical researchers and staff members, including research coordinators and others.

---

[10] See **Chapter 2**, **Section 2.3.2** for a more detailed discussion of exempt research categories under the pre-2018 Common Rule and 2018 Common Rule.

[11] OHRP & FDA, *Institutional Review Board (IRB) Written Procedures: Guidance for Institutions and IRBs*, (May 2018), *available at* https://www.fda.gov/downloads/RegulatoryInformation/Guidances/UCM512761.pdf.

2. **IRB Member Composition:** Provide training for members (*e.g.*, principal investigator, research coordinators, who gains consent, staff interfacing with sponsors) and advocates for vulnerable populations; provide administrative support for the review of applications of approval, record keeping. Keep in mind it sometimes may be difficult to get qualified individuals to serve on the board and to ensure robust representation on the board (*e.g.*, diversity, expertise). Consider current federal wide assurance (FWA) and other certification of program.
3. **Other Institutional Support:** Determine the need for reporting within the organization, including potentially a bioethicist or legal counsel.
4. **Human Subjects Protection:** Compliance with the requirements of the informed consent process (see **Chapter 9** for a more detailed discussion about the informed consent process); protecting the confidentiality of research subjects' data and information; providing a hotline to report an issue or concern; assuring non-retaliation.
5. **Record Maintenance:** Develop good record maintenance, which will help with the timely generation of reports and response to complaints.
6. **Scheduling of Activities:** Develop and implement schedules regarding the collection, storage, use, maintenance, destruction, discontinuance, etc. of drugs, devices, biohazards, chemicals, hazardous materials, radiation, lasers, controlled substances, human embryonic stem cells, etc. that are being used in research.
7. **Special Research:** Consider and develop additional policies and procedures that may be required due to the nature of special research and activities and the significant risks posed by such research, if any. The "special" nature of the research could derive from, for example, participation by vulnerable subjects, unique or innovative research techniques, or research requiring specialized clinical experts or advocates.

The compliance plan must be capable of providing guidance for both proactive and reactive efforts. This may occur through a review of policies in place or an audit of process.

17.4 Common Deficiencies and Areas of Risk

Common areas of concern include documenting compliance generally, protecting vulnerable populations (such as pregnant women and prisoners), having a robust evaluation by a properly constituted and trained IRB, training and oversight of a valid informed consent process for prospective subjects, and protecting subjects' privileged information. Toward that end, experience has demonstrated the value of the following logs, checklists, worksheets, and data bases:

1. **Checklists** on eligibility criteria, regulatory documentation, single visit, study closeout, personnel training (initial, annual, CITI), and study startup elements.
2. **Logs** regarding study startup checklist items, delegation of authority, informed consent form version tracking, informed consent tracking by subject, enrollment,

adverse event, concomitant medication, device accountability, phone screening, protocol deviation, storage of retained body fluids/tissue sampling, self-monitoring, study-specific signature, study-specific training, subject compensation, training attendance, site monitoring, initial and follow-up training (*e.g.*, CITI),[12] correspondence with sponsor, study team modifications/modifications required by sponsor, vulnerable population studies, complaints, and billing issues. See logs included in the Exhibits associated with this chapter.

3. **Templates, notes, worksheets and flow charts** regarding corrective/preventive action,[13] informed consent process, meeting minutes, and telephone contacts.[14] OHRP offers a series of decision charts facilitating compliance review of IRB decision-making.[15]
4. **Databases** are available and commonly used to provide up-to-date information on serious adverse events (SAEs) and initial new drug (IND) safety reports. They provide useful tools and should be evaluated for their reliability as part of the IRB compliance plan.

Preventive measures include the development of an effective system/organization-wide communication network so that there is institutional buy-in and the creation of partnerships that can actively oversee the various research studies. Transparency in the review process and transparency in the way research is conducted can help correct deficiencies, educate personnel at all levels, create workable mechanisms for resolving conflict, and cultivate a solid working relationship with those responsible for billing within the system or department.

17.5 What Is At Stake: Penalties, Sanctions, and Restrictions

The FDA maintains a registry of all clinical investigators, contract research organizations, and IRBs related to investigational new drugs and investigational devices.[16] The FDA can issue a "Restrictions Imposed Letter" informing an IRB of restrictions imposed under 21 C.F.R. §56.103 and 56.120(b). In addition, recalcitrant IRBs and repeat offenders may also be subject

[12] In the event of an external regulatory audit, the information should be readily accessible and accurately maintained.

[13] Accurate and timely documentation is important because they help identify areas of concern, minimize risks, and prompt actions—taken either preventively or as corrective measures—to protect human subjects in research.

[14] The importance of accurate and timely documentation is critical given the number of research support staff (through delegation of shared responsibilities on a research team, staff turnover, shift changes, etc.) involved in the various activities of research (*e.g.*, answering a phone call, reading and filing correspondence).

[15] OHRP, Human Subjects Regulations Decision Chart (Feb. 16, 2016), https://www.hhs.gov/ohrp/regulations-and-policy/decision-charts/index.html.

[16] FDA, Clinical Investigator Status (Biologics), https://www.fda.gov/BiologicsBloodVaccines/GuidanceComplianceRegulatoryInformation/ComplianceActivities/ucm165743.htm; FDA, Bioresearch Monitoring Information System (BMIS), (information source is FDA Forms 1571 and 1572), https://www.fda.gov/Drugs/InformationOnDrugs/ucm135162.htm; FDA, Clinical Investigator Inspection Search, https://www.accessdata.fda.gov/scripts/cder/cliil/index.cfm.

to an administrative IRB disqualification action.[17] A warning letter offers an informal advisory from the FDA, but the agency is not committed to a course of action by the letter, although failure to attend to the continuing violation is likely to result in agency enforcement action.[18] For a discussion of the FDA's approach with regard to wrongful acts and unreliability of data, see the FDA's Application Integrity Policy.[19] Another possible FDA response is debarment of an individual or an institution in which notice and hearing are provided.[20]

HHS regulations in 42 C.F.R. Part 93 outline compliance requirements and provide procedures for investigations, administrative actions, due process, and settlement in the event of a finding of research misconduct. HHS debarment regulations are set forth in 45 C.F.R. Part 76. The Department of Justice and the HHS Office of Inspector General are tasked with investigating[21] and prosecuting alleged misconduct. The Office of Research Integrity (ORI) website provides descriptions of behavior and actions taken by clinical investigators. Federal law also encourages and protects whistleblowers.[22] The research misconduct investigation process is discussed in more detail in **Chapter 18**.

Another area of significant potential penalties involves incidents of incorrect billing resulting in overpayments.[23] It is imperative to identify such mistakes so that corrections can be made and the system brought to conformance. It is advisable to work closely with those submitting claims so as to become familiar with corporate payment functions, as well as the compensation and billing portions of sponsor documents. A detailed discussion of clinical trial billing may be found at **Chapter 13**.

It is important to include a word about competing perspectives in the context of regulatory compliance for clinical research activities. Conflicts of interest are common given potentially varied objectives of regulators, drug companies and other vendors, patients and their advocates, and providers. A thorough discussion of conflicts of interest may be found at **Chapter 12**. Having a compliance plan that is complete with a robust audit will help in detecting issues and effectively working to mitigate the impact of varying interests.

---

[17] FDA, Institutional Review Boards—Restrictions Imposed Letters and Disqualification Proceedings, https://www.fda.gov/ScienceResearch/SpecialTopics/RunningClinicalTrials/ComplianceEnforcement/ucm369514.htm. Note that the clinical investigator disqualification proceedings database allows for access to names of individuals who have been subject to an administrative clinical investigator disqualification action. See also FDA, Clinical Investigators, Disqualification Proceedings, https://www.fda.gov/ICECI/EnforcementActions/ucm321308.htm.

[18] FDA, Warning Letters, https://www.fda.gov/ICECI/EnforcementActions/WarningLetters/default.htm.

[19] FDA, Application Integrity Policy, https://www.fda.gov/ICECI/EnforcementActions/ApplicationIntegrityPolicy/default.htm.

[20] FDA, Notice of Opportunity for Hearing (NOOH)—Proposal to Debar, https://www.fda.gov/RegulatoryInformation/FOI/ElectronicReadingRoom/ucm143240.htm; *see also* FDA, Debarment List (Drug Product Applications), https://www.fda.gov/ICECI/EnforcementActions/FDADebarmentList/default.htm.

[21] Dep't. of Health and Human Svcs., Ofc. of Research Integrity, http://ori.hhs.gov/.

[22] Federal Whistleblower Protection Act of 1989, Pub.L. 101-12 (Apr. 10, 1989), *available at* https://www.gpo.gov/fdsys/pkg/STATUTE-103/pdf/STATUTE-103-Pg16.pdf.

[23] A discussion of repayment and disclosure responsibilities is beyond the scope of this chapter, but it is an important component of resolution.

Chapter 18

Scientific Misconduct in Clinical Research

Thomas D. Shrack[1]

Introduction

Scientific misconduct in clinical research happens all the time, and the consequences can be damaging—to the institution where it occurred, to the investigator's career, and even to patients who have agreed to participate in research. As a result, institutions engaged in clinical research must be vigilant regarding their research programs. They must also know how to appropriately respond to and address allegations of scientific misconduct in a timely, thorough, and impartial manner so as to avoid harm to patients or sanctions to the institution and to maintain, or if necessary, restore public faith in science and health care.

18.1 Public Health Service and Food and Drug Administration Policy

For clinical research involving human subjects in the U.S., there are two separate sets of governing regulations and policies, promulgated by the Public Health Service (PHS) and the Food and Drug Administration (FDA). For the conduct of federally-funded clinical research, the Basic Health and Human Services Policy for Protection of Human Research Subjects (usually referred to as the Pre-2018 Common Rule as result of its adoption and use by more than 15 federal agencies, departments, and commissions), set forth at Title 45 of the Code of Federal Regulations, Part 46 controls.[2] For research intended to support an application for permission to market a new or equivalent drug, device or biologic, the FDA's regulations control.[3]

The Pre-2018 Common Rule was developed by the Department of Health and Human Services (HHS) to establish standards for research conducted or supported by the federal government, and is based on the Belmont Report, issued by the National Commission for the Protection of Human Services of Biomedical and Behavioral Research, which summarizes ethical principles and guidelines for research involving human subjects.[4] Compliance with the

[1] With significant assistance and support from Hall Render Killian Heath & Lyman attorney Melissa L. Markey and Ascension Health attorney Maryn T. Johnson and Hall Render Killian Heath & Lyman law clerks Kimberly Panian, Jordan Tanoury, Taylor Daily, and Macauley Rybar.

[2] Basic HHS Policy for Protection of Human Research Subjects, 45 C.F.R. pt. 46 (2009), *available at* https://www.hhs.gov/ohrp/regulations-and-policy/regulations/45-cfr-46/index.html.

[3] *See generally* 21 C.F.R. 50, 54, 56, 312, 812, 814.

[4] *See The Belmont Report*, accessible at https://www.hhs.gov/ohrp/regulations-and-policy/belmont-report/index.html.

Pre-2018 Common Rule is regulated by the Office of Human Research Protections (OHRP), an agency in HHS. Research misconduct in the context of research supported by Common Rule agencies is investigated by the Office of Research Integrity (ORI), an agency in the HHS Office of the Secretary. Although OHRP and ORI have different areas of focus, the agencies do maintain open lines of communication.

FDA regulations governing research involving human subjects are very similar to the Pre-2018 Common Rule, but there are differences. The FDA refers to research misconduct that occurs in the context of the approval process for a drug, device, or biologic as "fraud," which the FDA regulates by policy. Investigations of misconduct in research relating to FDA-regulated drugs, devices, or biologics are conducted through the FDA Office of Regulatory Affairs, and may involve the Office of Enforcement or Office of Criminal Investigations.

18.2 Defining Research and Scientific Misconduct

In order to evaluate an allegation of scientific misconduct, an institution must first determine whether the behavior in question occurred while engaged in clinical research, and then whether the behavior fits within the PHS or FDA definitions of research misconduct.

The Belmont Report states that "the term 'research' designates an activity designed to test an hypothesis, permit conclusions to be drawn, and thereby to develop or contribute to generalizable knowledge (expressed, for example, in theories, principles, and statements of relationships). . . ."[5] "Research" is defined in the PHS misconduct regulations as:

> a systematic experiment, study, evaluation, demonstration or survey designed to develop or contribute to general knowledge (basic research) or specific knowledge (applied research) relating broadly to public health by establishing, discovering, developing, elucidating or confirming information about, or the underlying mechanism relating to, biological causes, functions or effects, diseases, treatments, or related matters to be studied.[6]

OHRP also provides a chart intended to assist in the identification of activities that constitute research.[7]

In place of the term "research," FDA regulations define "clinical investigation" as "any experiment in which a drug is administered or dispensed to, or used involving, one or more human subjects . . . except for the use of a marketed drug in the course of medical practice."[8] Use of drugs, devices, or biologics not approved by the FDA for any indication in the U.S. is

[5] THE NAT'L COMM'N FOR THE PROT. OF HUMAN SUBJECTS OF BIOMEDICAL & BEHAVIORAL RESEARCH, THE BELMONT REPORT: ETHICAL PRINCIPLES AND GUIDELINES FOR THE PROTECTION OF HUMAN SUBJECTS OF RESEARCH (Apr. 18, 1979), *available at* https://www.hhs.gov/ohrp/regulations-and-policy/belmont-report/index.html.

[6] 42 C.F.R. § 93.222 (2017).

[7] OFFICE FOR HUMAN RESEARCH PROTECTIONS, *Is An Activity Research Involving Human Subjects?* (2016), *available at* https://www.hhs.gov/ohrp/regulations-and-policy/decision-charts/index.html.

[8] 21 C.F.R. § 312.3 (2017).

by definition a clinical investigation, as the only permissible use is investigational. In addition, use of an approved drug, device, or biologic for an unapproved indication will be considered a clinical investigation if the data will be submitted to the FDA in support of an application for approval of marketing that drug, device, or biologic for the new indication.

Research misconduct is narrowly defined in the PHS regulations as fabrication, falsification, or plagiarism in proposing, performing, or reviewing research, or reporting the results of research.[9] Fabrication is the creation of fictitious data or results and representing them as the actual outcome of the experiment. Falsification occurs when data is changed or omitted, or when research materials, equipment, or methods are modified from standard and result in an inaccurate research record. Plagiarism is the appropriation of another person's ideas, processes, results, or words without giving appropriate credit.[10] To constitute misconduct, the falsification, fabrication, or plagiarism must be shown to have been a "significant departure from accepted practices" of research[11] and must have been intentional, knowing, or reckless.[12]

The PHS rule clearly defines fabrication, falsification, and plagiarism.[13] Fabrication is defined as the "making up data or results and recording or reporting them."[14] Some examples of data fabrication are creating fictitious study participants (often called ghost patients), reporting more experiments than were actually conducted, inventing false data points, or creating, "out of whole cloth," drug logs or laboratory notebooks.

Falsification is "manipulating research materials, equipment, or processes, or changing or omitting data or results such that the research is not accurately represented in the research record."[15] Examples of falsification include: (i) duplicating test results with different subject names; (ii) duplicating subjects (enrolling the same subject multiple times using different subject identifiers); (iii) misrepresenting dates to match visits required by the protocol; and (iv) back-dating consents or altering laboratory test results to match values required by the protocol. At times, investigators have found falsification where the researcher "spiked" cell cultures or other research materials to obtain the desired result.[16]

Plagiarism is "the appropriation of another person's ideas, processes, results, or words without giving appropriate credit."[17] The ORI includes within the definition of plagiarism the "theft or misappropriation of intellectual property and the substantial unattributed textual

---

[9] 42 C.F.R. § 93.103 (2017).

[10] *Id.*

[11] 42 C.F.R.§ 93.104(a) (2017).

[12] *Id.* at § 93.104(b).

[13] 42 C.F.R. § 93.103

[14] 42 C.F.R. § 93.103(a).

[15] *Id.* at § 93.103(b).

[16] *See, e.g.*, OFFICE OF RESEARCH INTEGRITY, HANDLING MISCONDUCT—INQUIRY ISSUES: ORI RESPONSES TO ISSUES ARISING FROM INQUIRIES AND INVESTIGATIONS, *available at* https://ori.hhs.gov/ori-responses-issues (last visited July 2, 2018).

[17] 42 C.F.R. § 93.103(c) (2007).

copying of another's work."[18] Theft or misappropriation of intellectual property occurs when one researcher uses the ideas or methods of another without consent, while textual copying of another's work is "verbatim or near-verbatim copying of sentences and paragraphs which materially mislead the ordinary reader regarding the contributions of the author."[19] ORI typically does not pursue situations in which the copied material is limited, unless the reader would be misled.[20] It is worth noting that allegations that another researcher claimed authorship without basis, or disputes between collaborators regarding ownership of ideas, or "minor copying of text, including commonly used descriptions of methodology," typically will not support a finding of PHS research misconduct.[21]

Research misconduct encompasses a wider range of activities under FDA policy, including falsification of data, untrue statements of material fact, bribery, and illegal gratuities in any aspect of research leading to submissions to the FDA.[22] The FDA's definition of research misconduct, sometimes referred to as fraud, also includes falsification in proposing, designing, conducting, supervising, reviewing, or reporting of research.[23] The FDA may find research misconduct based on action or failure to act, such as failure to report adverse events or other important information if that failure adversely impacts the value of the science or reliability of the research. Further, the FDA may find that deliberate non-compliance with FDA regulations, good research, or clinical practices, or violation of institutional policies constitutes misconduct.[24]

It is just as important to know what does not constitute scientific misconduct. Sloppiness, honest disputes of fact or opinion, honest errors, and good-faith authorship disputes do not rise to the level of research misconduct. Most protocol violations are not misconduct, although some protocol violations are so significant and have such a serious impact on the quality of the research that the FDA may find misconduct. Even unethical behavior and violations of human subject protection regulations are typically not research misconduct.

---

[18] *See* OFFICE OF RESEARCH INTEGRITY, ORI POLICY ON PLAGIARISM, *available at* https://ori.hhs.gov/ori-policy-plagiarism (last visited July 2, 2018).

[19] *Id.*

[20] *Id.* (Noting how it is important for researchers to be aware that journals may have more stringent definitions and requirements with respect to attribution of sources).

[21] Chris B. Pascal, *Scientific Misconduct and Research Integrity for the Bench Scientist,* 224 PROC. SOC'Y FOR EXPERIMENTAL BIOLOGY & MED. 220, 220-30 (2000).

[22] FDA, Fraud, Untrue Statements of Material Facts, Bribery, and Illegal Gratuities, §120.100 CPG 7150.09 (Jul. 1, 1991), *available at* https://www.fda.gov/ICECI/ComplianceManuals/CompliancePolicyGuidanceManual/ucm073837.htm.

[23] *See* Fraud, Untrue Statements of Material Facts, Bribery, and Illegal Gratuities; Final Policy, 56 Fed. Reg. 46191 (Sept. 10, 1991), *available at* https://www.fda.gov/ICECI/EnforcementActions/ApplicationIntegrity-Policy/ucm134741.htm.

[24] *See generally* FDA, Application Integrity Policy, *available at* https://www.fda.gov/downloads/ICECI/EnforcementActions/ApplicationIntegrityPolicy/ucm072631.pdf.

18.3 Misconduct Under PHS Rules

Research misconduct may be committed by anyone involved in the conduct of clinical research, including principal investigators, sub-investigators, research staff, clerical staff, students, interns, and personnel associated with the contract research organization or the research sponsor. ORI has jurisdiction when allegations of scientific misconduct involve research subject to PHS regulations. Typically, ORI will respond to such allegations only if the misconduct occurred within six years of the date the agency or the institution receives the allegation.[25]

There are exceptions to this statute of limitations. For instance, allegations of research misconduct that the agency or institution received prior to the effective date of the PHS rule are excluded from the six-year limit.[26] In addition, if a researcher continues to use fabricated, falsified, or plagiarized data or research records "through the citation, republication or other use for the potential benefit of the [respondent]," or if ORI or the institution believes that alleged misconduct, if proven, would "possibly have a substantial adverse effect on the health or safety of the public," the six-year limit will not apply.[27]

Because PHS agencies typically award grants and cooperative agreements to institutions and not to principal investigators, those institutions have the primary responsibility for ensuring that research is conducted in accordance with law. PHS requires institutions that receive PHS funding to: (i) foster a culture of compliance and integrity; (ii) have written policies and procedures for addressing allegations of research misconduct that comply with the PHS regulations; (iii) respond to each allegation of research misconduct in a "fair, thorough, competent and objective" manner; and (iv) take steps to protect the positions and reputations of complainants, witnesses, and committee members, and to protect them from retaliation.[28]

Further, institutions that receive PHS funding for research are required by PHS regulations to maintain written policies and procedures that comply with the PHS rules for inquiring into and investigating allegations of research misconduct.[29] Institutions must provide PHS with assurance that they: (i) have such policies and will make their personnel involved in PHS-supported research aware of them; (ii) will evaluate any credible allegation of research misconduct involving PHS-supported research; and (iii) will comply with their policies and the PHS regulations when evaluating allegations of misconduct.[30] Institutions must also submit annual reports to ORI detailing their compliance with PHS regulations regarding scientific misconduct.[31]

[25] 42 C.F.R. § 93.105.

[26] 42 C.F.R. § 93.105(b)(3).

[27] *Id.* at § 93.105(b)(2).

[28] 42 C.F.R. § 93.300.

[29] 42 C.F.R. § 93.301.

[30] *Id.*

[31] *Id.* at § 93.302.

18.3.1 Receiving Allegations and Initiating an Inquiry

Upon receipt of a "sufficiently credible and specific" allegation, which, if true, would constitute scientific misconduct as defined by PHS, an institution must open an inquiry.[32] The purpose of this inquiry is not to answer the question of whether research misconduct actually occurred, but solely to determine whether sufficient evidence exists to support an investigation. Accordingly, the inquiry will determine whether "a reasonable basis" exists for finding that the action in question involves PHS support and whether there is evidence that indicates "that the allegation may have substance."[33]

Once an inquiry has been initiated, the responsible institution must promptly notify the subject of the allegation(s) and must "promptly take all reasonable and practical steps to obtain custody of the research records and evidence needed to conduct the research misconduct proceeding."[34] All relevant research records and evidence must be inventoried and stored in a secure location, "except that where the research records or evidence encompass scientific instruments shared by a number of users, custody may be limited to copies of the data or evidence on such instruments, so long as those copies are substantially equivalent to the evidentiary value of the instruments."[35]

Institutions have sixty calendar days to complete scientific misconduct inquiries, unless "circumstances clearly warrant a longer period."[36] Institutions must document the reasons for a review period that exceeds sixty days. Upon completion of a scientific misconduct inquiry, an institution must advise the subject of the allegation whether the institution has concluded that an investigation is warranted.[37] The individual who made the allegation may be notified as well, but the institution is not required to do so. The subject of the allegation must be provided with a copy of the inquiry report, the institution's applicable policies and procedures, and an opportunity to comment on the report.[38]

18.3.2 When Investigation Is Warranted

When an institution's scientific misconduct inquiry has determined that the alleged behavior or action involves PHS support and evidence exists that indicates "that the allegation may have substance,"[39] the institution has thirty days to notify ORI of its intent to open an investigation. The institution must provide ORI with a copy of the inquiry report, which must describe the allegations that gave rise to the inquiry, the details of any affected PHS funding,

[32] *Id.* at § 93.307(a).

[33] *Id.* at § 93.307(d).

[34] *Id.* at § 93.307(b).

[35] *Id.*

[36] *Id.* at § 93.307(g).

[37] *Id.* at § 93.308(a), (b).

[38] *Id.* at § 93.307(f).

[39] *Id.* at § 93.307(d).

the basis for the institution's decision to open the investigation, and any comments from the subject of the allegation regarding the inquiry report.[40] The institution also must provide ORI with its policies on scientific misconduct, if requested.[41]

An institution has thirty days to commence a scientific misconduct investigation after it determines that one is necessary.[42] Before doing so, it must notify the subject of the allegation of the pending investigation and of the institution's obligation to promptly notify the subject of the allegation in writing of any new allegations of misconduct that arise during the investigation.[43] At this time, as well, the institution must secure any additional records or evidence that have not already been sequestered.[44]

18.3.3 Investigation Procedure

Accurate and complete records of the investigation must be maintained by the institution, and they must establish the thoroughness and objectivity of the investigation, demonstrating that relevant documents and evidence were examined in an impartial manner, including participation of persons with appropriate scientific expertise who do not have conflicts of interest with those involved with the inquiry or investigation.[45] Interviews of anyone who has been reasonably identified as having information regarding any relevant aspects of the investigation conducted during the investigation should be recorded, and a transcription of the interview should be provided to the interviewee for correction.[46] All significant issues and leads relevant to the investigation must be pursued diligently, including any evidence of additional instances of possible research misconduct.[47] Finally, the institution must prepare and provide a draft final report to the subject of the allegation, who shall be given thirty days to comment.[48]

The institution has 120 days from commencement of an investigation to complete all aspects, including the submission of a final report of the investigation to ORI. An institution may request an extension past 120 days in writing from ORI, which has the discretion to approve or decline the request.[49] The final report must describe in detail the allegations and the affected PHS-supported activities, and identify and summarize the records and evidence reviewed. The report also must include a statement of findings for each allegation, specifying:

- the nature of the misconduct (*i.e.*, falsification, fabrication, or plagiarism);

---

[40] *Id.* at § 93.309.

[41] *Id.*

[42] *Id.*

[43] *Id.* at § 93.310.

[44] *Id.* at § 93.309.

[45] *Id.* at § 93.310.

[46] *Id.*

[47] *Id.*

[48] *Id.* at § 93.312.

[49] *Id.* at § 93.311.

- whether the misconduct was committed intentionally or in reckless disregard of whether it was misconduct;
- facts and the analysis that support the conclusion, including consideration of the merits of any reasonable explanation by the subject of the investigation;
- specific PHS-supported projects affected by that allegation;
- any publications that require correction or retraction;
- the individual responsible for the misconduct;
- any request by the respondent for PHS support that is currently pending; and
- any comments on the final report issued by respondent and complainant.[50]

In addition, the final report to ORI must state whether the investigation found research misconduct, whether the institution accepts those findings, and describe any pending or completed administrative actions against the subject of the investigation.[51] Though not required to do so, upon completion of the investigation and final report, the institution may grant the subject of the investigation an opportunity to appeal the institution's findings.[52] Any such appeal must be completed within 120 days of the request, though an extension can be requested from ORI.

When an institution closes an inquiry or investigation prior to completion for any reason, including an admission of guilt from, or a settlement with, the subject of the inquiry or investigation, the institution must notify ORI, which will either approve the closure, require the institution to continue the investigation, refer the case to another HHS agency for further action, or take other appropriate action.[53] Unless custody has been transferred to HHS upon HHS's request, or ORI has advised the institution in writing that it no longer needs to retain the records, the institution must retain the records associated with the inquiry, investigation, and appeal, if applicable, for at least seven years after the completion of the proceeding, including any proceedings within HHS.[54]

18.3.4 Notifying ORI

In cases of alleged scientific misconduct, an institution is required to keep ORI notified of specific events and timelines. As noted previously, an institution must notify ORI when an investigation is opened; when the final report of an investigation is completed (even if no misconduct was identified); if an investigation or an appeal will exceed permitted time; or when the institution plans to close a case at the inquiry, investigation, or appeal stage based on an admission of guilt or settlement with the respondent.

[50] *Id.* at § 93.313.

[51] *Id.* at § 93.315.

[52] *Id.* at § 93.314

[53] *Id.* at § 93.316.

[54] *Id.* at § 93.317.

In addition, an institution also must notify ORI if it reasonably believes that:

- the health or safety of the public is at risk, including an immediate need to protect human or animal subjects;
- HHS resources or interests are threatened;
- research activities should be suspended;
- there is reasonable evidence of possible violations of civil or criminal law;
- federal action is required to protect the interests of those involved in the research misconduct proceeding;
- the public may find out about the research misconduct proceeding before the investigation, inquiries, etc. are completed, thereby prompting HHS to take appropriate steps to safeguard evidence and protect the rights of those involved; or
- the research community or public should be informed.[55]

18.3.5 ORI's Authority

ORI may respond directly to or take action regarding any allegation of research misconduct at any time before, during, or after an institution's response to the matter. ORI may independently review allegations and make its own finding of research misconduct.[56] ORI can forward allegations of research misconduct to other HHS agencies or components, or recommend that HHS perform an inquiry or investigation or issue findings and take all appropriate actions in response to such inquiry, investigation, or findings.[57]

ORI can impose administrative sanctions on an institution for failure to comply with the regulations, and can also recommend to HHS that a person or institution be suspended or debarred from receiving federal funds.[58] In addition, ORI can request additional information, review an institution's assurance and policies, and provide technical and procedural assistance to the institution.[59] If ORI believes that criminal or civil fraud may have occurred, it must refer the matter to the Department of Justice (DOJ), the HHS Office of Inspector General (OIG), or other appropriate investigative body, and may assist them or other federal, state, or local offices involved in investigating research misconduct allegations or related matters.[60]

When ORI makes a finding of research misconduct and determines that administrative action is appropriate, it will notify the subject of the misconduct finding via a charge letter that specifies the findings of ORI, describes the basis for those findings, sets forth proposed administrative actions, and describes the rights that the subjects of the misconduct have to

---

[55] *Id.* at § 93.318

[56] *Id.* at § 93.400.

[57] *Id.*

[58] *Id.*

[59] *Id.*

[60] *Id.* at § 93.401.

appeal.[61] If debarment or suspension is proposed, the HHS debarring official[62] will send a notice of proposed debarment or suspension along with the charge letter.

18.3.6 Imposition of Sanctions

Following a finding of scientific misconduct, HHS may impose administrative actions, including:

- retraction or clarification of the research record;
- letter of reprimand;
- special certification or assurance requirements;
- suspension or termination of PHS funding or support;
- restriction of specific activities or expenditures of PHS funding or support;
- supervision requirements over use of PHS funding or support;
- certification of attribution or authenticity in all requests for PHS support and in all reports to PHS;
- prohibition against serving in an advisory role for PHS agencies;
- recovery of PHS funds; and
- suspension or debarment.[63]

To determine the appropriate administrative action, HHS will consider aggravating and mitigating factors such as:

- the intent or recklessness of the respondent;
- whether the misconduct was isolated or demonstrated a pattern of dishonest conduct;
- the impact of the misconduct on the research record, research subjects, other researchers, institutions, or the public health or welfare;
- whether the subject of the finding has accepted responsibility by admitting the misconduct, cooperating with the misconduct proceedings, demonstrating remorse and awareness of the seriousness of the misconduct, and taking steps to correct or prevent any recurrence of the misconduct;
- any attempt to intimidate or retaliate by the subject of the finding; and
- whether the subject of the finding is presently responsible to conduct PHS-supported research.[64]

Institutions must foster a research environment that discourages misconduct in all research and that deals forthrightly with possible misconduct associated with PHS supported research.

---

[61] *Id.* at § 93.405.

[62] *Id.* at § 93.206.

[63] *Id.* at § 93.407.

[64] *Id.* at § 93.408.

ORI can find that an institution has not met this requirement if it finds the institution lacks required policies, fails to respond appropriately to allegations, fails to properly report to ORI regarding investigations, fails to cooperate with ORI's investigation, or engages in "other actions or omissions that have a material, adverse effect on reporting and responding to allegations of misconduct."[65] ORI may provide a non-compliant institution with technical support "if the deficiencies do not substantially affect compliance" with the misconduct regulations, or it may take actions that include issuing a letter of reprimand, placing the institution on special review status, or imposing an institutional integrity agreement or suspension/debarment of the institution by HHS.[66]

18.3.7 Appeal of Findings and Actions

The subject of a scientific misconduct finding has the right to contest that finding and the subsequent administrative actions, including any debarment or suspension action, by requesting a hearing within 30 days of receipt of the charge letter.[67] The request must be in writing to ORI and the Chair of HHS's Departmental Appeals Board (DAB); admit or deny each finding of misconduct and each factual assertion made in support of the finding; accept or challenge each proposed administrative action; provide detailed, substantive reasons for each denial or challenge; and identify any legal issues or defenses the subject of the finding intends to raise, as well as any mitigating factors he or she wants ORI and the DAB Chair to consider. Any findings or actions not denied or challenged will be deemed admitted or accepted.[68]

The DAB Chair, in consultation with HHS's Chief Administrative Law Judge, will designate an Administrative Law Judge (ALJ) to determine whether the hearing request should be granted and, if granted, preside over the hearing.[69] The ALJ must grant a hearing request if he or she determines there is a genuine dispute of facts material to the finding of research misconduct or the proposed HHS administrative action. A "general denial or assertion of error . . . is not sufficient to establish a genuine dispute."[70] If the ALJ grants the hearing request, the subject of the scientific misconduct finding may waive the opportunity for an in-person proceeding and agree to the ALJ's review of the administrative record only, though the subject of the scientific misconduct finding may request an opportunity to submit additional pleadings and documentation.[71]

During the hearing, the parties will be the subject of the scientific misconduct finding and ORI; the institution is only a party to the hearing if ORI has named it as a respondent. Each party has the right to legal representation. The subject of the scientific misconduct finding is

[65] *Id.* at § 93.412.

[66] *Id.* at § 93.413.

[67] *Id.* at §§ 93.500, 501.

[68] *Id.*

[69] *Id.* at § 93.502.

[70] *Id.* at §§ 93.503, 504.

[71] *Id.*

responsible for covering costs of his or her counsel. Each party also has the right to supplement the record with pleadings, documents, testimony, and oral presentations.[72]

The ALJ's authority and the procedure for conduct of the hearing, in general, are consistent with traditional administrative law provisions and set forth in the PHS rule.[73] The ALJ must issue a ruling setting forth findings and conclusions of fact within 60 days after receipt of the last submission from the parties. The ruling will be provided to the parties and to the U.S. Assistant Secretary for Health (ASH); the ruling represents the ALJ's recommendation to the ASH, and the ASH may accept, modify or reject it.[74] The ALJ's recommendations will become a final agency action unless the ASH advises the parties within 30 days that the ASH intends to review the record. In order to modify or reject the ALJ's ruling, the ASH must determine the ALJ's findings and conclusions, in whole or in part, to be clearly erroneous or arbitrary and capricious.[75] The determination of the ASH is final, though if the ASH recommends debarment or suspension, the decision of the HHS debarring official[76] shall be final.

18.4 FDA's Policy on Scientific Misconduct

FDA addresses allegations of scientific misconduct through its policy entitled "Fraud, Untrue Statements of Material Facts, Bribery, and Illegal Gratuities" (the Fraud Policy), issued on September 10, 1991.[77] The Fraud Policy applies to "any person . . . who submits to FDA data or other information to influence or support an agency decision regarding approval to market an FDA-regulated product," referred to in the policy as an applicant.[78] The policy further defines an application as "any application, petition, amendment, supplement, or other submission made by an applicant to an agency review process in support of the approval or marketing of a regulated product."[79] Among the review processes listed are new drug and new animal drug approvals, biological product and establishment licensing, premarket notification, classification, and premarket approval of medical devices, food additive petitions, and color additive petitions.[80]

The FDA has noted that the Fraud Policy is for use when there is intent to defraud, such as through the submission of falsified or fabricated data, and also when intent is absent, as a pattern of errors by an applicant involving material subject matter may raise a significant question regarding the general reliability of data in applications from that applicant.[81]

---

[72] *Id.* at § 93.505.

[73] *Id.* at §§ 93.506-93.521.

[74] *Id.* at § 93.523.

[75] *Id.*

[76] *Id.* at § 93.206.

[77] FDA Final Fraud Policy, 56 Fed. Reg. 46191 (Sept. 10, 1991), *supra* note 23.

[78] *Id.* (Terminology).

[79] *Id.*

[80] *Id.*

[81] *Id.*

The FDA will conduct investigations under the Fraud Policy to identify all instances of wrongful acts and to determine the extent to which the wrongful acts may have affected approved or pending applications. If an applicant is found to have submitted fraudulent applications, made untrue statements of material facts, or given or promised bribes or illegal gratuities in the process of filing an FDA application, FDA may find reason to question the integrity of some or all of the applicant's FDA submissions.[82]

If the wrongful acts of an applicant have raised a significant question regarding the reliability of data in some or all of the applicant's pending applications, FDA ordinarily will conduct validity assessments of those applications and suspend substantive review of the applications during these assessments. If the FDA determines that the criteria for approval cannot be met because of unresolved questions regarding reliability of data, it will not approve the application.[83] An applicant cannot submit an amended application with corrected data—it is required to submit any corrected data in a new application, the truthfulness and accuracy of which must be certified by the president, chief executive officer, or other official most responsible for the applicant's operations.[84] All new applications are placed at the end of the review and approval queue.

Further, the FDA may recall marketed products and may request new testing of critical products, such as those that are difficult to manufacture or that have narrow therapeutic ranges. FDA may pursue other actions, including seizure, injunction, civil penalties, and criminal prosecution as necessary and appropriate.[85]

Under the Fraud Policy, in order to establish the reliability of data submitted to FDA, applicants who engage in wrongful acts will need to:

- Cooperate fully with FDA and any other federal investigations in the investigation of wrongful acts and their effects on the safety, effectiveness, or quality of relevant products;
- Identify and remove from authority on FDA-related matters all individuals who were involved in the wrongful acts;
- Conduct an internal review to identify all wrongful acts associated with the applicant's FDA applications, including any discrepancies between manufacturing conditions identified in approved applications and manufacturing conditions during actual production; and
- Develop and implement a corrective action operating plan to assure the safety, effectiveness, and quality of their products.[86]

[82] *Id.* (Validity Assessment).

[83] *Id.*

[84] *Id.*

[85] *Id.*

[86] *Id.* (Corrective Actions).

The corrective action plan must be designed to ensure that wrongful acts and other violations of law do not happen again. The corrective action plan must be signed by the president, chief executive officer, or other official most responsible for the applicant's operations, and must be submitted to FDA. The FDA will inspect the applicant to ensure implementation of the corrective action plan.[87]

---

[87] *Id.*

Exhibits & Sample Forms

Exhibit 2.3.2(a)—Sample Exempt Research Checklist

Research activities are exempt from regulations for the protection of human research subjects when the only involvement of human subjects falls within one or more of the categories listed below. Historically, these exempt categories did not apply to research involving prisoners; however, the 2018 Common Rule Requirements modify this position slightly by providing that the exemptions may be applied to research involving prisoners if the research is aimed at a broader population and only incidentally includes prisoners.

Directions: This form is to be completed and submitted to the IRB (or other person or body within the institution empowered to make exemption determinations) only when the investigator plans a research project which, in the investigator's judgment, is exempt from IRB review. The IRB (or other relevant person or body within the institution) will then determine whether the activity is exempt under the Federal Regulations. **Check the appropriate category that applies to your research project and underline or highlight the specific section within the category. Respond to the questions on the second page hereof. Please note that this checklist discusses the exemption categories as revised by the 2018 Requirements, identifying which aspects of each existing exemption category were modified and identifying new exemption categories introduced. Importantly, modifications introduced by the 2018 Requirements cannot be relied upon by institutions until the general compliance date of the rule, which at the time of this writing remained uncertain. The numbering of the exemption categories below corresponds to the numbering found in the 2018 Final Rule.**

(1) Research conducted in established or commonly accepted educational settings, involving normal educational practices, such as (i) research on regular and special education instructional strategies, or (ii) research on the effectiveness of or the comparison among instructional techniques, curricula, or classroom management methods. The 2018 Requirements added a requirement that the research is not likely to impact adversely students' opportunity to learn required educational content or the assessment of educators who provide instruction.

(2) Research involving the use of educational tests (cognitive, diagnostic, aptitude, achievement), survey procedures, interview procedures or observation of public behavior provided that at least one of the following criteria is met, the third of which was added by the 2018 Requirements:

(i) information obtained is recorded in such a manner that the identity of human subjects cannot readily be ascertained, directly or through identifiers linked to the subjects;

(ii) any disclosure of the human subjects' responses outside the research would not reasonably place the subjects at risk of criminal or civil liability or be damaging to the subjects' financial standing, employability, educational advancement, or reputation; or

(iii) for research subject to the 2018 Requirements, the information is recorded by the investigator in such a manner that the identity of the human subjects can readily be ascertained, directly or through identifiers linked to the subjects, and an IRB performs a "limited IRB review." A "limited IRB review" is a new concept introduced by the 2018 Requirements that requires that the IRB's review be limited to determining that there are adequate provisions to protect the privacy of subjects and maintain the confidentiality of data. The 2018 Requirements provide that the Common Rule agencies will issue further guidance to assist IRBs in making this assessment.

Subparagraphs (i) and (ii) above may be applied to research that is subject to 45 C.F.R. part 46, Subpart D (Additional Protections for Children) only when the investigator(s) does not participate in the activities being observed. Subparagraph (iii) above does not apply to research that is subject to Subpart D.

(4) This exemption contains four categories of exempt "secondary research," the third and fourth of which were introduced in the 2018 Requirements. To qualify for any of the categories contained in this exemption, the research must be "secondary research," meaning that the identifiable private information or identifiable biospecimens involved in the research must initially have been collected during some other primary or initial activity. Notably, under the 2018 Requirements, the identifiable private information or identifiable biospecimens under study need not be in existence at the time that the research begins.

(a) Research involving the collection or study of identifiable private information or identifiable biospecimens, if these sources are publicly available or if the information, which may include information about biospecimens, is recorded by the investigator in such a manner that the identity of the subjects cannot readily be ascertained directly or through identifiers linked to the subjects, the investigator does not contact the subjects, and the investigator will not re-identify the subjects.

(b) Research uses of identifiable health information when such uses are regulated under the HIPAA Privacy Rule for the purposes of "health care operations," "research" or "public health activities and purposes," as such terms are defined in the HIPAA Privacy Rule.

(c) Research that is conducted by, or on behalf of, a federal department or agency using government-generated or government-collected information obtained for nonresearch activities, if the information is stored in a manner that complies with certain federal government standards.

(5) Research and demonstration projects which are conducted by or subject to the approval of Department or Agency heads, and which are designed to study, evaluate, or otherwise examine: (i) Public benefit or service programs; (ii) procedures for obtaining benefits or services under those programs; (iii) possible changes in or alternatives to those programs or procedures; or (iv) possible changes in methods or levels of payment for benefits or services under those programs. The 2018 Requirements add an additional requirement that each federal department or agency conducting research and demonstration projects qualifying for this exemption establish on a publicly available website a list of all such research and demonstration projects <u>before</u> the research begins.

(6) Taste and food quality evaluation and consumer acceptance studies, (i) if wholesome foods without additives are consumed or (ii) if a food is consumed that contains a food ingredient at or below the level and for a use found to be safe, or agricultural chemical or environmental contaminant at or below the level found to be safe, by the Food and Drug Administration or approved by the Environmental Protection Agency or the Food Safety and Inspection Service of the U.S. Department of Agriculture.

The following new exemption categories were introduced by the 2018 Requirements. The numbering applies to the numbering of each exemption category in the 2018 Requirements.

(3) Benign behavioral interventions in conjunction with the collection of information from an adult subject through verbal or written responses or audiovisual recording if the subject prospectively agrees to the intervention and information collection and <u>at least</u> one of the following criteria is met:

(i) the information obtained is recorded by the investigator in such a manner that the identity of the human subjects cannot readily be ascertained;

(ii) any disclosure of the human subjects' responses outside the research would not reasonably place the subjects at risk of criminal or civil liability or be damaging to the subjects' financial standing, employability, educational advancement, or reputation; or

(iii) the information obtained is recorded in an identifiable format, but an IRB conducts a review limited to determining that there are adequate provisions to protect the privacy of subjects and maintain the confidentiality of data.

A "benign behavioral intervention" is defined as an intervention that is brief in duration, harmless, painless, not physically invasive, not likely to have a significant adverse lasting impact on the subjects, and the investigator has no reason to think the subjects will find the intervention offensive or embarrassing. This exemption cannot be used for research involving deception, unless the subject authorizes the deception through a prospective agreement to participate in research in which the subject is informed that he or she will be deceived. This exemption category cannot be used for research subject to 45 C.F.R. Part 46, Subpart D (Additional Protections for Children).

(7) Storage or maintenance for "secondary research" for which broad consent is required. This exemption permits identifiable private information or identifiable biosepcimens *to be stored for secondary research uses*, such as storage in a data repository or biobank, provided that the subject provides "broad consent" to the storage and the IRB conducts a "limited IRB review" to determine that (i) a broad consent has been obtained; (ii) a broad consent is appropriately documented; and (iii) if a change is made for research purposes in the way the identifiable private information or identifiable biospecimens are stored or maintained, there are adequate provisions to protect the privacy of the subject or to maintain the confidentiality of data.

(8) Secondary research for which broad consent is required. This exemption permits identifiable private information or identifiable biospecimens *to be used for secondary research purposes* if (i) the subject provided broad consent for the secondary research use of identifiable private information or identifiable biospecimens, (ii) an IRB conducts a "limited IRB review" to determine that there are adequate provisions to protect the privacy of subjects and maintain the confidentiality of data and to determine whether the research is within the scope of the broad consent obtained from the subject; and (iii) the investigator does not include returning individual research results to subjects as part of the study plan. This exemption could be used to permit the *use* of information or biospecimens stored pursuant to the exemption immediately above or it could be used to permit use of information and biospecimens stored under other mechanisms.

NOTE: A COMMON RULE DEPARTMENT OR AGENCY RETAINS FINAL AUTHORITY AS TO WHETHER A PARTICULAR HUMAN SUBJECTS RESEARCH STUDY CONDUCTED OR SUPPORTED BY THAT DEPARTMENT OR AGENCY IS EXEMPT FROM THE COMMON RULE.

Exempt Research Description

1. **Provide a brief description, in lay terms, of the purpose of the proposed project and the procedures to be used.**
   a. Please state the eligibility (inclusion/exclusion) criteria:
   b. Will subjects be compensated for participation?

2. **Explain how confidentiality will be protected.**

***Answer the following for all categories except categories 4 and 8 on the Exempt Research Checklist*:**

3. **Describe how subjects will be recruited.**
   a. Explain how subject selection will not unfairly target a particular population.

Exhibit 2.3.2(b)—Sample Exempt Research Checklist

Facility: ______________________________

Principal Investigator: ______________________________

Title of Research Project: ______________________________

If the ONLY involvement of human subjects will be in one or more of the following categories AND all the answers in one or more categories are 'True', the research may be eligible for exemption. However, the research must be declared exempt by the IRB (or other person or body charged by the institution with making exemption determinations) on the basis of the following answers. **Please note that the checklist below applies the exemption categories as revised by the 2018 Requirements; however, modifications introduced by the 2018 Requirements cannot be relied upon by institutions until the general compliance date of the rule, which at the time of this writing remained uncertain. All regulatory citations are to the 2018 Requirements.**

	Checklist Statements	True	Not True	Regulation
[ ]	**Category 1 - For Educational Settings:**			
1	The research will only be conducted in established or commonly-accepted educational settings including but not limited to schools and colleges. (May include other sites where educational activities regularly occur.)	[ ]	[ ]	45 C.F.R. 46.104(d)(1)
2	The research will involve only normal educational practices, such as (i) research on regular and special education instructional strategies, or (ii) research on the effectiveness of or the comparison among instructional techniques, curricula, or classroom management methods, **AND** the research is not likely to impact adversely (i) students' opportunity to learn required educational content or (ii) the assessment of educators who provide instruction.	[ ]	[ ]	45 C.F.R. 46.104(d)(1)

	Checklist Statements	True	Not True	Regulation
3	The research will <u>not</u> involve individuals as participants who are known to be prisoners except if the research is aimed at involving a broader subject population that only incidentally includes prisoners.	[ ]	[ ]	45 C.F.R. 46.104(b)(2)
4	The research is not subject to FDA regulations.	[ ]	[ ]	
[ ]	**Category 2 - For Educational Tests, Surveys, Interviews, Public Behavior Observation:**			
5	The research will involve only the use of educational tests (cognitive, diagnostic, aptitude, achievement), survey procedures, interview procedures or observation of public behavior.	[ ]	[ ]	45 C.F.R. 46.104(d)(2)
	Address statement 6 only if the research will involve children as participants. If children will NOT participate, check N/A and continue with statement 7.	[ ] **[ ] N/A**	[ ]	45 C.F.R. 46.104(b)(3)
6	The procedures will be limited to the use of educational tests (cognitive, diagnostic, aptitude, achievement) or observation of public behavior where the investigator will NOT participate in the activities being observed.			
7	The information obtained from educational tests, survey procedures, interview procedures or observation of public behavior will be recorded in such a manner that human subjects CANNOT be identified, directly or through identifiers linked to the subjects.	[ ]	[ ]	45 C.F.R. 46.104(d)(2)(i)
	'True' to <u>either</u> statement 7, 8, or 9 will qualify for exemption provided that statements 10 and 11 are true, <u>except that statement 9 cannot be used when the research involves children.</u>			

	Checklist Statements	True	Not True	Regulation
8	Any disclosure of the human subjects' responses outside the research could NOT reasonably place the subjects at risk of criminal or civil liability or be damaging to the subjects' financial standing, employability, educational advancement, or reputation.	[ ]	[ ]	45 C.F.R. 46.104(d)(2)(ii)
9	The information obtained is recorded by the investigator in such a manner that the identity of the human subjects can readily be ascertained, directly or through identifiers linked to the subjects, and an IRB conducts a limited IRB review to make the determination required by 45 C.F.R. § 46.111(a)(7).	[ ]	[ ]	45 C.F.R. 46.105(d)(2)(iii)
10	The research will not involve individuals as participants who are known to be prisoners except if the research is aimed at involving a broader subject population that only incidentally includes prisoners.	[ ]	[ ]	45 C.F.R. 46.104(b)(2)
11	The research is not subject to FDA regulations.	[ ]	[ ]	
[ ]	**Category 3 - Research Involving Benign Behavioral Interventions**			
12	The research does not involve children.	[ ]	[ ]	45 C.F.R. 46.104(b)(3)
13	The research involves only benign behavior interventions in conjunction with the collection of information from an adult subject through verbal or written responses (including data entry) or audiovisual recording if the subject prospectively agrees to the intervention and information collection.	[ ]	[ ]	45 C.F.R. 46.104(d)(3)(i)

Checklist Statements	True	Not True	Regulation
14 The information obtained is recorded by the investigator in such a manner that the identity of the human subjects cannot readily be ascertained, directly or through identifiers linked to the subjects. ***'True' to either statements 14, 15, or 16 will qualify for exemption provided that statements 17 through 20 are true.***	[ ]	[ ]	45 C.F.R. 46.104(d)(3)(i)(A)
15 Any disclosure of the human subjects' responses outside the research would not reasonably place the subjects at risk of criminal or civil liability or be damaging to the subjects' financial standing, employability, educational advancement, or reputation.	[ ]	[ ]	45 C.F.R. 46.104(d)(3)(i)(B)
16 The information obtained is recorded by the investigator in such a manner that the identity of the human subjects can readily be ascertained, directly or through identifiers linked to the subjects, and an IRB conducts a limited IRB review to make the determination required by 45 C.F.R. §46.111(a)(7).	[ ]	[ ]	45 C.F.R. 46.104(d)(3)(i)(C)
17 The interventions are brief in duration, harmless, painless, not physically invasive, not likely to have a significant adverse lasting impact on the subjects, and the investigator has no reason to think the subjects will find the interventions offensive or embarrassing.	[ ]	[ ]	45 C.F.R. 46.104(d)(3)(ii)
18 The research does <u>not</u> involve deception unless the subject authorizes the deception through a prospective agreement to participate in research in circumstances in which the subject is informed that he or she will be unaware of or misled regarding the nature or purposes of the research.	[ ]	[ ]	45 C.F.R. 46.104(d)(4)
19 The research will <u>not</u> involve individuals as participants who are known to be prisoners except if the research is aimed at involving a broader subject population that only incidentally includes prisoners.	[ ]	[ ]	45 C.F.R. 46.104(b)(2)

	Checklist Statements	True	Not True	Regulation
20	The research is not subject to FDA regulations.	[ ]	[ ]	
[ ]	**Category 4 - Secondary Research for Which Consent is Not Required:**			
21	The research consists solely of "secondary research". ("Secondary research" means that the identifiable private information or identifiable biospecimens used in the research were or will be gathered during some other "primary" or "initial" activity, such as clinical care or another research study).	[ ]	[ ]	45 C.F.R. 46.104(d)(4)
22	The sources of the data, documents, records or specimens are publicly available **OR** the information will be recorded by the investigator in such a manner that participants cannot be readily identified either directly or through identifiers (such as a code) linked to them, the investigator does not contact the subjects, and the investigator will not re-identify subjects. ***'True' to either statements 22, 23, or 24 will qualify for exemption provided that statements 25 and 26 are true.***	[ ]	[ ]	45 C.F.R. 46.104(d)(4)(i)-(ii)
23	The research involves only information collection and analysis involving the investigator's use of identifiable health information when such use is regulated under the HIPAA Privacy Rule for purposes of "health care operations," "research," or "public health activities and purposes" as those terms are defined in the HIPAA Privacy Rule.	[ ]	[ ]	45 C.F.R. 46.104(d)(4)(iii)

	Checklist Statements	True	Not True	Regulation
24	The research is conducted by, or on behalf of, a Federal department or agency using government-generated or government-collected information obtained for nonresearch activities, if the research generates identifiable private information that is or will be maintained on information technology that is subject to and in compliance with section 208(b) of the E-Government Act of 2002, 44 U.S.C. § 3501, if all of the identifiable private information collected, used, or generated as part of the activity will be maintained in systems of records subject to the Privacy Act of 1974, 5 U.S.C. § 552a, and, if applicable, the information used in the research was collected subject to the Paperwork Reduction Act of 1995, 44 U.S.C. § 3501 *et seq*.	[ ]	[ ]	45 C.F.R. 46.104(d)(4)(iv)
25	The research will <u>not</u> involve individuals as participants who are known to be prisoners except if the research is aimed at involving a broader subject population that only incidentally includes prisoners.	[ ]	[ ]	45 C.F.R. 46.104(b)(2)
26	The research is not subject to FDA regulations.	[ ]	[ ]	
[ ]	**Category 5 - For Public Benefit or Service Programs (Federal):**			
27	The project is a research or demonstration project conducted by or subject to the approval of a (federal) Department or Agency head and which is designed to study, evaluate, improve or otherwise examine: (i) public benefit or service programs; (ii) procedures for obtaining benefits or services under those programs; (iii) possible changes in or alternatives to those programs or procedures; or (iv) possible changes in methods or levels of payment for benefits or services under those public benefit or service programs.	[ ]	[ ]	45 C.F.R. 46.101(d)(5)

	Checklist Statements	True	Not True	Regulation
28	The research project has been listed on a publicly accessible Federal Website that lists the research and demonstration projects that the relevant Federal department or agency supports under this provision.	[ ]	[ ]	45 C.F.R. 46.101(d)(5)(i)
29	The research will <u>not</u> involve individuals as participants who are known to be prisoners except if the research is aimed at involving a broader subject population that only incidentally includes prisoners.	[ ]	[ ]	45 C.F.R. 46.104(b)(2)
30	The research is not subject to FDA regulations.	[ ]	[ ]	
[ ]	**Category 6 - For Taste and Food Quality and Consumer Acceptance Studies:**			
31	The research involves only a taste and food quality evaluation or a food consumer acceptance study in which (i) wholesome foods without additives will be consumed **<u>OR</u>** (ii) food will be consumed that contains a food ingredient, agricultural chemical or environmental contaminant that is at or below the level found to be safe by the Food and Drug Administration or is approved by the Environmental Protection Agency or the Food Safety and Inspection Service of the U.S. Department of Agriculture.	[ ]	[ ]	45 C.F.R. 46.104(d)(6);
32	The research will <u>not</u> involve individuals as participants who are known to be prisoners, except if the research is aimed at involving a broader subject population that only incidentally includes prisoners.	[ ]	[ ]	45 C.F.R. 46.104(b)(2)
[]	**Category 7 - Storage or Maintenance for Secondary Research for Which Broad Consent is Required**	[ ]	[ ]	

	Checklist Statements	True	Not True	Regulation
33	The identifiable private information or identifiable biospecimens to be stored have been or will be collected for secondary research. ("Secondary research" means that the identifiable private information or identifiable biospecimens used in the research were or will be gathered during some other "primary" or "initial" activity, such as clinical care or another research study).	[ ]	[ ]	45 C.F.R. 46.104(d)(7)
34	The investigator has obtained from the research subjects a "broad consent" that meets the requirements for "broad consent" found in the Common Rule.	[ ]	[ ]	45 C.F.R. 46.104(d)(7); 45 C.F.R. 46.116(d)
35	The IRB has conducted a limited review to make the following determinations: (i) Broad consent for storage, maintenance, and secondary research use of identifiable private information or identifiable biospecimens is obtained in accordance with the requirements of 45 C.F.R. **§ 46.116(a)(1)-(4), (a)(6), and (d)**; (ii) broad consent is appropriately documented or waiver of documentation is appropriate, in accordance with 45 C.F.R. § 46.117; **AND** (iii) if there is a change made for research purposes in the way the identifiable private information or identifiable biospecimens are stored or maintained, there are adequate provisions to protect the privacy of subjects and to maintain the confidentiality of data.	[ ]	[ ]	45 C.F.R. 46.104(d)(7); 45 C.F.R. 46.111(a)(8)
36	The research will **not** involve individuals as participants who are known to be prisoners, except if the research is aimed at involving a broader subject population that only incidentally includes prisoners.			45 C.F.R. 46.104(b)(2)
[ ]	**Category 8 - Secondary research for which broad consent is required**			

	Checklist Statements	True	Not True	Regulation
37	The research is secondary research. ("Secondary research" means that the identifiable private information or identifiable biospecimens used in the research were or will be gathered during some other "primary" or "initial" activity, such as clinical care or another research study).			45 C.F.R. 46.104(d)(8)
38	The investigator has obtained from the research subjects a "broad consent" that meets the requirements for "broad consent" found in the Common Rule.			45 C.F.R. 46.104(d)(8)(i); 45 C.F.R. 46.116(d)
39	Broad consent has been documented in accordance with the requirements of 45 C.F.R. § 46.117.			45 C.F.R. 46.104(d)(8)(ii)
40	<u>The IRB conducts a limited review to make the following determinations: (i) there are adequate provisions to protect the privacy of subjects and to maintain the confidentiality of data; and (ii) the research to be conducted is within the scope of the broad consent obtained for the research.</u>			45 C.F.R. 46.104(d)(8)(iii); 45 C.F.R. 46.111(a)(7)
41	The research plan does not include returning individual research results to study subjects.			45 C.F.R. 46.104(d)(8)(iii)
42	The research will <u>not</u> involve individuals as participants who are known to be prisoners, except if the research is aimed at involving a broader subject population that only incidentally includes prisoners.			45 C.F.R. 46.104(b)(2)
[ ]	**Emergency Use of an Unapproved Test Article (*i.e.*, a drug, device or biologic that is not FDA-approved)**			
	The activity involves emergency use of an investigational drug, device or biologic. The emergency use must be reported to the IRB within five business days. Any subsequent use of the investigational drug, device or biologic is subject to IRB review.	[ ]	[ ]	21 C.F.R. 56.104(c); 21 C.F.R. Part 56
	The activity does not meet the DHHS definition of "research."	[ ]	[ ]	45 C.F.R. 46.102(*l*); 21 C.F.R. Part 56

Signature of Principal Investigator: ______________________________

____

Printed Name ______________________________

____

Date

FOR THE IRB REVIEWER ONLY:

Is the activity exempt? YES [ ] NO [ ]

Which exemption category or categories apply to the activity? ______________

Signature of IRB Reviewer:

____

Printed Name ______________________________

Date

Exhibit 5.4.1—Sample Continuing Review Notice Letter

DO NOT DISCARD THIS LETTER—TIMELY RESPONSE IS REQUIRED

<Date of letter>

RE: Continuing Review Notice Regarding Study Number ________: <(Sponsor)>

Dear ________:

Our records show that continuing review of your study listed above is due on or before _________. The federal regulations require the IRB to perform a continuing review of your research at least once every 12 months. **Failure to complete a continuing review/closure form may delay re-approval of your study and could result in a suspension. All suspensions are promptly reported to the FDA or applicable regulatory body.** The IRB cannot grant extensions or temporary approval. Unless your study is re-reviewed and re-approved within 12 months from the date of last approval by the IRB, **federal regulations require the IRB to immediately suspend its approval.** Should suspension occur, all subject accrual must cease as of the date of suspension. Additionally, research related procedures for follow-up or other reasons can no longer be conducted of subjects who are enrolled in the study. Enclosed for your review are the IRB Requirements of Continuing Review of Research.

If you wish to continue the study, complete a continuing review application form. If your study requires full board review, it must be submitted by *<deadline for submission>*. It is your responsibility to submit this report in sufficient time to permit the IRB to complete a meaningful continuing review of the research.

Please contact _______________ at ______ if you have any questions or require further information. If you would like to have the renewal form mailed to you, please e-mail ___________ and it will be forwarded to you.

Sincerely,

Exhibit 5.4.2—IRB Requirements for Continuing Review of Research

What are the Regulatory Requirements for Continuing Review?

DHHS (45 C.F.R. 46) and FDA (21 C.F.R. 56) regulations require the IRB to perform Continuing Review of research at intervals appropriate to the degree of risk but *not less* than once per year. It is the responsibility of all investigators to submit an Application for Continuing Review in sufficient time to permit the IRB to complete a meaningful Continuing Review of the research.

What is the Purpose of Continuing Review?

The primary purpose of Continuing Review is to ensure that **1)** selection of subjects is equitable; **2)** the risk/benefit relationship of the research remains acceptable; **3)** the consent document contains information that is accurate, complete and up-to-date; and **4)** adequate safeguards for human subjects are in place. In addition, at this institution, some of the information that is requested will be reviewed by the Research Office for purposes of institutional oversight.

How Much Detail is Necessary for the Continuing Review?

The following are guidelines for completing the Application for Continuing Review. The IRB relies upon the investigator to provide all necessary information in sufficient detail to permit the Board to fulfill its Federal and institutional mandates to ensure that on-going human subject research continues to be justified. The status of the study determines what information is necessary for IRB review.

Why is Continuing Review by the IRB just as important as Initial Review.

Initial review and approval of research requires the IRB to make a judgment based largely upon background data and a risk/benefit analysis provided by the investigator. Continuing Review and re-approval of on-going research, however, serves to verify the correctness of the decisions made by both the investigator and the IRB using the study results to date and other relevant new information to make this judgment. Continuing Review is designed to help ensure that the rights and welfare of subjects continue to be fully protected in on-going research.

In order to facilitate IRB re-review of your project and to avoid unnecessary delays, your Application for Continuing Review must be completed according to the instructions. Please include sufficient detail to allow the IRB to perform a thorough Continuing Review. **Failure to provide this detail may delay re-approval of your project and could result in a suspension of the research. All suspensions will be promptly reported to the FDA or applicable regulatory body.** The IRB cannot grant extensions or temporary approval. Should suspension occur, all subject accrual must cease as of the date of suspension. Research related procedures can no longer be done on human subjects who are enrolled in the study for follow-up or other reasons. If suspension is a health hazard to the subjects, the IRB will grant an exception upon receipt of written justification.

Submission Deadline: Your Application for Continuing Review must be submitted on time so that expiration of IRB approval does not occur. **Unless your project is re-reviewed and re-approved within twelve (12) months from the date the protocol was last reviewed by the IRB, Federal Regulations require the IRB *immediately* suspend its approval.** The IRB staff sends out a request for submission of the Application for Continuing Review at 30, 60 and 90 day intervals prior to the month in which it must be reviewed. The deadline for submission is noted in the IRB letter.

Submission Documents: Submit one copy of your Application for Continuing Review, consent forms, and any written materials that have been reused or have not been approved by the IRB.

After IRB review of your Application for Continuing Review, you will be given an approval letter to continue. An original of each version of the IRB approved consent/assent form(s) should be kept on file. If you are making copies from the original consent form, make sure any outdated forms are destroyed and the currently approved version is being used.

Exhibit 8.3—Humanitarian Use Device Information Sheet

- A Humanitarian Use Device (HUD) is a device that is "intended to benefit patients in the treatment or diagnosis of a disease or condition that affects or is manifested in fewer than 8,000 individuals in the United States per year."[1]
  - The HUD is approved by the FDA for use for a specific indication.
- The HUD is FDA-approved under the Humanitarian Device Exemption (HDE).
  - The HDE application is similar to a premarket approval (PMA) application, but exempt from the effectiveness requirements of a PMA.
  - An approved HDE authorizes marketing of a HUD.
- The HUD is not considered "investigational" nor is use of the device considered "research."
  - However, the federal statute and implementing regulations require IRB review and approval before a HUD is used.
  - There is an exception for emergency situations in which the physician determines that approval cannot be obtained in time to prevent serious harm or death to the patient.[2]
- The IRB is responsible for the initial as well as continuing review of the HUD.
  - For initial review, the IRB is required to perform a full board review.
  - For continuing review, the IRB may use the expedited review process, unless the IRB determines that a full board review should be performed.
- The IRB does not need to review and approve each individual use of a HUD.
  - As long as the HUD is used within the FDA approved indication, the IRB may approve the use of the device without further restrictions, or if it so desires, the IRB can require approval of the device on a case-by-case basis.
- The HUD regulations do not require informed consent because an HDE provides for marketing approval and the use of the HUD does not constitute research or an investigation which would normally require specific informed consent.
  - However, guidance issued by the FDA on July 8, 2010, states there is nothing in the federal regulations that prohibits an institution from requiring prospective informed consent.[3]
  - The guidance states that most HDE holders have developed patient information packets that includes information to assist a patient in making an informed decision about the use of the device, which should be provided to patients.

---

1 21 C.F.R. §§ 814.3(n), 814.100(a),(b).

2 *See* 21 C.F.R. § 814.124(a). Within five days after use of the device, the physician would then provide written notification to the chair of the IRB of such use, including identification of the patient, the date the device was used, and the reason for the use.

3 Humanitarian Device Exemption (HDE) Regulation: Questions and Answers: Guidance for HDE Holders, Institutional Review Board (IRBs), Clinical Investigators, and Food and Drug Administration Staff, FDA (July 8, 2010), *available at* https://www.fda.gov/downloads/MedicalDevices/DeviceRegulationandGuidance/GuidanceDocuments/UCM110203.pdf (update for compliance with the 21st Century Cures Act is pending.)

- Such patient information packets contain a discussion of the potential risks and benefits of the device, as well as any procedures associated with the use of the HUD.
- The guidance also states that the HUD labeling must contain a statement that the device is a humanitarian use device for which effectiveness for the labeled indication has not been demonstrated.
- It is up to the individual IRB to determine whether specific informed consent should be obtained.

Exhibit 8.4—Sample Informed Consent for Off-Label Use of a Drug or Device

Name of Patient: ______________________________ Date: __________________

When a drug or device is approved for medical use by the Food and Drug Administration (FDA), the manufacturer produces a "label" to explain its use. Once a device/medication is approved by the FDA, physicians may use it "off-label" for other unapproved purposes if they are well-informed about the product, base its use on firm scientific method and sound medical evidence, and maintain records of its use and effects.

[State purpose of the off-label drug/device.]

[State alternatives to the off-label drug or device.]

[State known risks, complications and side effects of the off-label drug/device.]

I understand that **[state drug/device]** was approved by the FDA for **[state approval purpose/conditions]**. Nevertheless, I understand and agree to the off-label use of **[state drug/device]** for the treatment/management of my **[state patient's condition]**. Furthermore, I understand the safety and efficacy of this off-label use has not been established by adequate and well-controlled clinical trials. I am willing to accept the potential risks that my physician has discussed with me, and I acknowledge that there may be other, unknown risks and that the long term effects and risks of **[state drug/device]** are not known. I also acknowledge that my physician has reviewed the use of **[state drug/device]** with me in detail, and answered all of my questions.

Authorization and Consent:

My signature below means that I have read this informed consent, I have had the opportunity to ask questions, and all of my questions have been answered. I hereby authorize my physician (and/or persons designated by him/her) to use the **[state drug or device]** in connection with my medical treatment.

I CERTIFY THAT I HAVE READ AND FULLY UNDERSTAND THE CONSENT FORM. I FURTHER CERTIFY ALL THE BLANKS IN THIS FORM WERE FILLED IN AT THE TIME I SIGNED.

Signature: ____________________________________ Date: __________________

Witness: ______________________________________ Date: __________________

Exhibit 9.0.1—Sample Informed Consent Checklist, Pre-2018 Common Rule and FDA

Consent Document:

1. Are the eight basic elements of informed consent included? (**Section 9.3.1**) ___ Yes ___ No
2. Are the additional elements of consent included when appropriate? (**Sections 9.3.2 and 9.3.3**) ___ Yes ___ No
3. Will the consent be understandable to an individual with a 6th grade education? ___ Yes ___ No
4. Has the Principal Investigator requested waiver or alteration of informed consent? (**Section 9.8.2**) ___ Yes ___ No
5. Does the study meet the requirements for waiver or alteration of consent? (**Section 9.8.2**) ___ Yes ___ No
6. Is a Certificate of Confidentiality (CoC) applicable to the research, and if so, is a description of the CoC protections included in the consent document? (**Section 9.1**) ___ Yes ___ No

Eight Required Basic Elements of Informed Consent (Section 9.3.1):

1. Statement that the study involves research, an explanation of the purposes of the research and the expected duration of the subject's participation, a description of the procedures to be followed, and identification of any procedures that are experimental.
2. Description of any reasonably foreseeable risks and discomforts to the subject.
3. Description of any benefits to the subject (direct benefits) or to others (indirect benefits to others with similar health problems or to society at large) to be reasonably expected from the research.
4. Disclosure of any appropriate alternative procedures or courses of treatment that might be advantageous for the subject.
5. Statement describing the extent, if any, to which confidentiality of records identifying the subject will be maintained, including appropriate HIPAA language (unless contained in a separate Authorization), and noting the possibility that the FDA may inspect the records, if applicable.
6. For research involving more than minimal risk, an explanation as to whether any compensation or medical treatments are available if injury occurs and, if so, what they consist of, or where further information may be obtained, and whom to contact in the case of an injury.

7. An explanation as to whom to contact for answers to pertinent questions about the research and the research subject's rights.

8. Statement that participation is voluntary, refusal to participate will involve no penalty or loss of benefits to which the subject is otherwise entitled, and that the subject may discontinue participation at any time without penalty or loss of benefits to which the subject is otherwise entitled.

Six Additional Elements of Informed Consent (must be included when appropriate) (Section 9.3.2):

1. A statement that the particular treatment or procedure may involve risks to the subject (or to the embryo or fetus if the subject is or may become pregnant) which are currently unforeseeable.

2. Anticipated circumstances under which the subject's participation may be terminated unilaterally by the investigator.

3. Additional costs to the subject that may result from research participation.

4. The consequences of withdrawal from the research (adverse health/welfare effects, if any) and procedures for orderly termination of the subject's participation.

5. Statement that significant new findings developed during the course of the research which may relate to the subject's willingness to continue to participate will be provided to the subject.

6. Approximate number of subjects involved in the study.

Additional Informative Elements (Sections 9.3.3 and 9.1):

1. For FDA-regulated clinical trials that will be posted on the website www.ClinicalTrials.gov, the following statement must be provided to each subject of such trial in the informed consent document:

    A description of this clinical trial will be available on http://www.ClinicalTrials.gov, as required by U.S. law. This Web site will not include information that can identify you. At most, the Web site will include a summary of the results. You can search this Web site at any time.

2. For research to which a Certificate of Confidentiality (CoC) from NIH applies, include a description of the CoC protections. NIH provides the following suggested language that should be edited as necessary for the study population:

    This research is covered by a Certificate of Confidentiality from the National Institutes of Health. The researchers with this Certificate may not disclose or use information, documents, or biospecimens that may identify you in any federal, state, or local civil, criminal, administrative, legislative, or other action, suit, or proceeding, or be used as evidence, for example, if there is a court subpoena, unless you have consented for this use. Information, documents, or biospecimens protected by this Certificate cannot be disclosed to anyone else who is not connected with the research except, if there is a federal, state, or local law that requires disclosure (such as to report child abuse or communicable diseases but not for federal, state, or local civil, criminal, administrative, legislative, or other proceedings, see below); if you have consented to the disclosure, including for your medical treatment; or if it is used for other scientific research, as allowed by federal regulations protecting research subjects.

[INCLUDE IF APPLICABLE:] The Certificate cannot be used to refuse a request for information from personnel of the United States federal or state government agency sponsoring the project that is needed for auditing or program evaluation by [*THE AGENCY*] which is funding this project or for information that must be disclosed in order to meet the requirements of the federal Food and Drug Administration (FDA). You should understand that a Certificate of Confidentiality does not prevent you from voluntarily releasing information about yourself or your involvement in this research. If you want your research information released to an insurer, medical care provider, or any other person not connected with the research, you must provide consent to allow the researchers to release it.

[INCLUDE IF APPLICABLE (if researcher intends to disclose information covered by a Certificate, such as potential child abuse, or intent to hurt self or others in response to specific federal, state, or local laws).] The Certificate of Confidentiality will not be used to prevent disclosure as required by federal, state, or local law of *[list what will be reported, such as child abuse and neglect, or harm to self or others]*.

[INCLUDE IF APPLICABLE (if researcher intends to disclose information covered by a Certificate, with the consent of research participants).] The Certificate of Confidentiality will not be used to prevent disclosure for any purpose you have consented to in this informed consent document *[restate what will be disclosed, such as including research data in the medical record]*.

3. Payments (incentives and/or expense reimbursements), if any.

4. Disclosure of financial interests of investigator(s), institution, or IRB members.

5. When relevant, information about subjects who become pregnant while enrolled in the study; possible effects of the study intervention on the pregnancy; whether pregnant partners of subjects will be contacted.

Requirements for Waiver of Informed Consent/Authorization (Section 9.8.2):

Under the pre-2018 Common Rule and FDA policy,[4] an IRB may (i) approve a consent procedure that does not include, or that alters, some or all of the elements of informed consent otherwise required by federal regulation, or (ii) waive the requirements to obtain informed consent altogether, if the IRB finds and documents that:

1. The research involves no more than minimal risk to the subjects;
2. The waiver or alteration will not adversely affect the rights and welfare of the subjects;
3. The research could not practicably be carried out without the waiver or alteration; ***and***
4. Whenever appropriate, the subjects will be provided with additional pertinent information after participation.

A waiver is possible if a study investigates certain aspects of public benefit or service programs, where the research or demonstration project is to be conducted by or subject to the approval of state or local government officials and is designed to study, evaluate, or otherwise examine:

1. public benefit or service programs;
2. procedures for obtaining benefits or services under those programs;
3. possible changes in or alternatives to those programs or procedures; ***or***
4. possible changes in methods or levels of payment for benefits or services under those programs; ***and***
5. the research could not practicably be carried out without the waiver or alteration.

In addition, HIPAA requires that the IRB find and document the following when a waiver will include a waiver of Authorization for the use or disclosure of protected health information (PHI) in connection with the research project:

1. The use of disclosure of PHI must involve no more than minimal risk to the privacy of individuals, based on at least the presence of the following elements:

---

[4] Per July 2017 FDA guidance, FDA will not object to use of the pre-2018 Common Rule regulations regarding waiver and alteration of informed consent until FDA promulgates its own regulations.

The FDA regulations also allow extremely limited emergency exceptions to standard informed consent requirements, applicable only in certain emergency life-threatening situations where standard therapies are unproven or unsatisfactory and significant administrative burdens are met by the relevant investigators and IRB. HHS-supported research also allows a parallel exception through a Secretarial waiver of the standard informed consent requirements in such emergency situations.

i. an adequate plan to protect identifiers from improper use and disclosure;

ii. an adequate plan to destroy the identifiers at the earliest opportunity consistent with the conduct of the research, unless there is a health or research justification for retaining the identifiers or such retention is otherwise required by law;

iii. adequate written assurances that the PHI will not be reused or disclosed to any other person or entity, except:

(a) as required by law;

(b) for authorized oversight of the research study, ***or***

(c) for other research for which the use and disclosure of the PHI would be permitted under the Privacy Rule;

2. The research could not practicably be conducted without the waiver or alteration; ***and***

3. The research could not practicably be conducted without access to and use of the PHI.

Exhibit 9.0.2—Sample Study-Specific Informed Consent Checklist, 2018 Common Rule

Consent Document:

1. Does the informed consent begin with a summary of key information? (**Section 9.2**, in the "Added by the 2018 Common Rule" section) ___ Yes ___ No
2. Is the informed consent information, overall, provided in enough detail, and organized and presented sufficiently, to assist the subject in understanding the reasons why or why not to participate in the study? (**Sections 9.2 and 9.3.1–9.3.3**) ___ Yes ___ No
3. Does the informed consent provide the information a reasonable person would want to have in order to make an informed decision about whether to participate, and is the subject provided an opportunity to discuss that information? (**Sections 9.2 and 9.3.1–9.3.3**) ___ Yes ___ No
4. Are the nine basic elements of informed consent included? (**Section 9.3.1**) ___ Yes ___ No
5. Are the additional elements of consent included when appropriate? (**Sections 9.3.2 and 9.3.3**) ___ Yes ___ No
6. Will the consent be understandable to an individual with a 6th grade education? ___ Yes ___ No
7. Has the Principal Investigator requested waiver or alteration of informed consent? (**Section 9.8.2**) ___ Yes ___ No
8. Does the study meet the requirements for waiver or alteration of consent? (**Section 9.8.2**) ___ Yes ___ No
9. Is a Certificate of Confidentiality (CoC) applicable to the research, and if so, is a description of the CoC protections included in the consent document? (**Section 9.1**) ___ Yes ___ No

Nine Required Basic Elements of Informed Consent (Section 9.3.1):

1. Statement that the study involves research, an explanation of the purposes of the research and the expected duration of the subject's participation, a description of the procedures to be followed, and identification of any procedures that are experimental.
2. Description of any reasonably foreseeable risks and discomforts to the subject.
3. Description of any benefits to the subject (direct benefits) or to others (indirect benefits to others with similar health problems or to society at large) to be reasonably expected from the research.

4. Disclosure of any appropriate alternative procedures or courses of treatment that might be advantageous for the subject.

5. Statement describing the extent, if any, to which confidentiality of records identifying the subject will be maintained, including appropriate HIPAA language (unless contained in a separate Authorization), and noting the possibility that the FDA may inspect the records, if applicable.

6. For research involving more than minimal risk, an explanation as to whether any compensation or medical treatments are available if injury occurs and, if so, what they consist of, or where further information may be obtained, and whom to contact in the case of an injury.

7. An explanation as to whom to contact for answers to pertinent questions about the research and the research subject's rights.

8. Statement that participation is voluntary, refusal to participate will involve no penalty or loss of benefits to which the subject is otherwise entitled, and that the subject may discontinue participation at any time without penalty or loss of benefits to which the subject is otherwise entitled.

9. One of the following statements about any research that involves the collection of identifiable private information or identifiable biospecimens:

   i. A statement that identifiers might be removed from the identifiable private information or identifiable biospecimens and that, after such removal, the information or biospecimens could be used for future research studies or distributed to another investigator for future research studies without obtaining additional informed consent from the subject or the legally authorized representative (if such a transfer is a possibility); ***or***

   ii. A statement that the subject's information or biospecimens collected as part of the research, even if identifiers are removed, will not be used or distributed for future research studies.

Nine Additional Elements of Informed Consent (must be included when appropriate) (Section 9.3.2):

1. A statement that the particular treatment or procedure may involve risks to the subject (or to the embryo or fetus if the subject is or may become pregnant) which are currently unforeseeable.

2. Anticipated circumstances under which the subject's participation may be terminated unilaterally by the investigator.

3. Additional costs to the subject that may result from research participation.

4. The consequences of withdrawal from the research (adverse health/welfare effects, if any) and procedures for orderly termination of the subject's participation.

5. Statement that significant new findings developed during the course of the research which may relate to the subject's willingness to continue to participate will be provided to the subject.

6. Approximate number of subjects involved in the study.

7. A statement that the subject's biospecimens (even if identifiers are removed) may be used for commercial profit, and whether or not the subject will share in this profit.

8. A statement regarding whether clinically relevant research results will be disclosed to subjects, and if so, under what conditions.

9. For research involving biospecimens, whether the research will (if known) or might include whole genome sequencing.

Additional Informative Elements (Sections 9.3.3 and 9.1):

1. For FDA-regulated clinical trials that will be posted on the website www.ClinicalTrials.gov, the following statement must be provided to each subject of such trial in the informed consent document:

    A description of this clinical trial will be available on http://www.ClinicalTrials.gov, as required by U.S. law. This Web site will not include information that can identify you. At most, the Web site will include a summary of the results. You can search this Web site at any time.

2. For research to which a Certificate of Confidentiality (CoC) from NIH applies, include a description of the CoC protections. NIH provides the following suggested language that should be edited as necessary for the study population:

    This research is covered by a Certificate of Confidentiality from the National Institutes of Health. The researchers with this Certificate may not disclose or use information, documents, or biospecimens that may identify you in any federal, state, or local civil, criminal, administrative, legislative, or other action, suit, or proceeding, or be used as evidence, for example, if there is a court subpoena, unless you have consented for this use. Information, documents, or biospecimens protected by this Certificate cannot be disclosed to anyone else who is not connected with the research except, if there is a federal, state, or local law that requires disclosure (such as to report child abuse or communicable diseases but not for federal, state, or local civil, criminal, administrative, legislative, or other proceedings, see below); if you have consented to the disclosure, including for your medical treatment; or if it is used for other scientific research, as allowed by federal regulations protecting research subjects.

[INCLUDE IF APPLICABLE:] The Certificate cannot be used to refuse a request for information from personnel of the United States federal or state government agency sponsoring the project that is needed for auditing or program evaluation by [*THE AGENCY*] which is funding this project or for information that must be disclosed in order to meet the requirements of the federal Food and Drug Administration (FDA). You should understand that a Certificate of Confidentiality does not prevent you from voluntarily releasing information about yourself or your involvement in this research. If you want your research information released to an insurer, medical care provider, or any other person not connected with the research, you must provide consent to allow the researchers to release it.

[INCLUDE IF APPLICABLE (if researcher intends to disclose information covered by a Certificate, such as potential child abuse, or intent to hurt self or others in response to specific federal, state, or local laws):] The Certificate of Confidentiality will not be used to prevent disclosure as required by federal, state, or local law of [*list what will be reported, such as child abuse and neglect, or harm to self or others*].

[INCLUDE IF APPLICABLE (if researcher intends to disclose information covered by a Certificate, with the consent of research participants):] The Certificate of Confidentiality will not be used to prevent disclosure for any purpose you have consented to in this informed consent document [*restate what will be disclosed, such as including research data in the medical record*].

3. Payments (incentives and/or expense reimbursements), if any.
4. Disclosure of financial interests of investigator(s), institution, or IRB members.
5. When relevant, information about subjects who become pregnant while enrolled in the study; possible effects of the study intervention on the pregnancy; whether pregnant partners of subjects will be contacted.

Requirements for Waiver of Informed Consent/Authorization:

Under the pre-2018 Common Rule and FDA policy[1], an IRB may (i) approve a consent procedure that does not include, or that alters, some or all of the elements of informed consent otherwise required by federal regulation, or (ii) waive the requirements to obtain informed consent altogether, if the IRB finds and documents that:

1. The research involves no more than minimal risk to the subjects;
2. The waiver or alteration will not adversely affect the rights and welfare of the subjects;
3. If the research involves using identifiable private information or identifiable biospecimens, the research could not practicably be carried out without using such information or biospecimens in an identifiable format; (**<u>NOTE:</u>** this element does **not** need to be met for FDA-regulated research that is not also regulated by the 2018 Common Rule. This element is not contained in the pre-2018 Common Rule, which is the version of the Common Rule that FDA states can be used without objection until FDA promulgates its own regulations.)
4. The research could not practicably be carried out without the waiver or alteration; ***and***
5. Whenever appropriate, the subjects will be provided with additional pertinent information after participation.

A waiver is possible if a study investigates certain aspects of public benefit or service programs, where the research or demonstration project is to be conducted by or subject to the approval of state or local government officials and is designed to study, evaluate, or otherwise examine:

1. public benefit or service programs;
2. procedures for obtaining benefits or services under those programs;
3. possible changes in or alternatives to those programs or procedures; ***or***
4. possible changes in methods or levels of payment for benefits or services under those programs; ***and***
5. the research could not practicably be carried out without the waiver or alteration.

---

[1] Per July 2017 FDA guidance, FDA will not object to the use of the pre-2018 Common Rule regulations regarding waiver and alteration of informed consent until FDA promulgates its own regulations. Thus, only elements 1, 2, 4, and 5, above, need to be met for FDA-regulated research that is not also regulated by the 2018 Common Rule.

The FDA regulations also allow extremely limited emergency exceptions to standard informed consent requirements, applicable only in certain emergency life-threatening situations where standard therapies are unproven or unsatisfactory and significant administrative burdens are met by the relevant investigators and IRB. HHS-supported research also allows a parallel exception through a Secretarial waiver of the standard informed consent requirements in such emergency situations.

In addition, HIPAA requires that the IRB find and document the following, when a waiver will include a waiver of Authorization for the use or disclosure of protected health information (PHI) in connection with the research project:

1. The use of disclosure of PHI must involve no more than minimal risk to the privacy of individuals, based on, at least the presence of the following elements:

   i. an adequate plan to protect identifiers from improper use and disclosure;

   ii. an adequate plan to destroy the identifiers at the earliest opportunity consistent with the conduct of the research, unless there is a health or research justification for retaining the identifiers or such retention is otherwise required by law;

   iii. adequate written assurances that the PHI will not be reused or disclosed to any other person or entity, except:

      (a) as required by law;

      (b) for authorized oversight of the study, ***or***

      (c) for other research for which the use and disclosure of the PHI would be permitted under the Privacy Rule;

2. The research could not practicably be conducted without the waiver or alteration; ***and***

3. The research could not practicably be conducted without access to and use of the PHI.

Exhibit 9.0.3 — Sample Broad Consent Checklist, 2018 Common Rule

Consent Document:

1. Does the consent apply only to the storage, maintenance, and secondary research use of identifiable private information and identifiable biospecimens that were collected for a study other than the proposed research or for non-research purposes? **(Section 9.3.4)** ___ Yes ___ No

2. Does the informed consent provide the information a reasonable person would want to have in order to make an informed decision about whether to participate, and is the subject provided an opportunity to discuss that information? **(Sections 9.2 and 9.3.4)** ___ Yes ___ No

3. Are the ten basic elements of broad consent included? **(Section 9.3.4)** ___ Yes ___ No

4. Are the two additional elements of consent included when appropriate? **(Section 9.3.4)** ___ Yes ___ No

5. Will the consent be understandable to an individual with a 6th grade education? ___ Yes ___ No

6. Is a Certificate of Confidentiality (CoC) applicable to the research, and if so, is a description of the CoC protections included in the consent document? **(Section 9.1)** ___ Yes ___ No

Note: No alteration of broad consent elements is permitted. If broad consent is refused, waiver of consent may not be obtained.

Ten Required Basic Elements of Broad Consent (Section 9.3.4):

1. General description of types of research that may be conducted with the subject's information or biospecimens, including sufficient information such that a "reasonable person" would expect the consent would permit the types of research conducted.
2. Description of information or biospecimens that might be used for research, whether they will be shared, types of institutions or researchers that might use them for research.
3. Description of any reasonably foreseeable risks and discomforts to the subject.
4. Description of any benefits to the subject (direct benefits) or to others (indirect benefits to others with similar health problems or to society at large) to be reasonably expected from the research.
5. Description of period of time information or biospecimens may be stored and maintained, and period of time they may be used for research (both periods may be "indefinitely").

6. Statement describing the extent, if any, to which confidentiality of records identifying the subject will be maintained, including appropriate HIPAA language (unless contained in a separate Authorization), and noting the possibility that the FDA may inspect the records, if applicable.
7. Statement that the subject will not be provided details of specific research studies, and that the subject might have chosen not to consent to some such research (Note: this statement need not be included if the subject will be provided details about specific studies).
8. Statement that the subject will not be provided clinically relevant research results (Note: this statement need not be included if it is known that the subject will be provided with clinically relevant research results).
9. Statement that participation is voluntary, refusal to participate will involve no penalty or loss of benefits to which the subject is otherwise entitled, and that the subject may discontinue participation at any time without penalty or loss of benefits to which the subject is otherwise entitled.
10. Explanation of whom to contact with questions about the subject's rights, or storage and use of subject's information and biospecimens, and whom to contact in case of research-related harm.

Two Additional Elements of Informed Consent (must be included when appropriate) (Section 9.3.4):

1. A statement that the subject's biospecimens (even if identifiers are removed) may be used for commercial profit, and whether or not the subject will share in this profit.
2. For research involving biospecimens, whether the research will (if known) or might include whole genome sequencing.

Certificate of Confidentiality Language (if appropriate) (Section 9.1):

For research, to which a Certificate of Confidentiality (CoC) from NIH applies, include a description of the CoC protections. NIH provides the following suggested language that should be edited as necessary for the study population:

> This research is covered by a Certificate of Confidentiality from the National Institutes of Health. The researchers with this Certificate may not disclose or use information, documents, or biospecimens that may identify you in any federal, state, or local civil, criminal, administrative, legislative, or other action, suit, or proceeding, or be used as evidence, for example, if there is a court subpoena, unless you have consented for this use. Information, documents, or biospecimens protected by this Certificate cannot be disclosed to anyone else who is not connected with the research except, if there is a federal, state, or local law that requires disclosure (such as to report child abuse or communicable diseases but not for federal, state, or local civil, criminal, administrative, legislative, or other proceedings, see below); if you have consented to

the disclosure, including for your medical treatment; or if it is used for other scientific research, as allowed by federal regulations protecting research subjects.

[INCLUDE IF APPLICABLE:] The Certificate cannot be used to refuse a request for information from personnel of the United States federal or state government agency sponsoring the project that is needed for auditing or program evaluation by [*THE AGENCY*] which is funding this project or for information that must be disclosed in order to meet the requirements of the federal Food and Drug Administration (FDA). You should understand that a Certificate of Confidentiality does not prevent you from voluntarily releasing information about yourself or your involvement in this research. If you want your research information released to an insurer, medical care provider, or any other person not connected with the research, you must provide consent to allow the researchers to release it.

[INCLUDE IF APPLICABLE (if researcher intends to disclose information covered by a Certificate, such as potential child abuse, or intent to hurt self or others in response to specific federal, state, or local laws):] The Certificate of Confidentiality will not be used to prevent disclosure as required by federal, state, or local law of [*list what will be reported, such as child abuse and neglect, or harm to self or others*].

[INCLUDE IF APPLICABLE (if researcher intends to disclose information covered by a Certificate, with the consent of research participants):] The Certificate of Confidentiality will not be used to prevent disclosure for any purpose you have consented to in this informed consent document [*restate what will be disclosed, such as including research data in the medical record*].

[INCLUDE IF APPLICABLE (if researcher intends to disclose information covered by a Certificate, such as potential child abuse, or intent to hurt self or others in response to specific federal, state, or local laws):] The Certificate of Confidentiality will not be used to prevent disclosure as required by federal, state, or local law of [*list what will be reported, such as child abuse and neglect, or harm to self or others*].

[INCLUDE IF APPLICABLE (if researcher intends to disclose information covered by a Certificate, with the consent of research participants):] The Certificate of Confidentiality will not be used to prevent disclosure for any purpose you have consented to in this informed consent document [*restate what will be disclosed, such as including research data in the medical record*].

Exhibit 9.3.1—Sample Informed Consent, Pre-2018 Common Rule and FDA

- THIS IS A SAMPLE CONSENT FORM AND IS NOT INTENDED FOR VERBATIM USE.
- IT MUST BE MODIFIED TO FIT EACH INDIVIDUAL STUDY.
- ALL MEDICAL TERMINOLOGY SHOULD BE DISCLOSED TO THE SUBJECT IN LAY TERMS.
- CONSIDER USING A PLAIN LANGUAGE WRITING STYLE, WITH A FOCUS ON DESCRIBING WHAT IS IMPORTANT TO THE SUBJECT.
- INCLUDE REVISION DATE AND PAGE NUMBER IN THE FOOTER.

[NAME OF INSTITUTION WHERE STUDY IS TAKING PLACE]

SUBJECT INFORMED CONSENT
AND
AUTHORIZATION FOR USE AND DISCLOSURE OF HEALTH INFORMATION

Title of Protocol:

Name and Contact Information of Principal Investigator:

Study Sponsor:

Please read this document carefully.

You are asked to take part in a research study to [insert brief description of purpose]. Taking part in this research study is voluntary.

Before you decide, you should know why the research is being done, how you may benefit from it, any risk to you, and what it involves. Please read this form carefully and take your time to decide. Please ask questions about anything that is unclear to you or that you do not understand.

If anything is unclear or you would like further information, please contact the study team. You may take an unsigned copy of this form home with you to read again. Take your time to think and talk about it with your family and friends before making your decision.

[Include if appropriate: "A description of this clinical study is available on http://www.ClinicalTrials.gov, as required by U.S. law. This Web site will not include information that can identify you. At most, the Web site will include a summary of the results. You can search this Web site at any time."]

If you would like further information, please contact the study team.

INFORMATION ABOUT THE STUDY

Before you decide to take part in this study, please take as much time as you need to ask any questions and discuss this study with the study team, or with family, friends or your personal physician or other health professionals.

1. **Purpose ("Why is this study being done?"):**

   (Why is the study being performed and what use may be made of the results. Avoid technical jargon and use language understandable to the person signing the consent.)

2. **Description of Study and Procedure ("What happens during the study, and what is done at study visits?"):**

   (Describe the specific procedures involved in the study, including invasive techniques, expected duration of participation, restriction on normal activities, the possibility of receiving placebo medications in a double-blind trial, and any experimental procedures. A visit-by-visit description of the study is preferred. For some more involved studies, the description of the study and the description of the study procedures may more appropriately be broken into two sections.)

3. **Study Sponsor ("Who is paying for this study?"):**

   (Include information about the study sponsor(s), and disclose whether any members of the study team have financial relationships with the study sponsor or otherwise may benefit from the subject's participation in the study.)

4. **Approximate Number of Subjects ("How many people are taking part in this study?"):**

   (Include the approximate number of subjects to be enrolled in each study arm, if appropriate.)

5. **Duration of Study ("How long will I be in the study?"):**

   (Describe the duration of study participation, including specific information about each study visit and the procedures in which the subject will participate.)

6. **Eligibility Criteria ("What will I have to do to be able to participate?"):**

   (Describe the eligibility criteria, including actions the subject must take to remain eligible for study participation (*e.g.*, avoid alcohol, certain drugs or medications, etc.).)

7. **Risks of Research Participation ("What are the risks to me from being in the study?"):**

   (List reasonably foreseeable risks or side effects and measures taken to minimize any hazards or discomforts, including reproductive risks. Include statement that some risks are currently unforeseeable, if appropriate.)

8. **Benefits of Research Participation ("What are the benefits of being in the study?"):**

   (Describe any therapeutic benefits to the subject as a result of participation in the study. If there are no direct benefits, state that the subject may not receive any benefit by taking part in this research study. However, the information gained from participation may help medical science and other patients in the future.)

9. **Alternatives to Research Participation ("What are my options other than being in the study?"):**

   (List alternative treatments that are available to the subject's condition. Include, if appropriate, that the subject could obtain the research intervention outside of the research context.)

10. **Significant New Findings ("Will I be told about new information learned that may affect whether I want to stay in the study?"):**

    (Consider a statement such as the following: "The research team will inform you of any significant new information about any of the drugs or treatments you are receiving, or any other new medical treatment for your condition, while you are participating in this study.")

11. **Confidentiality of Research-Related Information ("What happens to the information collected about me?"):**

    (Describe privacy protections for subjects, and confidentiality protections for subjects' information, biospecimens, and research data. Include how the information and biospecimens will be stored (*e.g.*, identifiable, coded, or de-identified form); transmitted and shared; and relevant data security protections. Describe who may access the information, biospecimens, data, including appropriate regulatory authorities such as OHRP, FDA, foreign/state/local authorities, if any.

    Consider including statements such as the following, when appropriate:

    - "Complete confidentiality cannot be promised, but every effort will be made to keep the records as confidential as possible within the limits of the law. All data and medical information obtained about you as an individual will be considered important and held in confidence. If you decide to leave the study at any time, the sponsor may still use your information collected up to that point, as the law allows."

    - "Research-related personal health information that can identify you is protected by the federal privacy and security regulations issued under the Health Insurance Portability and Accountability Act (HIPAA). Your information may be provided as described above through the length of the research study, unless you revoke this Authorization for such use and disclosure. Your personal information may no longer be protected under these laws when shared with others as described above. Other privacy laws may apply to this information."

- "Clinical trial information from this study may be disclosed in the U.S. government registry databank (located at www.clinicaltrials.gov) in order to comply with requirements of the U.S. Federal Food, Drug and Cosmetic Act (FD&C) and Public Health Service (PHS) Act, and no personal identifiable information will be provided as a result of this disclosure."
- "***The information authorized for release may include records that may indicate the presence of a communicable or noncommunicable disease required to be reported pursuant to [state] law.***")

If a Certificate of Confidentiality from the National Institutes of Health (NIH) applies to the research, include a description of the Certificate's protections, as appropriate. The sample language from NIH, below, should be modified as appropriate for the research and the research population:

> This research is covered by a Certificate of Confidentiality from the National Institutes of Health. The researchers with this Certificate may not disclose or use information, documents, or biospecimens that may identify you in any federal, state, or local civil, criminal, administrative, legislative, or other action, suit, or proceeding, or be used as evidence, for example, if there is a court subpoena, unless you have consented for this use. Information, documents, or biospecimens protected by this Certificate cannot be disclosed to anyone else who is not connected with the research except, if there is a federal, state, or local law that requires disclosure (such as to report child abuse or communicable diseases but not for federal, state, or local civil, criminal, administrative, legislative, or other proceedings, see below); if you have consented to the disclosure, including for your medical treatment; or if it is used for other scientific research, as allowed by federal regulations protecting research subjects.
>
> **[INCLUDE IF APPLICABLE:]** The Certificate cannot be used to refuse a request for information from personnel of the United States federal or state government agency sponsoring the project that is needed for auditing or program evaluation by [*THE AGENCY*] which is funding this project or for information that must be disclosed in order to meet the requirements of the federal Food and Drug Administration (FDA). You should understand that a Certificate of Confidentiality does not prevent you from voluntarily releasing information about yourself or your involvement in this research. If you

want your research information released to an insurer, medical care provider, or any other person not connected with the research, you must provide consent to allow the researchers to release it.

[*INCLUDE IF APPLICABLE (if researcher intends to disclose information covered by a Certificate, such as potential child abuse, or intent to hurt self or others in response to specific federal, state, or local laws)*:] The Certificate of Confidentiality will not be used to prevent disclosure as required by federal, state, or local law of [*list what will be reported, such as child abuse and neglect, or harm to self or others*].

[*INCLUDE IF APPLICABLE (if researcher intends to disclose information covered by a Certificate, with the consent of research participants)*:] The Certificate of Confidentiality will not be used to prevent disclosure for any purpose you have consented to in this informed consent document [*restate what will be disclosed, such as including research data in the medical record*].

12. **Costs of Research Participation ("Who pays for the treatment and tests I receive?"):**

    (Explain what costs will be incurred for procedures that are solely related to the study and who is responsible for payment of study-related costs. Consider a statement such as the following:

    "Any costs that are part of your usual medical care for your condition are your responsibility or, where appropriate, the responsibility of your health insurance company or Medicare. If your health insurance company or Medicare requires any co-payment, co-insurance, or deductible, you will be responsible for making that payment.")

13. **Compensation for Study Participation ("Will I be compensated?")**

    (State here whether this study offers compensation (*e.g.*, check payments, gift cards, or other items) for participation (*e.g.*, time and inconvenience). If compensation is offered, state the type, amount, and timing of payment. For research involving more than minimal risk, provide an explanation as to whether any compensation is offered.)

14. **Research-Related Illness or Injury ("What if I am hurt by this study?"):**

    (Consider a statement such as the following:

    "Should you become ill or are injured as a direct result of your study participation or should you experience study related reactions, you should contact [INSERT CONTACT FOR THE HUMAN SUBJECTS PROTECTION OFFICE OR RESEARCH TEAM] at [INSERT TELEPHONE NUMBER, EMAIL, ETC.]. In the event of physical injury or physical illness related to the study, no monetary compensation or subsidized medical treatment will be routinely provided to you by any person involved in this study including the research team, [institution], or [study sponsor]. Any immediate medical treatment, however, that may be necessary will be provided and you [INSERT "WILL" or "WILL NOT", AS APPROPRIATE] be billed for this treatment. There are no plans to provide you with other compensation as a result of illness or injury resulting from your research participation.")

15. **Voluntary Participation and Withdrawal of Participation ("Can I decline to participate and can I stop participating in the study? Can I be removed from the study?"):**

(Include information about the subject's ability to withdraw from research, and the circumstances, if any, under which the investigator might unilaterally terminate the subject's participation. Include information about what happens to the information and biospecimens about the subject that already have been collected. Consider a statement such as the following:

"Your participation in this study is voluntary and you are free to withdraw or refuse participation at any time without penalty or adversely affecting your future care at this institution. Withdrawal will not cause a loss of benefits to which you might otherwise be entitled. Any questions you have pertaining to the research have been and will be answered by the principal investigator, *Dr.* ________________ *at* ______________. If you have any questions about your rights as a research subject, you may contact the Human Subjects Protection Office at *[Institution]* at *[Phone Number]*.

The study team has the right to take you out of the study at any time with or without your agreement. The Sponsor has the right to direct your study doctor to take you out of the study at any time with or without your agreement. These decisions will be made if, for example:

- It is in your best medical interest to stop your participation
- You do not follow instructions
- The study is canceled.")

16. **Storage, Sharing, and Future Research Use of Biospecimens and Data ("What happens to the information and biospecimens collected about me?")**

(If appropriate, include a discussion of what biospecimens and data will be stored by the study team; how long will the biospecimens and data be stored; any possible sharing of biospecimens and data; potential future research use of biospecimens and data; whether biospecimens and data will be stored and used in an identifiable form; risks of storage and sharing of biospecimens and data.)

17. **Signatures:**

I have read the information provided to me about this study and have been given the opportunity to discuss the information and to ask questions. I consent to participate in this study.

____

Subject's Printed Name

______________________________ ____________________

Subject Signature Date

WHEN SUBJECT IS INCOMPETENT TO GIVE CONSENT:

I have read the explanation about this study and have been given the opportunity to discuss it and to ask questions. I am legally authorized to make research decisions on behalf of the adult participant unable to consent and have the authority to provide consent to this study.

______________________________ ____________________

Signature of Legally Authorized Representative Date

____

Printed Name of Legally Authorized Representative

______________________________ ____________________

Signature of Individual Obtaining Consent Date

______________________________ ____________________

Witness Signature Date

Exhibit 9.3.2—Sample Study-Specific Informed Consent, 2018 Common Rule

- THIS IS A SAMPLE CONSENT FORM AND IS NOT INTENDED FOR VERBATIM USE.
- IT MUST BE MODIFIED TO FIT EACH INDIVIDUAL STUDY.
- ALL MEDICAL TERMINOLOGY SHOULD BE DISCLOSED TO THE SUBJECT IN LAY TERMS.
- CONSIDER USING A PLAIN LANGUAGE WRITING STYLE, WITH A FOCUS ON DESCRIBING WHAT IS IMPORTANT TO THE SUBJECT.
- INCLUDE REVISION DATE AND PAGE NUMBER IN THE FOOTER.

[NAME OF INSTITUTION WHERE STUDY IS TAKING PLACE]

SUBJECT INFORMED CONSENT

AND

AUTHORIZATION FOR USE AND DISCLOSURE OF HEALTH INFORMATION

Title of Protocol:

Name and Contact Information of Principal Investigator:

Study Sponsor:

Please read this document carefully

You are asked to take part in a research study to [insert brief description of purpose]. Taking part in this research study is voluntary.

Before you decide, you should know why the research is being done, how you may benefit from it, any risk to you, and what it involves. Please read this form carefully and take your time to decide. Please ask questions about anything that is unclear to you or that you do not understand.

If anything is unclear or you would like further information, please contact the study team. You may take an unsigned copy of this form home with you to read again. Take your time to think and talk about it with your family and friends before making your decision.

[Include if appropriate: "A description of this clinical study is available on http://www.ClinicalTrials.gov, as required by U.S. law. This Web site will not include information that can identify you. At most, the Web site will include a summary of the results. You can search this Web site at any time."]

If you would like further information, please contact the study team.

KEY INFORMATION

This summary gives you important information about the research to help you decide if you want to participate in the study. More information about these topics is available in the rest of the document.

[*Include a summary of key information a subject would want to know before agreeing to participate in research. This should include, at a minimum, (1) the fact that consent is being sought for research and that participation is voluntary; (2) the purposes of the research, the expected duration of the prospective subject's participation, the procedures to be followed in the research, and the identification of procedures that are experimental; (3) the reasonably foreseeable risks or discomforts to the prospective subject; (4) the benefits to the prospective subject or to others that may reasonably be expected from the research; and (5) appropriate alternative procedures or courses of treatment, if any, that might be advantageous to the prospective subject. Suggested headings could include:*

WHY THIS STUDY IS BEING DONE

WHAT WILL HAPPEN TO ME DURING THE STUDY

HOW LONG WILL THE STUDY WILL TAKE

MAIN RISKS OF BEING IN THE STUDY

MAIN BENEFITS OF BEING IN THE STUDY

ALTERNATIVES TO BEING IN THE STUDY

OTHER INFORMATION YOU MAY WANT TO CONSIDER]

INFORMATION ABOUT THE STUDY

Before you decide to take part in this study, please take as much time as you need to ask any questions and discuss this study with the study team, or with family, friends or your personal physician or other health professionals.

1. **Purpose ("Why is this study being done?"):**

   (Why is the study being performed and what use may be made of the results. Avoid technical jargon and use language understandable to the person signing the consent.)

2. **Description of Study and Procedure ("What happens during the study, and what is done at study visits?"):**

   (Describe the specific procedures involved in the study, including invasive techniques, expected duration of participation, restriction on normal activities, the possibility of receiving placebo medications in a double-blind trial, and any experimental procedures. A visit-by-visit description of the study is preferred. For some more involved studies, the description of the study and the description of the study procedures may more appropriately be broken into two sections.)

3. **Study Sponsor ("Who is paying for this study?"):**

   (Include information about the study sponsor(s), and disclose whether any members of the study team have financial relationships with the study sponsor or otherwise may benefit from the subject's participation in the study.)

4. **Approximate Number of Subjects ("How many people are taking part in this study?"):**

   (Include the approximate number of subjects to be enrolled in each study arm, if appropriate.)

5. **Duration of Study ("How long will I be in the study?"):**

   (Describe the duration of study participation, including specific information about each study visit and the procedures in which the subject will participate.)

6. **Eligibility Criteria ("What will I have to do to be able to participate?"):**

   (Describe the eligibility criteria, including actions the subject must take to remain eligible for study participation (*e.g.*, avoid alcohol, certain drugs or medications, etc.).)

7. **Risks of Research Participation ("What are the risks to me from being in the study?"):**

   (List reasonably foreseeable risks or side effects and measures taken to minimize any hazards or discomforts, including reproductive risks. Include statement that some risks are currently unforeseeable, if appropriate.)

8. **Benefits of Research Participation ("What are the benefits of being in the study?"):**

   (Describe any therapeutic benefits to the subject as a result of participation in the study. If there are no direct benefits, state that the subject may not receive any benefit by taking part in this research study. However, the information gained from participation may help medical science and other patients in the future.)

9. **Alternatives to Research Participation ("What are my options other than being in the study?"):**

(List alternative treatments that are available to the subject's condition. Include, if appropriate, that the subject could obtain the research intervention outside of the research context.)

10. **Significant New Findings ("Will I be told about new information learned that may affect whether I want to stay in the study?"):**

    (Consider a statement such as the following: "The research team will inform you of any significant new information about any of the drugs or treatments you are receiving, or any other new medical treatment for your condition, while you are participating in this study.")

11. **Confidentiality of Research-Related Information ("What happens to the information collected about me?"):**

    (Describe privacy protections for subjects and confidentiality protections for subjects' information, biospecimens, and research data. Include how the information and biospecimens will be stored (*e.g.*, identifiable, coded, or de-identified form); transmitted and shared; and relevant data security protections. Describe who may access the information, biospecimens, data, including appropriate regulatory authorities such as OHRP, FDA, foreign/state/local authorities, if any.

    Consider including statements such as the following, when appropriate:

    - "Complete confidentiality cannot be promised, but every effort will be made to keep the records as confidential as possible within the limits of the law. All data and medical information obtained about you as an individual will be considered important and held in confidence. If you decide to leave the study at any time, the sponsor may still use your information collected up to that point, as the law allows."

    - "Clinical trial information from this study may be disclosed in the U.S. government registry databank (located at www.clinicaltrials.gov) in order to comply with requirements of the U.S. Federal Food, Drug and Cosmetic Act (FD&C) and Public Health Service (PHS) Act, and no personal identifiable information will be provided as a result of this disclosure."

    - "Research-related personal health information that can identify you is protected by the federal privacy and security regulations issued under the Health Insurance Portability and Accountability Act (HIPAA). Your information may be provided as described above through the length of the research study, unless you revoke this Authorization for such use and disclosure. Your personal information may no longer be protected under these laws when shared with others as described above. Other privacy laws may apply to this information."

- ***"The information authorized for release may include records which may indicate the presence of a communicable or noncommunicable disease required to be reported pursuant to [state] law."***)

If a Certificate of Confidentiality from the National Institutes of Health (NIH) applies to the research, include a description of the Certificate's protections, as appropriate. The sample language from NIH, below, should be modified as appropriate for the research and the research population:

> This research is covered by a Certificate of Confidentiality from the National Institutes of Health. The researchers with this Certificate may not disclose or use information, documents, or biospecimens that may identify you in any federal, state, or local civil, criminal, administrative, legislative, or other action, suit, or proceeding, or be used as evidence, for example, if there is a court subpoena, unless you have consented for this use. Information, documents, or biospecimens protected by this Certificate cannot be disclosed to anyone else who is not connected with the research except, if there is a federal, state, or local law that requires disclosure (such as to report child abuse or communicable diseases but not for federal, state, or local civil, criminal, administrative, legislative, or other proceedings, see below); if you have consented to the disclosure, including for your medical treatment; or if it is used for other scientific research, as allowed by federal regulations protecting research subjects.
>
> **[INCLUDE IF APPLICABLE:]** The Certificate cannot be used to refuse a request for information from personnel of the United States federal or state government agency sponsoring the project that is needed for auditing or program evaluation by [*THE AGENCY*] which is funding this project or for information that must be disclosed in order to meet the requirements of the federal Food and Drug Administration (FDA). You should understand that a Certificate of Confidentiality does not prevent you from voluntarily releasing information about yourself or your involvement in this research. If you want your research information released to an insurer, medical care provider, or any other person not connected with the research, you must provide consent to allow the researchers to release it.
>
> ***[INCLUDE IF APPLICABLE (if researcher intends to disclose information covered by a Certificate, such as potential child abuse, or intent to hurt self or others in response to specific federal, state, or local laws):]*** The Certificate of Confidentiality will not be used to prevent disclosure as required by federal, state, or local law of [*list what will be reported, such as child abuse and neglect, or harm to self or others*].

[INCLUDE IF APPLICABLE (if researcher intends to disclose information covered by a Certificate, with the consent of research participants):] The Certificate of Confidentiality will not be used to prevent disclosure for any purpose you have consented to in this informed consent document [*restate what will be disclosed, such as including research data in the medical record*].

12. **Costs of Research Participation ("Who pays for the treatment and tests I receive?"):**

    (Explain what costs will be incurred for procedures that are solely related to the study and who is responsible for payment of study-related costs. Consider a statement such as the following:

    Any costs that are part of your usual medical care for your condition are your responsibility or, where appropriate, the responsibility of your health insurance company or Medicare. If your health insurance company or Medicare requires any co-payment, co-insurance, or deductible, you will be responsible for making that payment.")

13. **Compensation for Study Participation ("Will I be compensated?")**

    (State here whether this study offers compensation (*e.g.*, check payments, gift cards, or other items) for participation (*e.g.*, time and inconvenience). If compensation is offered, state the type, amount, and timing of payment. For research involving more than minimal risk, provide an explanation as to whether any compensation is offered.)

14. **Research-Related Illness or Injury ("What if I am hurt by this study?"):**

    (Consider a statement such as the following:

    "Should you become ill or are injured as a direct result of your study participation or should you experience study related reactions, you should contact [INSERT CONTACT FOR THE HUMAN SUBJECTS PROTECTION OFFICE OR RESEARCH TEAM] at [INSERT TELEPHONE NUMBER, EMAIL, ETC.]. In the event of physical injury or physical illness related to the study, no monetary compensation or subsidized medical treatment will be routinely provided to you by any person involved in this study including the research team, [institution], or [study sponsor]. Any immediate medical treatment, however, that may be necessary will be provided and you [INSERT "WILL" or "WILL NOT", AS APPROPRIATE] be billed for this treatment. There are no plans to provide you with other compensation as a result of illness or injury resulting from your research participation.")

15. **Voluntary Participation and Withdrawal of Participation ("Can I decline to participate and can I stop participating in the study? Can I be removed from the study?"):**

(Include information about the subject's ability to withdraw from research, and the circumstances, if any, under which the investigator might unilaterally terminate the subject's participation. Include information about what happens to the information and biospecimens about the subject that already have been collected. Consider a statement such as the following:

"Your participation in this study is voluntary and you are free to withdraw or refuse participation at any time without penalty or adversely affecting your future care at this institution. Withdrawal will not cause a loss of benefits to which you might otherwise be entitled. Any questions you have pertaining to the research have been and will be answered by the principal investigator, *Dr.* ________________ *at* ______________. If you have any questions about your rights as a research subject, you may contact the Human Subjects Protection Office at *[Institution]* at *[Phone Number]*.

The study team has the right to take you out of the study at any time with or without your agreement. The Sponsor has the right to direct your study doctor to take you out of the study at any time with or without your agreement. These decisions will be made if, for example:

- It is in your best medical interest to stop your participation
- You do not follow instructions
- The study is canceled.")

16. **Storage, Sharing, and Future Research Use of Biospecimens and Data ("What happens to the information and biospecimens collected about me?")**

(If appropriate, include a discussion of what biospecimens and data will be stored by the study team; how long will the biospecimens and data be stored; any possible sharing of biospecimens and data; potential future research use of biospecimens and data; whether biospecimens and data will be stored and used in an identifiable form; risks of storage and sharing of biospecimens and data).

If the research is regulated by the Common Rule and involves the collection of identifiable private information or identifiable biospecimens, one of the following statements **must** be included:

- A statement that identifiers might be removed from the identifiable private information or identifiable biospecimens and that, after such removal, the information or biospecimens could be used for future research studies or distributed to another investigator for future research studies without obtaining additional informed consent from the subject or the legally authorized representative (if such a transfer is a possibility); ***or***

- A statement that the subject's information or biospecimens collected as part of the research, even if identifiers are removed, will not be used or distributed for future research studies.)

17. **Commercial Profit from Biospecimens ("Will my biospecimens be used for commercial profit?')**

    (If appropriate, include a statement that the subject's biospecimens (even if identifiers are removed) may be used for commercial profit (*e.g.*, creation of a cell line), and whether or not the subject will share in this profit.)

18. **Return of Research Results ("Will I get information about the study results?")**

    (If appropriate, include a statement regarding whether clinically relevant research results will be disclosed to subjects, and if so, under what conditions.)

19. **Whole Genome Sequencing ("Will the study involve whole genome sequencing?")**

    (If appropriate, include a statement, for research involving biospecimens, whether the research will (if known) or might include whole genome sequencing. Include a lay description of whole genome sequencing.)

Continue to next page for signatures.

20. **Signatures:**

I have read the information provided to me about this study and have been given the opportunity to discuss the information and to ask questions. I consent to participate in this study.

____

Subject's Printed Name

______________________________ ____________________

Subject Signature Date

WHEN SUBJECT IS INCOMPETENT TO GIVE CONSENT:

I have read the explanation about this study and have been given the opportunity to discuss it and to ask questions. I am legally authorized to make research decisions on behalf of the adult participant unable to consent and have the authority to provide consent to this study.

______________________________ ____________________

Signature of Legally Authorized Representative Date

____

Printed Name of Legally Authorized Representative

______________________________ ____________________

Signature Of Individual Obtaining Consent Date

______________________________ ____________________

Witness Signature Date

Exhibit 9.3.3—Sample Broad Consent, 2018 Common Rule[1]

- THIS IS A SAMPLE CONSENT FORM AND IS NOT INTENDED FOR VERBATIM USE.
- IT MUST BE MODIFIED TO FIT EACH INDIVIDUAL SITUATION.
- ALL MEDICAL TERMINOLOGY SHOULD BE DISCLOSED TO THE SUBJECT IN LAY TERMS.
- CONSIDER USING A PLAIN LANGUAGE WRITING STYLE, WITH A FOCUS ON DESCRIBING WHAT IS IMPORTANT TO THE SUBJECT.
- INCLUDE REVISION DATE AND PAGE NUMBER IN THE FOOTER.
- **NO ALTERATION OF BROAD CONSENT ELEMENTS IS PERMITTED.**
- **IF BROAD CONSENT IS REFUSED, CONSENT MAY NOT BE WAIVED.**

[NAME OF INSTITUTION WHERE STUDY IS TAKING PLACE]

BROAD CONSENT FOR STORAGE, MAINTENANCE, AND SECONDARY RESEARCH USE OF IDENTIFIABLE INFORMATION AND IDENTIFIABLE BIOSPECIMENS

AND

AUTHORIZATION FOR USE AND DISCLOSURE OF PHI FOR FUTURE RESEARCH PURPOSES

Please read this document carefully

WHAT ARE WE ASKING YOU TO DO?

We are asking for your consent to allow your identifiable information and identifiable biospecimens originally collected for one purpose (such as for your medical care or another research study) to be stored and used in a wide range of different types of research studies in the future. Research using personal health information (such as information about your health status, medical test results, and what medical conditions you have), and biospecimens (for example, blood or other body tissues) has led to important advances in medicine, science, and other areas. As explained in this form, we hope to make it easier for researchers to use your information and biospecimens.

---

1 Based largely on SACHRP August 2, 2017, recommendations to HHS Secretary, "Attachment D - Recommendations for a Broad Consent Template," found at https://www.hhs.gov/ohrp/sachrp-committee/recommendations/attachment-d-august-2-2017/index.html.

If you are willing to give your consent to the research use of your identifiable information and identifiable biospecimens, your information and biospecimens may be stored indefinitely, and researchers may use your identifiable information or identifiable biospecimens in many different research studies, over a long period of time (likely indefinitely), without asking your permission again for any specific study covered by this form. If you do not consent to this, researchers in most cases will have to ask your permission to use your identifiable information or identifiable biospecimens in any other research study.

WHAT WILL HAPPEN TO MY IDENTIFIABLE INFORMATION OR IDENTIFIABLE BIOSPECIMENS IF I GIVE CONSENT?

If you give consent, [Name of Repository/Biobank/Institution/Institutional Department or Division] will store, use and share your identifiable information and/or identifiable biospecimens, and may do so for the purpose of medical, scientific, and other research, now and into the future, for as long as they are needed for this purpose [or specific a shorter period]. We may share your identifiable information and identifiable biospecimens with other research, academic, and medical institutions, other researchers, drug and device companies, biotechnology companies, and others.

WHAT TYPES OF RESEARCH MAY BE DONE WITH MY IDENTIFIABLE INFORMATION OR IDENTIFIABLE BIOSPECIMENS?

If you give consent, there are no plans to tell you about any of the specific research studies that will be done with your identifiable information and identifiable biospecimens, or the purposes of the research studies that use your identifiable information and identifiable biospecimens. Possible future research may include, for example:

- Studying the causes and progression of different diseases and conditions
- Developing and testing methods to diagnose and treat different diseases and conditions
- Whole genome sequencing (meaning that your entire personal genetic code will be identified)
- Specific genetic research looking at diseases and medical conditions that are passed on in families and among populations larger than families
- Research that creates cell lines by growing cells from your biospecimens in a laboratory – including cells that can be used to create different types of tissue
- Research that includes changing the genes in cells or putting human cells into animals
- Research about drug abuse and alcoholism diagnosis and treatment
- Research about mental health diagnosis and treatment
- Research about developmental disabilities
- Research about HIV and sexually transmitted diseases
- Research about induced termination of pregnancy [abortion]

- Family planning and reproductive health research

[Add here any statements required by applicable state law to conduct research in the categories above]

It is possible that, if asked, you might not have agreed to the specific research studies which will be done using your identifiable information and identifiable biospecimens.

The results of research done on your identifiable information and identifiable biospecimens will not be put into your medical records. It is possible, but unlikely, that testing on your biospecimens could show that you have a medical condition (like tuberculosis or HIV), that the laws in your state say must be reported to public health departments, with information that identifies you. This is required anytime someone is found to have a condition that must be reported, whether this is found in medical care or in a research study.

[If applicable: "The following types of research will not be conducted using your identifiable biospecimens and identifiable information: (List any types of sensitive or genetic research that will not be conducted)."]

[If applicable: "At least the following types of research (as well as other types not listed here) will be conducted using your identifiable biospecimens and identifiable information: (List any types of known research activities not covered by the above list)."]

ARE THERE ANY RISKS TO ME?

The main risk in giving consent is to the confidentiality of the information about you. We will do our best to protect the confidentiality of your information, and prevent your information from going to people who should not have it, including by removing information that could be used easily to identify you. The risk that your identifiable information or identifiable biospecimen will go to someone who should not get it is very small.

Your identifiable information or identifiable biospecimens could be used in a research project to which you might not agree to participate, if you were asked specifically about it. The examples listed above should give you a good idea of the kinds of research projects that might be done. Also, a research ethics committee will make sure that this broad consent covers the research studies planning to use identifiable information or identifiable biospecimens from you.

[If appropriate: PRIVACY AND YOUR PROTECTED HEALTH INFORMATION

The personal information that can identify you is protected by federal privacy and security regulations issued under the Health Insurance Portability and Accountability Act (HIPAA). This section of this form advises you on your rights under these regulations.

If you give consent, we may share your identifiable information and identifiable biospecimens with researchers in the future, as described above. We may also share your identifiable information with regulatory authorities that oversee research, including the Food and Drug

Administration (FDA) and the U.S. Department of Health and Human Services Office for Human Research Protections (OHRP), and with committees and people here at [institution/entity] and in other places whose job is to review and oversee research.

Your medical information and records, once given to parties who are not bound by laws, such as the HIPAA regulations, that protect your identifiable information may no longer be protected from being used and shared without your consent.

This permission will last as long as we have a scientific and research need to use and share your identifiable information (including identifiable health information) and identifiable biospecimens.

If results of studies done with your identifiable information or identifiable biospecimens are published, your name will not be used in those publications.]

[If appropriate: CERTIFICATE OF CONFIDENTIALITY

This research is covered by a Certificate of Confidentiality from the National Institutes of Health. The researchers with this Certificate may not disclose or use information, documents, or biospecimens that may identify you in any federal, state, or local civil, criminal, administrative, legislative, or other action, suit, or proceeding, or be used as evidence, for example, if there is a court subpoena, unless you have consented for this use. Information, documents, or biospecimens protected by this Certificate cannot be disclosed to anyone else who is not connected with the research except, if there is a federal, state, or local law that requires disclosure (such as to report child abuse or communicable diseases but not for federal, state, or local civil, criminal, administrative, legislative, or other proceedings, see below); if you have consented to the disclosure, including for your medical treatment; or if it is used for other scientific research, as allowed by federal regulations protecting research subjects.

[INCLUDE IF APPLICABLE:] The Certificate cannot be used to refuse a request for information from personnel of the United States federal or state government agency sponsoring the project that is needed for auditing or program evaluation by [*THE AGENCY*] which is funding this project or for information that must be disclosed in order to meet the requirements of the federal Food and Drug Administration (FDA). You should understand that a Certificate of Confidentiality does not prevent you from voluntarily releasing information about yourself or your involvement in this research. If you want your research information released to an insurer, medical care provider, or any other person not connected with the research, you must provide consent to allow the researchers to release it.

[INCLUDE IF APPLICABLE (if researcher intends to disclose information covered by a Certificate, such as potential child abuse, or intent to hurt self or others in response to specific federal, state, or local laws):] The Certificate of Confidentiality will not be used to prevent disclosure as required by federal, state, or local law of [*list what will be reported, such as child abuse and neglect, or harm to self or others*].

[INCLUDE IF APPLICABLE (if researcher intends to disclose information covered by a Certificate, with the consent of research participants):] The Certificate of Confidentiality will not be used to prevent disclosure for any purpose you have consented to in this informed consent document [*restate what will be disclosed, such as including research data in the medical record*].]

ARE THERE ANY BENEFITS?

You will not personally benefit from agreeing to consent. Research with your identifiable information and identifiable biospecimens may help others by improving our understanding of health and disease, improving health care and making safer or more effective medical therapies, and developing new scientific knowledge.

CAN I DECLINE TO PARTICIPATE?

You do not have to agree to allow your identifiable information and identifiable biospecimens to be stored for future research use, or to be used in future research. If you decide not to allow your identifiable information and identifiable biospecimens to be used in the research, this will not cause a penalty to you or adversely affect your future care at this institution. You will not lose any benefits to which you might otherwise be entitled.

CAN I CHANGE MY MIND ABOUT PARTICIPATING?

You can change your mind about allowing your identifiable information and identifiable biospecimens to be used in the research, but there are some limits. If you change your mind, contact [Name or office] at [Phone Number]. [Repository/Biobank/Institution/Institutional Department or Division] will not begin new research uses of your identifiable information or identifiable biospecimens, but your specimens will continue to be used in studies that started before you changed your mind. If your identifiable information and identifiable biospecimens have already been given to another researcher, person, institution, or company, it may not be possible to limit their continued and new uses.

WILL IT COST ANYTHING?

There are no costs to you.

WILL I RECEIVE COMPENSATION?

If you give consent, your identifiable information and identifiable biospecimens may be used to create products or to deliver services, including some that may be sold and/or make money for others. If this happens, there are [no plans] [or insert plans] to tell you, or to pay you, or to give any compensation to you or your family. Most uses of biospecimens or information do not lead to commercial products or to profit for anyone.

Regardless of whether you say "yes" or "no" on this form, or whether you don't respond at all, if your de-identified information and de-identified biospecimens are used to create products or deliver services, there are no plans to pay you or give any compensation to you and your family. [Alternatively, include a statement that the subject will share in such commercial profit.]

WILL I LEARN MORE ABOUT MY HEALTH?

There are no plans to tell you about any specific research studies that might be done with your identifiable information or identifiable biospecimens, and there are no plans to give you any results from these studies. [Alternatively, include a statement that clinically relevant research results, including individual research results, will be disclosed to the subject in all circumstances].

WHO DO I CONTACT WTH QUESTIONS?

If you have any questions about this broad consent, please contact [Name] at [Phone Number].

You may discuss your rights as a person who has agreed to, refused, or declined to respond to an offer of broad consent with [Name] at [Phone Number].

WHO DO I CONTACT IF I AM HARMED?

If you want to report or have questions about an injury that you believe you or others have suffered as a result of your agreeing to this broad consent, please contact [Name] at [Phone Number].

Please ask us to explain anything in this form that you do not clearly understand. Please think about this broad consent and/or discuss it with family or friends before making a decision.

IF YOU AGREE TO CONSENT:

- Your identifiable information and identifiable biospecimens will be stored, used and shared for the kinds of future research described in this broad consent form, without anyone asking your permission for each new study.
- Identifying information may also be removed from your information and biospecimens, allowing them to be used for any future research or other purpose.

IF YOU DO NOT AGREE TO CONSENT:

- The researchers and institutions identified above will not store, use or share your identifiable information and identifiable biospecimens for the research described in this broad consent form.
- Researchers could come to you again later and ask to store, use and share your identifiable information or biospecimens for research.

STATEMENT OF AGREEMENT

I agree to give my consent to the storage and research uses of my identifiable information and identifiable biospecimens. My participation is voluntary, and I may withdraw at any time without any penalty or loss of benefits to which I am entitled.

____

Your Printed Name

____ *

Legally Authorized Representative's Printed Name (if applicable)

____ ______________

Your Signature or Signature of Legally Authorized Representative Date

STATEMENT OF REFUSAL

I do not agree to provide consent.

____

Your Printed Name

____ *

Legally Authorized Representative's Printed Name (if applicable)

____ ______________

Your Signature or Signature of Legally Authorized Representative Date

* If the subject is incompetent to give consent, the legally authorized representative agrees that he/she has been provided with information sufficient to understand the broad consent, has had the opportunity to ask questions about the broad consent, and is legally authorized to provide research consent on behalf of the adult participant who is unable to provide consent.

Exhibit 10.2—Sample HIPAA Authorization

[NOTE: This exhibit reflects baseline requirements for general clinical research. If secondary research is being considered, refer to **Chapter 9** and its associated exhibits for a discussion of broad consent.]

HIPAA Authorization for use with Protocol Number ____________ Informed Consent

AUTHORIZATION TO USE AND DISCLOSE PROTECTED HEALTH INFORMATION

During this research study, your doctors, their staff, their agents and hospital personnel (collectively called the "Researchers") will be collecting health information about you that is called "protected health information" or "PHI." PHI is protected under a federal privacy law called the Health Insurance Portability and Accountability Act (HIPAA) (45 C.F.R. Parts 160 and 164). By signing this form, you are giving your written permission for the Researchers, as well as the study Sponsor [Insert Sponsor Name] and the Sponsor's agents and contractors (collectively called the "Sponsor Group") to use and disclose (share) your PHI for the purposes described below:

1. These are the types of your PHI that may be used and shared in the study:

- [State PHI elements that will be used and shared, *e.g.*, name, gender, initials, address, telephone number, date of birth, dates of hospitalization, social security number and insurance information;

- All information in your medical record, the results of physical exams and tests, your medical history and other data collected during the study;

- Insurance reimbursement information (*e.g.*, bills for hospital care, physicians services, laboratory tests, diagnostic procedures, drugs, etc.); and

- Information contained in your medical records prepared by other health care providers from whom you have sought medical care while taking part in the study.]

2. The Researchers may:

- [State how Researchers will use and disclose PHI, *e.g.*, Receive, use and share your PHI to conduct the study;

- Share your PHI with the Sponsor Group;

- Share your PHI, as required by law, and with representatives of government organizations, review boards, including the [Insert Institution Name] IRB, and others who are required to watch over the safety and effectiveness of medical products or the conduct of medical research; and

- Remove from your health information your name, and to the extent feasible, other information that could be used to identify you.]

3. The Sponsor Group may:

- [State how Sponsors will use and disclose PHI, *e.g.*, Receive, use and share your PHI to conduct the study and as required by law;
- Use and share your PHI as described in the Informed Consent form and in this Authorization;
- Use and share your insurance information (e.g., hospital and doctor bills, bills for laboratory test, diagnostic procedures, drugs, etc.) for reimbursement purposes;
- Share your PHI with representatives of US and foreign government agencies, review boards and others who watch over the safety and effectiveness of medical products and research activities;
- Use and share your PHI for internal reference, for comparison with other data, to help design subsequent trials, and in regulatory papers submitted to United States and foreign regulatory agencies for later developed products; and
- Remove from your health information, your name, and to the extent feasible, other information that could be used to identify you.]

4. Please note:

- After your PHI is given to someone other than the Researchers, federal privacy laws might not protect the PHI from further use or disclosure. However, the Researchers and Sponsor Group will protect your PHI by using and disclosing it only as permitted by you in this Authorization.
- You do not have to sign this Authorization, but if you do not, you will not be able to be in the study if the study involves treatment.
- Your medical treatment, payment for services, enrollment and eligibility for benefits will not be based on whether or not you sign this Authorization.
- This Authorization has no expiration (ending) date.

By signing this consent form, you authorize the use and disclosure of health information about you as described above. You have the right to revoke this authorization, in writing, at any time by sending written notification to [Insert Name and Address]. If you revoke your authorization for use and disclosure of health information for research purposes, you will be discontinued from the research. However, the principal investigator, hospital, sponsor and its researchers may still use and disclose health information that has already been obtained as permitted in this authorization to maintain the reliability of the research.

- If you withdraw this Authorization, your PHI that has already been shared may continue to be used and shared to maintain the integrity of the research.

- While the Study is taking place, you will not be allowed to see your health information that is created or collected during the study. After the study is finished; however, you may see this information if you ask your doctor, in writing.

- The results of the study may be published in scientific journals or presented at medical meetings, but your name and identity will not be disclosed in them.

PATIENT'S HIPAA AUTHORIZATION

By signing this Authorization form, I give my written permission for my Protected Health Information to be used and collected as described in this form. I have been given a copy of this signed Authorization.

____/__________

Signature of Participant Date

____

Printed Name of Participant

OR

____/__________

Signature of Legal Authorized Representative & their relationship Date

____

Printed name of Legal Authorized Representative & their relationship

Exhibit 10.3.1—Sample Waiver or Alteration of Authorization

REQUEST FOR WAIVER OR ALTERATION OF AUTHORIZATION FOR RESEARCH

Protocol Title:

____

____

Principal Investigator: _______________________________/___________________

Name Telephone

Request for waiver of authorization:

Request for alteration of authorization:

Describe alteration requested.

HIPAA requires that the Principal Investigator document for the IRB (or Privacy Board) the following information when a waiver or alteration of authorization will result in the use or disclosure of protected health information (PHI) (subject to accounting) in connection with the research project.

1. Describe the PHI to be collected in detail, including sources of the PHI.

____

____

____

2. Describe use and disclosure of PHI.

____

____

____

3. The use or disclosure of PHI involves no more than a minimal risk (not greater in probability or magnitude than those ordinarily encountered in daily life) to the privacy of individuals based on at least (a.) through (c.) below:

a. A plan to protect identifiers from improper use and disclosure. Describe the plan (use of confidentiality agreement, coding, etc.), including where PHI will be stored and who will have access (list all entities that might have access to the study's PHI, such as sponsors, FDA, data safety monitoring committees, and any others given authority by law).

b. An adequate plan to destroy identifiers at the earliest opportunity consistent with the conduct of the research unless there is a health or research justification for retaining identifiers, or such retention is otherwise required by law.

Describe the timing and procedure used to destroy all the data collected during the study (electronic, paper, audio/video, photography, etc.) consistent with HIPAA law, regulations and guidance:

If the identifiers collected during the study will not be destroyed, describe the health or research justification for retaining the identifiers or how such retention is otherwise required by law.

c. Written assurances that the PHI will not be reused or disclosed, except as required by law, for authorized oversight of the research study, or for other research uses permitted under HIPAA. List known exceptions.

d. Describe other privacy protections.

4. Explain why the research could not practicably be conducted without the waiver or alteration.

5. Explain why the research could not practicably be conducted without access to and use of the PHI.

____

____

____

6. HIPAA requires reasonable efforts to limit PHI to the minimum necessary to accomplish the intended purpose of the use, disclosure, or request. Explain why PHI obtained under the waiver/alteration is the minimum information needed to meet the research objectives.

____

____

____.

PRINCIPAL INVESTIGATOR REPRESENTATION

I seek the above-described waiver or alteration of research authorization. I hereby certify and provide written assurance that the above statements are true and that the above-referenced protected health information will not be re-used or disclosed to any other person or entity except as described above, unless specifically authorized by this IRB or Privacy Board or by the subject of the PHI.

____/______________________

Signature of Principal Investigator Printed Name Date

Exhibit 10.3.4—Sample Data Use Agreement

This Data Use Agreement (Agreement), effective as of this __ day of _____, 20__ (Effective Date), is entered into by and between __________________ (Recipient) and __________________ (Covered Entity). The purpose of this Agreement is for Covered Entity to provide Recipient with a Limited Data Set (LDS) of Protected Health Information (PHI) for research purposes.

1. Definitions. Unless otherwise specified in this Agreement, all capitalized terms used in this Agreement not otherwise defined have the meaning established for purposes of the "HIPAA Regulations" codified at Title 45 parts 160 through 164 of the United States Code of Federal Regulations, as amended from time to time.

2. Preparation of the LDS. Covered Entity shall provide Recipient a LDS in accordance with the HIPAA Regulations.

3. Permitted Uses. Recipient agrees to use and disclose the LDS solely for the research protocol entitled:

____

Protocol No.: ____

4. Permitted Users. The following individuals or class of individuals (including Recipient) are permitted to use/receive the LDS:

____

____

____

5. Minimum Necessary Data Fields in the LDS. The LDS shall include the data fields specified by the parties from time to time, which are the minimum necessary to accomplish the purposes set forth in Section 3 of this Agreement.

6. Responsibilities of Recipient. Recipient agrees to:

a. Use or disclose the LDS only as permitted by this Agreement or as required by law;

b. Use appropriate safeguards to prevent use or disclosure of the LDS other than as per-mitted by this Agreement or required by law;

c. Report to Covered Entity any use or disclosure of the LDS of which it becomes aware that is not permitted by this Agreement or required by law;

d. Require all Permitted Users that receive or have access to the LDS to agree in writing to the same restrictions and conditions on the use and/or disclosure including use of appropriate safeguards of the LDS that apply to Recipient under this Agreement and under applicable law; and

e. Ensure that all Permitted Users agree not to use the information in the LDS to identify or contact the individuals who are data subjects in the LDS or his/her relatives, employers or household members.

f. Ensure that electronic information is secured consistent with HIPAA requirements.

7. Term and Termination.

a. Term. The term of this Agreement shall commence as of the Effective Date and shall continue for so long as Recipient retains the LDS, unless sooner terminated as set forth in this Agreement.

b. Termination by Recipient. Recipient may terminate this agreement at any time by notifying the Covered Entity and returning or destroying the LDS.

c. Termination by Covered Entity. Covered Entity may terminate this agreement at any time by providing thirty (30) days prior written notice to Recipient or immediately in the event that recipient is in material breach of its terms.

d. Effect of Termination. The terms and conditions of this Agreement shall survive any termination of this Agreement under subsections c or d.

8. Miscellaneous.

a. Change in Law. The parties agree to negotiate in good faith to amend this Agreement to comport with changes in federal law that materially alter either or both parties' obligations under this Agreement. Provided however, that if the parties are unable to agree to mutually acceptable amendment(s) by the compliance date of the change in applicable law or regulations, either Party may terminate this Agreement as provided in section 7.

b. Construction of Terms. The terms of this Agreement shall be construed to give effect to applicable federal interpretative guidance regarding the HIPAA Regulations.

c. No Third Party Beneficiaries. Nothing in this Agreement shall confer upon any person other than the parties and their respective successors or assigns, any rights, remedies, obligations, or liabilities whatsoever.

d. Counterparts. This Agreement may be executed in one or more counterparts, each of which shall be deemed an original, but all of which together shall constitute one and the same instrument.

e. Headings. The headings and other captions in this Agreement are for convenience and reference only and shall not be used in interpreting, construing or enforcing any of the provisions of this Agreement.

Exhibit 17.0.1 — Study Startup Checklist

Study Title:

IRB #

Principal Investigator: **Sponsor:**

If investigator-initiated study, please use the IIT Management Checklist. Investigators holding an IND or IDE (Sponsor-Investigators) are advised to use the SI Trial Initiation Checklist.

Task	Date completed and initials	Comments
Study materials (*e.g.*, scientific protocol and consent) ☐ Obtain or develop the lay summary, scientific protocol and informed consent form with HIPAA authorization ☐ Obtain documentation on the study intervention if applicable (*e.g.*, investigator's brochure or package insert for drugs, device manual for devices, information on a dietary supplement) ☐ Identify study personnel		
Required submissions as applicable ☐ Office of Sponsored Programs for grants and contracts or Office of Grant Administration for studies ☐ Clinical and Translational Review Committee for cancer-related studies ☐ Institutional Review Board (IRB) via eIRB, Form A (WIRB Eligibility Checklist) for WIRB studies to WIRB listserv or contact IRB for other external IRBs ☐ Office for Clinical Research (OCR)for studies with billable items and services ☐ Office of Quality checklists (including nursing checklist) ☐ Conflict of Interest (COI) via eCOI ☐ Radiation safety and/or Biosafety, if applicable ☐ Investigational Drug Service, if applicable		
Hospital and Veterans Affairs (VA), after IRB approval ☐ Research Oversight Committee (ROC) ☐ VA Research and Development Committee ☐ Hospital ROC approval		

Task	Date completed and initials	Comments
Study personnel ☐ IRB approval for all personnel ☐ eCOI completion for applicable personnel ☐ Documented study-specific training for all personnel ☐ Delegation of authority log for all personnel ☐ Sponsor forms for all personnel (*e.g.*, financial disclosures)		
FDA documentation, if applicable ☐ 1572 for drug studies ☐ Investigator agreement for device studies		
Websites, if applicable ☐ Trial listed on clinicaltrials.gov ☐ Other for recruitment/advertising, as approved by the IRB		

Exhibit 17.0.2 — Delegation of Authority & Signature Log

Study Title:
IRB #: **Principal Investigator:**
Sponsor: **Study Site:**

Study team member	Title	Signature	Initials	Start date	Stop date	Activities (refer to code list below)	(*)PI Initials & date
							PI:__________ Date:
							PI:__________ Date:
							PI:__________ Date:
							PI:__________ Date:
							PI:__________ Date:

Activity codes (please amend activities as appropriate for your study):

A	Informed consent process	B	Eligibility assessment	C	Paper CRF/eCRF completion	D	Obtain medical history
E	Regulatory documentation	F	Concomitant medication review	G	Perform physical exam	H	Review lab and procedure results
I	Investigational product accountability	J	Investigational product storage	K	AE grading	L	AE attribution
M	AE reporting to sponsor and/or IRB	N	IRB submissions	O	Shipment and handling of samples	P	Other

(*) I have delegated the identified duties and will directly supervise the named personnel in the performance of protocol requirements.

____________________________ ____________________________

PI Signature **PI Initials**

Used with permission of the authors: Emory University, Margaret Huber, Maria Davila, Sharla Karlebach, and Stephanie De Rijke. The authors provide this material as an example and for informational purposes and do not suggest or represent that it complies with or will enable any third party to comply with all applicable laws or regulations.

Exhibit 17.0.3 — Informed Consent Form (ICF) Version Tracking Log

Study Title:

Principal Investigator: **Subject ID:**

List each document version and any subsequent version changes. Examples are included below.

ICF/HIPAA Version	ICF Approval Period	Comments
Main ICF version 1 (date)	*11/15/2010-11/14/2011*	
Sub-study ICF Version 1 (date)	*11/15/2010-11/14/2011*	
Sub-study ICF Version 2 (date)	*12/10/10-11/14/11*	*Added details regarding follow up contact*
HIPAA Authorization Version 1 (date)	*11/15/2010-11/14/2011*	

Exhibit 17.0.4 — Informed Consent Tracking Log by Subject

Study Title:	
IRB#	PI:

Instructions: List each IRB approved document and date subject signed. Examples are included below:

ICF/HIPAA authorization Version	Subject Number											
	101	102	103	104	105	106	107	108	109	110	111	112
Main ICF version 1 11/10/10. Approved 11/15/10-11/14/11	Subject signed 12/1/10 PI signed 12/1/10 *Page 13 missing subject's initials											
Sub-study ICF Version 1 11/10/10 Approved 11/15/10-11/14/11	Subject signed 12/1/10. *Missing PI signature											
Main ICF version 2 1/27/11 Approved 1/30/11-11/14/11	Pending subject reconsent.											

ICF/HIPAA authorization Version	Subject Number											
	101	102	103	104	105	106	107	108	109	110	111	112
Sub-study ICF Version 2 12/10/10 Approved 12/15/10-11/14/11	Pending subject reconsent.											
Assent version 1 11/10/10 Approved 11/15/10-11/14/11	N/A											
Date of 18th birthday if subject is 17 y.o. signing ICF	N/A											
HIPAA Authorization	12/1/2010											

Used with permission of the authors: Emory University, Margaret Huber, Maria Davila, Sharla Karlebach, and Stephanie De Rijke. The authors provide this material as an example and for informational purposes and do not suggest or represent that it complies with or will enable any third party to comply with all applicable laws or regulations.

Exhibit 17.0.5 — Subject Enrollment Log

Study Title:
IRB #: **Principal Investigator:**
Sponsor: **Study Site:**
IRB Approved Enrollment number *:

Subject ID and Initials		Subject Demographics		Date Subject signed ICF	Subject eligible? (yes/no)	If not eligible, Reason for Exclusion/ Comments	Subject final status **	Additional comments
		Gender	Age					
		M ☐ F ☐			Y ☐ N ☐		C ☐ WS ☐ WP ☐ S ☐	
		M ☐ F ☐			Y ☐ N ☐		C ☐ WS ☐ WP ☐ S ☐	
		M ☐ F ☐			Y ☐ N ☐		C ☐ WS ☐ WP ☐ S ☐	
		M ☐ F ☐			Y ☐ N ☐		C ☐ WS ☐ WP ☐ S ☐	
		M ☐ F ☐			Y ☐ N ☐		C ☐ WS ☐ WP ☐ S ☐	
		M ☐ F ☐			Y ☐ N ☐		C ☐ WS ☐ WP ☐ S ☐	
		M ☐ F ☐			Y ☐ N ☐		C ☐ WS ☐ WP ☐ S ☐	
		M ☐ F ☐			Y ☐ N ☐		C ☐ WS ☐ WP ☐ S ☐	
		M ☐ F ☐			Y ☐ N ☐		C ☐ WS ☐ WP ☐ S ☐	
		M ☐ F ☐			Y ☐ N ☐		C ☐ WS ☐ WP ☐ S ☐	
		M ☐ F ☐			Y ☐ N ☐		C ☐ WS ☐ WP ☐ S ☐	
		M ☐ F ☐			Y ☐ N ☐		C ☐ WS ☐ WP ☐ S ☐	
		M ☐ F ☐			Y ☐ N ☐		C ☐ WS ☐ WP ☐ S ☐	
		M ☐ F ☐			Y ☐ N ☐		C ☐ WS ☐ WP ☐ S ☐	

* Per IRB policy, an enrolled subject is anyone who signs a consent form. If the number of subjects enrolled is approaching the IRB approved enrollment number, the PI should consider submitting an amendment to the IRB to increase enrollment number.
** C= completed participation, WS: subject withdrew, WP= withdrawn by PI, S: screen failure

Used with permission of the authors: Emory University, Margaret Huber, Maria Davila, Sharla Karlebach, and Stephanie De Rijke. The authors provide this material as an example and for informational purposes and do not suggest or represent that it complies with or will enable any third party to comply with all applicable laws or regulations.

Exhibit 17.0.6 — Adverse Event Log

Study Title:
Principal Investigator:
Subject ID*:
Intervention Start Date*:
Intervention End Date*:
IRB #:
Initial Consent Date*:
Off Study Date*:

Adverse event	Start and stop dates	Serious	Grade**	Relationship to study	Anticipated	Action taken with the drug/device/ intervention	Other actions taken	Was the AE reported to the sponsor?	Was the AE reported to the IRB? ***	PI initials and date
	Start: Stop:	□ Yes □ No	□ Mild □ Moderate □ Severe □ Life Threatening □ Death	□ Not related □ Possibly related □ Probably related □ Unknown	□ Yes □ No	□ None □ Reduced □ Interrupted □ Discontinued □ Other		□ No □ Yes Date of report:	□ No □Yes Date of report:	
	Start: Stop:	□ Yes □ No	□ Mild □ Moderate □ Severe □ Life Threatening □ Death	□ Not related □ Possibly related □ Probably related □ Unknown	□ Yes □ No	□ None □ Reduced □ Interrupted □ Discontinued □ Other		□ No □ Yes Date of report:	□ No □Yes Date of report:	
	Start: Stop:	□ Yes □ No	□ Mild □ Moderate □ Severe □ Life Threatening □ Death	□ Not related □ Possibly related □ Probably related □ Unknown	□ Yes □ No	□ None □ Reduced □ Interrupted □ Discontinued □ Other		□ No □ Yes Date of report:	□ No □Yes Date of report:	
	Start: Stop:	□ Yes □ No	□ Mild □ Moderate □ Severe □ Life Threatening □ Death	□ Not related □ Possibly related □ Probably related □ Unknown	□ Yes □ No	□ None □ Reduced □ Interrupted □ Discontinued □ Other		□ No □ Yes Date of report:	□ No □Yes Date of report:	

* *If you expect multiple AEs per subject, create a log for each subject. If you don't expect many AEs on the study, delete the subject-specific header and add a column for Subject initials and ID. If you will maintain one log for the entire study, maintain the log with the regulatory documentation.*

***Revise this column to meet the grading requirements of the protocol (e.g., "1-5" vs "mild-severe").*

****To further document your assessment of this event and determine if it meets the IRB's reporting requirements, please complete the Reportable Event Assessment Form.*

Exhibit 17.0.7 — Concomitant Medication Log

Study Title:
Principal Investigator: **Subject ID:**
Initial Consent Date: **Intervention Start Date:** **Intervention End Date:** **Off Study Date:**

Medication	Start date	Stop date	Dose	Frequency	Route	Reason	Comments	Initials of person completing form

Exhibit 17.0.8 — Device Accountability Log

Study Title:
IRB #: **Principal Investigator:**
Sponsor: **Study Site:** **Device Name:**

DEVICE RECEIPT				DEVICE USE			DEVICE RETURN / REPAIR / DESTRUCTION					
Date Rec'd	Initials Receiver	Lot # / Serial or Model #	Device Type / Batch #	Date Used	Initials of Device Dispenser	Subject ID	RET= Returned DES= Destroyed REP= Repaired	Date	Initials	# of Units	Reason	Comments

Note: Retain a copy of the packing slips for all shipments received and sent.

Used with permission of the authors: Emory University, Margaret Huber, Maria Davila, Sharla Karlebach, and Stephanie De Rijke. The authors provide this material as an example and for informational purposes and do not suggest or represent that it complies with or will enable any third party to comply with all applicable laws or regulations.

Exhibit 17.0.9 — Phone Screening Log

Study Title:	
IRB Study #:	
Principal Investigator:	

NOTE:

- **You must have IRB review and approval of the screening script and questions to be asked.**
- **Do not document any personal information or identifiers on this form, i.e., name or birth date, etc. unless the IRB has approved a verbal consent and HIPAA authorization.**

Screen #	Subject ID	Date	Eligible Y / N	Brief Reason for Screen Failure	Person Conducting Screen

Used with permission of the authors: Emory University, Margaret Huber, Maria Davila, Sharla Karlebach, and Stephanie De Rijke. The authors provide this material as an example and for informational purposes and do not suggest or represent that it complies with or will enable any third party to comply with all applicable laws or regulations.

Exhibit 17.0.10 — Protocol Deviation Log

Study **Title:**

IRB #: **Principal Investigator:**

Sponsor: **Study Site:**

Date study team became aware	Date of deviation	Subject ID	Deviation code	Short description of deviation	Was the deviation reported to the sponsor? Y/N and date of report	Was the deviation reported to the IRB? Y/N and date of report*	Initials of person completing this form	PI initials and date

Deviation codes: 1= Eligibility 2= Informed consent 3= Drug/device error 4= Missed labs 5= Missed procedures 6= Prohibited medication 7= Event outside window 8= Other

** The PI must report to the IRB any circumstances where the PI becomes aware of a substantive deviation from the protocol that adversely affected at least one of the following: 1) the rights, welfare, or safety of subjects; 2) the subjects' willingness to continue participation; or 3) the integrity of the research data. If the protocol deviation/protocol non-compliance concerns study documentation associated with an FDA-regulated study or was a protocol deviation undertaken to prevent immediate hazard to a human subject, then the PI shall report the protocol deviation/protocol non-compliance to the IRB.*

Exhibit 17.0.11 — Storage of Retained Body Fluids/Tissue Sampling Log

Study Title:

IRB #

Principal Investigator: **Study contact name:**

Subject ID	Date subject provided consent	Date sample collected	Sample type, *e.g.*, plasma, full blood, urine, tissue, or DNA	Storage location *	Storage period from:	Storage period to: (Date samples are destroyed)	Initials of person collecting the samples

* *Please specify building, department, location and type of storage facility (e.g.-80°C, 4°C, room temperature, or liquid nitrogen).*

Exhibit 17.0.12 — Self-Monitoring Tool

Study Title:	
Investigator:	**IRB#:**

Instructions

This Self-Monitoring Tool is designed for use as part of the overall Data Safety Monitoring Plan (DSMP) to assess compliance with IRB policies and procedures and federal regulations and guidance governing research with human subjects, on a per-study basis. This form can be modified to include review of the specific human subject protection and data integrity risks of the trial. Site monitoring should be completed regularly once subjects have been enrolled.

If the IRB required the self-assessment, please send the completed form to the IRB through eIRB. For instructions of how to submit a RE, please go to: How to Submit a Reportable Event in eIRB (text instructions).

As you complete this form, please consider the IRB's reporting requirements for protocol deviations and noncompliance. IRB Policies & Procedures are posted at [website address], along with other helpful information.

If you have any questions or need help with this form, please feel free to contact ________________.

Section A: Regulatory Responsibilities

A-1 Are all staff working on the study listed on the IRB submission? ☐ Yes ☐ No

A-2 Is CITI certification and additional training current for all study team members? ☐ Yes ☐ No

A-3 Has the study maintained continuous active IRB approval?
☐ Yes ☐ No,

If no, were all activities that occurred during the lapse reported to the IRB?
☐ Yes ☐ No

A-4 IRB-approved subject sample size: _____

A-5 Number of subjects who signed consent (enrolled) to date: ______

A-6 If subjects withdrew, were these withdrawals reported to the IRB at continuing review?
☐ Yes ☐ No ☐ N/A

A-7 Have all study data collected in the past 30 days been entered into the study database as required by the protocol, contract, or standard operating procedure? ☐ Yes ☐ No

A-8 Is the IRB approved plan for storage & dispensation of the test article being followed?
☐ Yes ☐ No

A-9 If re-consent of subjects was required by IRB or sponsor, were all subjects appropriately re-consented?
☐ Yes ☐ No

A-10 Is the IRB approved DSMP being followed? ☐ Yes ☐ No

A-11 Is the data protection plan being followed, including use of encrypted devices? ☐ Yes ☐ No

Section B: Reporting Responsibilities

B-1 Are there reporting requirements (*e.g.* SAEs or deviations) to the sponsor or funding source? ☐ Yes ☐ No

If yes, were reports submitted as required?
☐ Yes ☐ No

B-2 Have all protocol deviations/protocol non-compliance and/or non-compliance with IRB Policies and Procedures, federal regulations, or funding requirements been reported to the IRB per their requirements? ☐ Yes ☐ No ☐ N/A

B-3 Have all events that require prompt reporting been reported to the IRB? ☐ Yes ☐ No ☐ N/A

Have all events that require periodic reporting been reported at the time of continuing review? ☐ Yes ☐ No ☐ N/A

Section C: Regulatory Documentation Review

Document	**Yes, No or N/A**	**Comments:** Note if an item is maintained in a location other than the regulatory binder and confirm documentation of the location in the regulatory binder
Investigator Brochures, package inserts, or device manuals with signature pages, if applicable		Current version/date ________________ Date submitted to IRB ________________
Protocol/protocol amendment with signature page, if applicable		Current version/date ________________ Date approved by IRB ________________ Current study approval period: ___________
ICF, HIPAA authorization form and, if applicable, revocation letter		Current ICF version/date ______________ Date approved by IRB ________________ Current authorization version/date________ Date approved by IRB ________________
Institutional Review Board reviews Documentation of IRB approval: protocol and amendments, continuing review, ICFs, trial information for subjects, advertisements, and other		Current study approval period: __________

Document	**Yes, No or N/A**	**Comments:** Note if an item is maintained in a location other than the regulatory binder and confirm documentation of the location in the regulatory binder
Investigator agreement or Form FDA 1572 signed by site PI with current listing of all sub-investigators & facilities		
CV, licenses and/or other relevant documents evidencing qualifications of investigators and sub investigators		
FDA Financial Disclosure Certification Forms (FDF) completed by each investigator		
Delegation of Authority (DOA) Log: may include site signature log		
Records of Study Specific training including updates for each individual listed on DOA Log		
Reportable Events: SAEs, UPs or non-compliance including safety reports, internal & external with documentation of review		Required reports to IRB, date:__________
Data and Safety Monitoring Committee Reports		Required reports to IRB, date:__________
Site Monitoring Log & Reports		Site monitoring completed, date:________ Required reports to CTAC, date:________
Investigational product IP documentation of disposition (dates, quantity, use by subjects, and return). Note if drug is managed by IDS.		
Screening and enrollment logs		
Laboratory Certifications/accreditations; normal lab values		
Ancillary Committee Approvals, if applicable		
Miscellaneous		

Does the PI hold an IND or IDE for this study? ☐ Yes ☐ No

If Yes, continue below to the Sponsor-Investigator Regulatory Documentation Review. If No, skip to section D.

Document	**Yes, No or N/A**	**Comments:** Note if an item is maintained in a location other than the regulatory binder and confirm documentation of the location in the regulatory binder
FDA submissions with accompanying 1571 Original application; FDA correspondence; amendments; IND Safety Reports (MedWatch); annual reports		IND Anniversary Date ____________ Current IND Annual Report __________ Date submitted to FDA ____________ Date submitted to IRB ____________

Document	Yes, No or N/A	Comments: Note if an item is maintained in a location other than the regulatory binder and confirm documentation of the location in the regulatory binder
Reportable Events: SAEs, UPs or non-compliance including Safety Reports, internal & external with documentation of review by the **S-I Adverse Event Assessment Form**		Required Reports to IRB, date: __________
clinicaltrials.gov information updated within past 6 months		Updated: ____________________________
Investigational product (IP) documentation copy of label(s) attached to IP; shipping records for IP (note if drug managed by IDS)		

Is this a multisite study where the PI holds the IND or IDE? ☐ Yes ☐ No

If Yes, continue below to the Multisite documentation review. If No, skip to section D.

Document	Yes, No or N/A	Comments: Note if an item is maintained in a location other than the regulatory binder and confirm documentation of the location in the regulatory binder
Site contact information sheet		
Signature pages: Protocol/protocol amendment signature page Investigator brochure/package insert/device manual signature pages Site signature log (to document entries on source documents)		
Agreements: Signed site agreement & any other agreement between involved parties		
IRB local IRB Composition; documentation of IRB approval (protocol and amendments, ICFs)		Current study approval period: __________ Current protocol version/date __________ Date approved by IRB ______________
ICF, HIPAA authorization and, if applicable, revocation letter		Current ICF version/date ____________ Date approved by IRB ______________ Current authorization version/date_______ Date approved by IRB ______________
Form FDA 1572 or Investigator Agreement signed by site PI listing all sub-investigators		
CV and license of site PI		
FDA Financial Disclosure Certification Forms (FDF) completed by each investigator listed on Form 1572 or Investigator agreement		
Records of sponsor provided training		

Document	**Yes, No or N/A**	**Comments:** Note if an item is maintained in a location other than the regulatory binder and confirm documentation of the location in the regulatory binder
Safety reports, with documentation of review & assessment by the IND/IDE sponsor & communication of safety information to participating investigators		Required reports to IRB, date: ____________________ FDA, date: ____________________ Participating investigators, date: ________
Laboratory Certifications/accreditations; normal lab values		
Investigational Product (IP) Copy of labels attached to IP; shipping records for IP (note if managed by IDS)		
Site monitoring reports & follow-up documentation		Site monitoring completed, date: ________ Required reports to CTAC, date: ________
Correspondence to individual site (including trial updates, updated product or safety information, teleconference minutes)		
Miscellaneous		

Section D: Subject Case History Review

Select 3 or more subject files.

First Subject

Subject ID#:

- Is there an original copy of informed consent form (ICF) and HIPAA authorization on file? ☐ Yes ☐ No
- Was the person who obtained informed consent authorized by the IRB to obtain consent for this study? ☐ Yes ☐ No
- Did the subject sign and date the ICF prior to the research procedures? ☐ Yes ☐ No
- Is there documentation of the consent process in the research record which includes that the subject received a copy of the ICF? ☐ Yes ☐ No
- Were the correct versions of the ICF and HIPAA used? ☐ Yes ☐ No
- Is each document properly completed with initials/signatures? ☐ Yes ☐ No
  - *If no, explain:*
- Was the subject registered in ERMS in the required timeframe? ☐ Yes ☐ No ☐ N/A
- Did the subject meet eligibility criteria? ☐ Yes ☐ No
- Is documentation of eligibility complete and in the record? ☐ Yes ☐ No
- Were subject visits conducted in the timeframe required by the protocol? ☐ Yes ☐ No
- Were all tests/procedures performed and documented according to the protocol? ☐ Yes ☐ No
- Did this subject experience any adverse events? ☐ Yes ☐ No
  - If yes, is there documentation of timely review and assessment? ☐ Yes ☐ No

- Has the data for this subject been entered into the study database within the required timeframe of the protocol or by the sponsor, but no later than 30 days? ☐ Yes ☐ No

Repeat for Subjects Two, Three, or more

Section E: Action Required

For any questions answered No above, determine if there are reporting requirements.

Do any findings require action? ☐ Yes ☐ No ☐ N/A

If yes, specify?

- Report to IRB
- Report to sponsor
- Report to funding source
- Other action

Section F: Corrective and Preventive Action Plan

For any questions answered No, also determine if a Corrective and Preventive Action (CAPA) Plan is required. If required, please describe the CAPA including the corresponding item identifier, e.g., A-4 CITI certification, as a header and implementation/completion dates.

Item Identifier:

Problem:

Root Cause:

Corrective Action:

Preventive Action:

____

Signature and date of study staff member completing this form

____

Signature and date of Investigator reviewing this form

____

Signature and date of Sponsor reviewing this form, if applicable

Please send this report to Clinical Trials Audit and Compliance (CTAC).

Date sent to CTAC: ____________

Used with permission of the authors: Emory University, Margaret Huber, Maria Davila, Sharla Karlebach, and Stephanie De Rijke. The authors provide this material as an example and for informational purposes and do not suggest or represent that it complies with or will enable any third party to comply with all applicable laws or regulations.

Exhibit 17.0.13 — Study Specific Signature Log

Study Title:
IRB #:
Principal Investigator: **Study Site:**

The purpose of a site signature log is to document the signatures and initials of all persons authorized to collect and record study data so that study documentation attributed to specific staff members may be verified.

Staff Name (Print or Type)	**Initials**	**Signature (include all signature versions below)**

Exhibit 17.0.14 — Study-Specific Training Log

Study Title:
IRB#
PI:

All study team members should be trained on the protocol and investigator's brochure or device manual, including any subsequent changes. Maintain copies of agendas, attendance logs and relevant training materials with this Study-Specific Training Form. Examples are included below.

Training description	**Trainer**	**Date completed and initials**	**Comments**
Protocol version 2.1	*Dr. Jones, Study PI*	*1/1/2012*	*Research nurse read protocol prior to training. PI discussed purpose, eligibility criteria, procedures, risks, informed consent, and investigational drug.*
Investigator Brochure version 9	*Sponsor's monitor*	*1/10/2012*	

Used with permission of the authors: Emory University, Margaret Huber, Maria Davila, Sharla Karlebach, and Stephanie De Rijke. The authors provide this material as an example and for informational purposes and do not suggest or represent that it complies with or will enable any third party to comply with all applicable laws or regulations.

Exhibit 17.0.15 — Subject Compensation Log

Study Title:	
IRB#:	Principal Investigator:
Study Site:	Sponsor:

Note: This log serves as documentation of subjects' compensation according to the IRB approved informed consent. Please keep a receipt of each payment with the subject's signature. Changes to payment type/amount require IRB approval.

Subject ID	Visit Date	Payment Amount	Payment Type	Payer Signature

Exhibit 17.0.16 — Training Attendance Log

Study Title:
IRB#
Training Topic:
Trainer:
Date:

Name (print legibly)	Signature

Store with study-specific training logs and educational materials.

Used with permission of the authors: Emory University, Margaret Huber, Maria Davila, Sharla Karlebach, and Stephanie De Rijke. The authors provide this material as an example and for informational purposes and do not suggest or represent that it complies with or will enable any third party to comply with all applicable laws or regulations.

Exhibit 17.0.17 — Site Monitoring Log

Study Title:
IRB#:
Principal Investigator:
Sponsor:

Visit date	Study team member signature	Monitor signature	Reason for visit	Date site received monitoring report*	Date site replied to monitoring report	Date site sent monitoring report to CTAC**

**Monitoring report maintained at site should be initialed and dated upon receipt and review.*

*** Within 10 days of receiving the report, study teams must submit all monitoring reports to the Clinical Trials Audit and Compliance (CTAC). Please include corrective and preventive actions in the body of the email.*

INDEX

[References are to sections and exhibits.]

[References are to sections and exhibits]

[References are to sections and exhibits]

[References are to sections and exhibits]

[References are to sections and exhibits]